Study Guide and Review of NEONATAL NURSING

Study Guide and Review of
NEONATAL NURSING

CAROLE KENNER, D.N.S., R.N., C.
Professor and Department Chair
Parent Child Health Nursing
College of Nursing and Health
University of Cincinnati
Cincinnati, Ohio

LAURIE PORTER GUNDERSON, Ph.D., R.N.
Associate Professor
College of Nursing and Health
University of Cincinnati
Cincinnati, Ohio

JUDY WRIGHT LOTT, D.N.S., N.N.R., R.N.
Director, Neonatal Nurse Practitioner Program
Children's Hospital Medical Center
Cincinnati, Ohio

STEPHANIE AMLUNG, M.S.N., R.N., C.
Clinical Nurse Specialist
Bethesda Hospital
Cincinnati, Ohio

W.B. SAUNDERS COMPANY
A Division of Harcourt Brace & Company
Philadelphia London Toronto Montreal Sydney Tokyo

W. B. SAUNDERS COMPANY
A Division of
Harcourt Brace & Company

The Curtis Center
Independence Square West
Philadelphia, Pennsylvania 19106

Illustrations of the heart courtesy of Ross Laboratories, Columbus, Ohio.

Study Guide and Review of Neonatal Nursing ISBN 0–7216–4204–7

Printed in the United States of America.

Last digit is the print number: 9 8 7 6 5 4 3 2

Preface

Neonatal nursing is a highly specialized field. The ever increasing demands placed on the nurse due to advanced technology have resulted in the need for greater expertise. Accountability coupled with the trend toward advanced education has caused more neonatal nurses to seek further certification. This study guide serves as a resource for those nurses who may wish to prepare for certification in neonatal intensive care or as a neonatal nurse practitioner. Those nurses who wish to test their knowledge of neonatal nursing are also helped.

The questions are in the format of those in certification examinations. None of the questions from this text are actual certification items, as these examinations are updated annually. The level of the questions in this study guide ranges from basic knowledge through to analysis and synthesis. The content of the questions is based on the text *Comprehensive Neonatal Nursing: A Physiologic Perspective* edited by Carole Kenner, Ann Brueggemeyer, and Laurie Porter Gunderson, published by the W.B. Saunders Company. Vignettes, some of which also appear in the text, give the test taker the opportunity to apply the nursing process to neonatal situations. Joyce M. Dohme, Helen Archer-Dusté, Marianne McGraw, and Sheila Southwell have generously provided these for study.

Two separate tests provide the opportunity to better evaluate the knowledge of the test taker. An annotated bibliography is included for those seeking further information on a particular subject.

Good luck and happy studying!

CAROLE KENNER
LAURIE PORTER GUNDERSON
JUDY WRIGHT LOTT
STEPHANIE AMLUNG

Instructions

The two test forms found in this guide are similar in content and level. They are meant to offer two opportunities for evaluation of neonatal nursing knowledge. Each question is a multiple choice with three options. Only one option is correct. The format for the questions resembles that for the certification examinations that are available. After completing one version of the test, the reviewer can check the responses with the answers found in the key. For further information on specific content, the reviewer is referred to the annotated bibliography.

Additional reading can be found in *Comprehensive Neonatal Nursing: A Physiologic Perspective,* edited by Carole Kenner, Ann Brueggemeyer, and Laurie Porter Gunderson.

Contents

REVIEW TEST

1

1. Neonatal nurses go through a staged process of professional development into the role. Characteristics of the beginning practitioner include:

   A. dependent decision-making.
   B. independent decision-making.
   C. needs repetitive, tedious tasks.

2. Single gene transmission refers to:

   A. mendelian inheritance.
   B. multifactorial inheritance.
   C. sex-linked inheritance.

3. Certification of the advanced practice nurse should:

   A. be related to state boards of nursing standards for advanced practice.
   B. reflect a congruency between program content and certification requirements.
   C. be required by law of all advanced practice nurses.

4. Collaboration assumes:

   A. the contribution of each member of the group is equal.
   B. each profession has something unique to contribute.
   C. some members may be beginning level professionals.

5. Organizational characteristics that suggest successful collaboration include:

   A. delegation of authority to a primary nurse.
   B. centralized decision making.
   C. low staff turnover.

6. Clinical ethics refers to:

   A. medical ethics.
   B. nursing ethics.
   C. practice ethics.

7. The four key elements of informed consent are:

   A. disclosure of accurate information, assurance information is understood, determination of voluntary participation, and competence of individual.
   B. disclosure of accurate information, outline of risks, assurance of confidentiality of information, and determination of voluntary participation.
   C. outline of risks, assurance of confidentiality, assurance information is understood, and a witness to the consent.

8. Expert neonatal nurses must be competent in a technical and theoretical sense. The hallmark of an expert neonatal nurse is:

   A. being able to care for a sick neonate independently.
   B. pursuing graduate level education.
   C. knowing the limits of professional knowledge.

Helen Archer-Dusté, MSN, RN & Sheila Southwell, MSN, MBA, RN

A 36-year-old, gravida 1, para 0, American woman, married to a Saudi Arabian, presented in labor at 36 weeks' gestation. She had two previous ultrasonograms that were interpreted as normal, and she had refused amniocentesis for prenatal diagnosis. The infant's father had returned to Saudi Arabia before delivery, and the mother planned to emigrate with the infant after birth.

At delivery, the male infant was found to have amniotic band disruption complex, an in utero breaking of the amnion causing it to wrap around body parts and restrict normal growth and development. He had a midfacial cleft involving the left orbit, nose, palate, and lip. He had only one skull bone (right parietal). The rest of the brain was covered only by dura, without leakage of cerebrospinal fluid. He also had a Dandy-Walker malformation of the brain, a posterior fossa cyst causing hydrocephalus and neurological deficit. He had minor amputation of the ends of some fingers. Other organs were intact on ultrasound evaluation. On the second day of life, the infant developed severe, life-threatening apnea and bradycardia episodes. The nurse caring for the patient seeks to clarify the infant's resuscitation ("code") status. The nurse should consider the following questions:

1. Who should be involved in the decision-making process?
2. What are the ethical questions raised in this case?
3. What ethical principles are pertinent to this deliberation?
4. What potential course of action can be identified?
5. What are the ethical and clinical consequences of each?
6. What informational factors would need to be reviewed with the parents?
7. What legal precedence has been established relative to the treatment plan?

THE FOLLOWING FOUR QUESTIONS ARE BASED ON THIS VIGNETTE.

9. The nurse who is most concerned about question 4 in this vignette is probably operating from a:

   A. metaethics perspective.
   B. normative ethics perspective.
   C. teleologic perspective.

10. The nurse who is uncomfortable with a Do Not Resuscitate order is probably operating from a:

    A. metaethics perspective.
    B. normative ethics perspective.
    C. teleologic perspective.

11. In this case, treatment could be withheld for the infant according to U.S. Baby Doe Regulations if the:

    A. infant is chronic and reversibly comatose.
    B. treatment would only prolong dying.
    C. treatment would improve survival but be inhumane.

12. Substantive standards in this case would include the nurse's and parents' consideration of the benefit or burden of their decision. This refers to:

    A. sanctity of life.
    B. quality of life.
    C. best interests.

13. Research is necessary for nursing practice to:
    A. evaluate new therapies scientifically.
    B. base care on observations only.
    C. uphold traditional models of care.

14. Malpractice describes:
    A. deviation from hospital policy.
    B. negligence of individuals who violate a standard.
    C. physician care that causes harm to an individual.

15. Accountable professionals practice prudently based on their education and experience. To ensure that a legal challenge can be successfully defended, one must practice according to:
    A. current standards of care.
    B. physician orders.
    C. routine nursing care protocol.

16. Incident reports should include all of the following information <u>EXCEPT</u>:
    A. facts surrounding the event.
    B. steps taken to assess for and alleviate any actual injury.
    C. conclusory and blaming statements about the event.

17. The purpose of institutional review boards (IRBs) is to:
    A. review research proposals to ensure protection for human subjects.
    B. review research proposals to determine allocation of federal funds.
    C. provide guidance to beginning nurse researchers.

18. H.E.L.L.P. syndrome is characterized by all of the following <u>EXCEPT</u>:
    A. hypoglycemia.
    B. elevated liver enzymes.
    C. low platelets.

A qualitative study was conducted to examine the phenomenon of the transition from hospital to home for new mothers and infants going home from a NICU. The study's research question was: What are the maternal responses to caring for the infant at home? The semistructured interview asked the following questions: (1) What has it been like for you having your infant at home? (2) Describe your infant. What problems or concerns have you had since your infant's discharge?

THE FOLLOWING FIVE QUESTIONS ARE BASED ON THIS RESEARCH.

19. The level of inquiry is:
    A. explanative-descriptive.
    B. comparative.
    C. experimental.

20. The purpose of this study is to:
    A. test a relationship.
    B. determine interventions for the mother.
    C. describe patterns of responses.

21. Data analysis for this study probably would be done by:
    A. paired T-tests.
    B. content analysis.
    C. Pearson's correlatives.

22. The sample mostly would like be:
    A. a matched sample.
    B. stratified random sample.
    C. convenience sample.

23. The study's specific objectives should be stated in the form of:
    A. a null hypothesis.
    B. a directional hypothesis.
    C. a research question.

24. ______ is established by consensus and conveys a sense of a common social tradition or acceptable behavior.
    A. Ethics
    B. Morality
    C. Normative ethics

25. When selecting a research instrument, the question, "Does the instrument or technique measure what it is supposed to measure?" refers to:
    A. reliability.
    B. validity.
    C. suitability.

26. Dissemination of information obtained from a study:
    A. is not as important as conducting the research.
    B. is important because it promotes a critical dialogue among professionals.
    C. should only be done through oral presentations or peer-reviewed journals.

27. Various clinical trials have been performed administering surfactant at different times during the neonate's course of therapy. When given in the delivery room, this is termed the prevention mode. When given later in the treatment course, it is termed:

    A. rescue surfactant replacement therapy.
    B. maintenance surfactant replacement therapy.
    C. prophylactic surfactant replacement therapy.

28. Why are infants/children with TOF at greater risk from consequences of fluid imbalances during minor illness such as gastroenteritis?

    A. disturbances of fluids/electrolytes, especially calcium, can cause decreased cardiac metabolism and lead to decreased cardiac function, precipitating frequent "tet" spells.
    B. polycythemia develops as a compensatory mechanism to increase the oxygen-carrying capacity of the blood. In the presence of decreased volume, the increased viscosity of the blood can impede cerebral circulation and increase risk for cerebral infarcts.
    C. volume overload will result in increased workload on the heart, increased metabolism, and increased oxygen demand, which may precipitate a "tet" spell.

Joyce M. Dohme, RNC, MSN

Sandy sat quietly by her baby Jessica's bedside. "You can hold her if you like," I said as I approached, reaching for her baby. "No, don't disturb her. I just want to watch her sleep," she replied. "I was just thinking of what she's been through. Poor little thing. But she's tough. She made it and is OK."

"It must have been tough for you, too, mother," I responded. She looked at me with surprise. "Mother. I guess I'm not used to hearing that. It sounds funny." "It feels strange to think of myself as someone's mother." "I haven't really done what a mother is supposed to do," she said reflectively.

"What does a mother do?" I asked.

"Well, you know, change diapers, get up at night to feed the baby, and take her for walks in the stroller," she replied.

"All I could do was touch and talk to her. You nurses really did all the mothering, doing her suctioning and gavage feedings and all that."

"That's nursing. That's not mothering. Your baby knows the difference," I said. She knew you even before she was born. She knew the sound of your voice, your touch, your smell. It was special when you were here with her, touching, taking to, and holding her."

"When she was born, I didn't think she was going to make it. I was so scared," she said.

THE FOLLOWING SEVEN QUESTIONS ARE BASED ON THIS VIGNETTE.

29. When Jessica was born eight weeks premature her parents, Sandy and Jim, knew an NICU stay would be required. To cope with their baby's separation, Sandy and Jim decided to ask Jessica's nurse how they could develop a plan to participate in Jessica's care. They felt the need to develop this plan because they felt unclear as to their role in the NICU. Parents who want to help develop a plan and adapt their roles to a social situation are following the tenets of:

    A. Social Structure Role Theory.
    B. Classic Role Theory.
    C. Symbolic Interaction Theory.

30. Sandy and Jim's expression of concern over their role in the NICU is an example of:

    A. role conflict.
    B. role ambiguity.
    C. role overload.

31. Sandy and Jim's need to become involved in Jessica's care is characteristic of role:

    A. reorganization.
    B. adaptation.
    C. change.

32. Nursing strategies to help integrate Sandy and Jim into the NICU would include:

    A. presenting information to Jim first so he can help Sandy to cope.

B. calling Jessica by pet names in front of the parents so they recognize a personal touch.
C. encouraging Sandy and Jim to bring in toys, clothes, or audiotapes for Jessica.

33. Caretaking of the premature Jessica was promoted by the nursing staff by all of the following EXCEPT:

A. positively reinforcing Sandy and Jim's caretaking attempts.
B. assessing Sandy and Jim's readiness to participate.
C. encouraging other family members to participate in the care.

34. The primary nurse noticed that Sandy would only minimally touch Jessica when encouraged. This type of behavior represents:

A. normal coping behavior.
B. maladaptive mothering behavior.
C. adaptive mothering behavior.

35. Jim would often stay at Jessica's bedside for 45 minutes to one hour. He would state that he wished he could spend more time. This behavior is:

A. abnormal coping behavior.
B. maladaptive fathering behavior.
C. adaptive fathering behavior.

36. All of the following are signs of respiratory difficulty in the neonate EXCEPT:

A. cyanosis and tachypnea.
B. grunting and retractions.
C. acrocyanosis and irregular respirations.

37. ______ is the state of having suffered a loss.

A. Bereavement
B. Grief
C. Sorrow

38. Rejection of the null hypothesis when it is in fact true refers to:

A. a type I error.
B. a type II error.
C. a beta error.

39. A thermoneutral state is defined as:

A. a normal temperature range.
B. an infant whose temperature is maintained through a heated and humidified incubator.
C. body temperature that is maintained with the lowest expenditure of energy and oxygen consumption.

CASE STUDY

Nancy and Bob gave birth to a 26-week-old infant named Julia. For the past three weeks, Julia has been in the NICU on ventilatory support. This afternoon, Jeanne, the primary nurse, noted Nancy to come into the unit, sit quietly at Julia's bedside, and stare. This behavior was different from Nancy's usual talking, touching, and stroking Julia. Jeanne asked Nancy what was wrong. She burst into tears. She said she was angry because Julia was making little progress. Bob had returned to his usual late night work routine, and their two-year-old, Willie, was throwing temper tantrums at home. All she could think about right now was Julia and how she might not live.

THE FOLLOWING EIGHT QUESTIONS ARE BASED ON THIS VIGNETTE.

40. Nancy is experiencing a:

A. grief response.
B. anxiety attack.
C. period of ambivalence.

41. Grief occurs:

A. with a real loss.
B. immediately after a death.
C. with an anticipated or real loss.

42. Nancy is in the ______ phase of grief.

A. acute
B. denial
C. bargaining

43. Jeanne should suggest to Nancy to:

A. recognize that she has Bob to help her.
B. recognize that Bob is grieving too.
C. recognize that she is neglecting Willie's needs.

44. Jeanne might suggest:
   A. Willie would be better off staying with his grandparents now.
   B. Willie would benefit from someone coming into the home to help.
   C. Willie needs both parents to turn their complete attention to him.

45. Jeanne should tell Nancy:
   A. that Bob's late night work schedule may be his way of coping.
   B. that she needs to confront Bob's behavior and get him to help her.
   C. to ignore Bob's behavior and concentrate on what helps her now.

46. Jeanne tried to assist Nancy by:
   A. encouraging her to recount the birth experience and Julia's transport.
   B. encouraging her to spend time at home and not to come to the NICU for a while.
   C. encouraging her to avoid trying to participate in Julia's care for a while.

47. Several weeks later Julia died. Nancy and Bob asked Jeanne if they should have a funeral. The appropriate response would be:
   A. "It is an unnecessary expense for you."
   B. "It may give you a feeling of support and relief."
   C. "It will add stress by facing the rest of the family."

48. The process of ______ refers to reduction division of the cells.
   A. meiosis
   B. mitosis
   C. symbiosis

49. Duchenne's muscular dystrophy is an example of:
   A. autosomal dominant.
   B. autosomal recessive.
   C. sex-linked recessive.

50. ______ is an enzymatic reaction that removes the glycoprotein coating from the spermatozoa and plasma proteins from the seminal fluid.
   A. Spermatogenesis
   B. Capacitation
   C. Acrosomal reaction

51. If the corpus luteum regresses well before the 16th week of gestation, the result will be:
   A. spontaneous abortion.
   B. an increase in placental growth.
   C. an increase in estrogen.

52. Documentation of the transport includes:
   A. information from the time of the first telephone contact through admission to the receiving hospital.
   B. information from the time the transport team reaches the referring hospital to the time they return to the receiving unit.
   C. information from the time of the first phone call until the team reaches the receiving unit.

53. Human placental lactogen (HPL) is produced by the placenta and acts as:
   A. a fetal growth hormone.
   B. a placental growth hormone.
   C. the basis of pregnancy tests.

54. Circulation of essential components across the placenta depends on:
   A. gestational age.
   B. presence of Wharton's jelly.
   C. amount of amniotic fluid.

55. Risk factors for placenta previa include:
   A. short umbilical cord.
   B. folic acid deficiency.
   C. closely spaced pregnancies.

56. The defined national standard by which a level II can be differentiated from a level III is set by:
   A. American Academy of Pediatrics.
   B. American College of Obstetrics and Gynecology.
   C. neither.

57. The ideal time to transport a fetus/neonate who is extremely premature to a tertiary center is:
   A. immediately after birth.
   B. when the infant is stabilized.
   C. before birth.

58. Helicopter air transports are advantageous if the distance is:
   A. 100 miles or less.

B. 100–250 miles.
C. over 250 miles.

59. Reverse transports occur when:

A. infants are taken from a level III to a level I for convalescing care.
B. infants are returned when stable to the referring hospital for convalescing care.
C. infants are returned to a level I or II unit for intermediate or convalescing care.

60. The ductus arteriosus is a wide muscular connection between the pulmonary artery and the aorta. The ductus arteriosus allows oxygenated blood from the placenta to bypass the lungs and enter the circulation. In the term newborn, the ductus arteriosus closes functionally around 15 hours of life. Closure in the preterm newborn is often delayed, resulting in shunting of blood and signs and symptoms of congestive heart failure. Why is failure of the ductus arteriosus to close a frequent complication in preterm neonates?

A. decreased pulmonary vascular resistance causes decreased oxygenation.
B. increased pulmonary venous congestion and decreased lung compliance.
C. decreased responsiveness of the muscle to increased oxygen saturation.

Joyce M. Dohme, RNC, MSN

Mrs. Y presented to labor and delivery at term with regular contractions approximately six to eight minutes apart, and membranes intact. Cervical exam indicated 3 cm dilation. Active labor progressed as expected. Fetal heart tones remained stable in the 130 to 140 range, with variability present and no periodic changes.

The nurse call came in 10 minutes later, accompanied by Mr. Y coming to get me. "Something's wrong!" he said. The uterine contraction tracing was showing increased, constant pressure. I palpated the uterine fundus to validate an "unending contraction." The fetal heart rate was in the 160 range, with minimum variability and occasional variable decelerations. I rolled Mrs. Y to her left side; placed a 100 percent O_2 face mask at 4 to 6 L/min. I summoned help. Mrs. Y's pulse had increased significantly; her blood pressure was slightly higher. I opened up the rate on her maintenance IV and checked the fetal heart tones. Bradycardia in the 100 range was present with no variability. Late decelerations were occurring with some contractions. I checked the cervix, which was 8 cm dilated, and searched gently for the pulsing of a prolapsed cord. The fetal heart tracing showed bradycardia at 60 bpm with no variability. Dark red blood trickled from the vagina. Vital signs showed maternal tachycardia and a widening pulse pressure. Mrs. Y looked pale and felt cool. She was in tremendous pain.

Baby Y was born by emergency C-section three minutes later. The baby was blue and limp, with no signs of life. Because of the presence of meconium, the pediatrician initiated resuscitation with direct suction below the cords, then 100 percent O_2 administration per positive pressure ventilation to the endotracheal tube with chest compressions.

Within the first minute, the infant's pulse was spontaneous and in the 60's range and increasing. Chest compressions were stopped, and positive pressure ventilation with 100 percent O_2 was continued for two more minutes. The baby was pink and trying to breath on her own, so constant positive airway pressure was given at 4 cm pressure while the adequacy of her effort was assessed. Apgar scores were 1(1) and 7(5). By 10 minutes, her score had risen to 8, and the team began to wean the O_2 content and prepare for transfer to the special care nursery (SCN).

THE FOLLOWING SEVEN QUESTIONS ARE BASED ON THIS VIGNETTE.

61. Development of the fetal cardiovascular system begins:

A. with implantation of the blastocyst into the decidua.
B. during the third week of gestation in the wall of the yolk sac.
C. by the end of the second week as the chorionic villi begin to form.

62. Baseline fetal heart rate (FHR) is defined as:
    A. FHR between contractions for at least a 10-minute period.
    B. FHR during contractions only.
    C. FHR between contractions including periodic changes.

63. _____ is a sign of fetal wellness and is seen as reassuring.
    A. Variability
    B. Deceleration
    C. Acceleration

64. Late decelerations are a result of:
    A. uteroplacental insufficiency.
    B. head compression.
    C. cord compression.

65. Treatment of late decelerations involves all of the following EXCEPT:
    A. decreasing uterine stimulation.
    B. administration of 5 or more liters of 100 percent O_2 per mask.
    C. decreasing IV fluids to correct maternal hypotension.

66. Overshoots of fetal heart rate can be caused by:
    A. catecholamine release of the myocardium.
    B. repeated hypoxic episodes that stress the fetus.
    C. decreased chemoreceptor stimulation.

67. Maternal blood loss or obstetric hemorrhage has been documented as one of the leading causes of maternal mortality. The nurse must be able to manage these potentially life-threatening situations. The primary goal for management of maternal hemorrhage is:
    A. immediate restoration of the blood volume and the oxygen-carrying capacity.
    B. prepare for emergency delivery.
    C. assess vital signs and monitor FHR closely.

68. Hypertension, sudden weight gain, and proteinuria are three classic symptoms associated with:
    A. gestational diabetes.
    B. PIH
    C. H.E.L.L.P.

69. To keep oxygen consumption to a minimum during the rewarming process, the incubator should be adjusted:
    A. 1 to 1.5° higher than the infant's temperature.
    B. 36.5 to 37° higher than the infant's desired temperature.
    C. at least 2° higher than the infant's desired temperature.

70. During the transition from intrauterine circulation to extrauterine circulation, an increase in blood oxygen content will cause the ductus arteriosus to close. The substance that maintains a patent ductus arteriosus is:
    A. dopamine.
    B. prostaglandins.
    C. dobutamine.

71. Secondary apnea refers to:
    A. a series of spontaneous deep gasps that become weaker and then stop, resulting in anoxia.
    B. rapid gasping with muscular effort and thrashing movements of the arms and legs.
    C. terminal apnea that results in death if the asphyxia is not reversed within several minutes.

72. The Apgar scoring can be used for assessment and evaluation of the newborn's cardiopulmonary function. The five signs, in order of importance, are:
    A. color, respiratory effort, pulse, reflex irritability, and tone.
    B. pulse, respiratory effort, tone (activity), reflex irritability (grimace), and color.
    C. pulse, color, tone, respiratory effort, and reflex irritability.

73. Cyanosis, early onset respiratory distress, and scaphoid abdomen are the classic triad of symptoms with:
    A. meconium aspiration.
    B. diaphragmatic hernia.
    C. pneumothorax.

74. An important point of neonatal stabilization in the delivery room is to:
    A. provide 100 percent oxygen to all infants during the stabilization period.

B. rapidly dry the infant to decrease the chance of iatrogenic hypothermia.
C. monitor rectal temperatures every 15 minutes until stabilization occurs.

75. Long-term responses to cold stress include:

A. poor growth patterns.
B. tachycardia.
C. peripheral vasoconstriction.

76. An ASD is a hole or opening in the atrial septum that develops as a result of improper septal formation early in fetal cardiac development. Symptoms of ASD typically appear when:

A. pulmonary vascular resistance begins to fall and right ventricular end-diastolic and right atrial pressures fall.
B. the difference between atrial pressure increases, causing a pressure gradient between the atria with resultant decreased pulmonary blood flow.

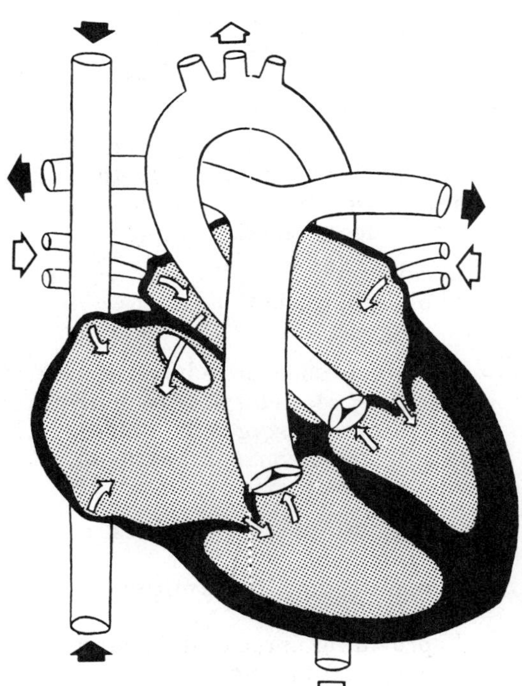

FIGURE 1 Atrial septal defect

C. right atrial pressure increases, causing systemic blood to shunt from the right to left atrium, sending mixed blood to aorta, causing systemic cyanosis.

77. Neonates who are large for gestational age may have difficulty maintaining thermoregulation. This can be due to:

A. hyperglycemia.
B. an increased oral intake.
C. insufficient brown fat stores.

78. The physical assessment obtained at birth is performed primarily to:

A. evaluate gestational age of the newborn.
B. evaluate adaptation to extra-uterine life.
C. facilitate bonding between the newborn and parents.

79. Incorporating gestational age assessments together with birth weight helps the examiner to determine if the infant's weight is appropriate for gestational age. An infant who is LGA falls into the weight percentile of:

A. >50th percentile.
B. >75th percentile.
C. >90th percentile.

80. While assessing the infant's skin and color status, the nurse observes a blush discoloration of the hands and feet. This can best be interpreted as:

A. patent ductus ateriosus.
B. cardiac dysfunction.
C. acrocyanosis.

81. Symptoms suggestive of atelectasis and pneumothorax include:

A. periodic breathing.
B. diminished breath sounds.
C. PMI at the fourth or fifth intercostal space.

82. Caregivers need to be skilled in assessing the infant's respiratory status while on high frequency ventilation. An important point the nurse needs to know in performing an accurate assessment for the infant requiring HFV is:

A. these infants do not require endotracheal suctioning.
B. auscultation of heart and breath sounds will be difficult because of the noise and constant vibration of HFV.
C. cardiopulmonary monitoring is not necessary with HFV because of increased respiratory rate and pulse oximeter usage.

83. Asymmetrical limbs are associated with all of the following EXCEPT:

A. maternal diabetes.
B. drug use.
C. hypocalcemia.

84. Erb-Duchenne paralysis is:

A. paralysis of the facial muscles.
B. paralysis of the upper portion of the arm.
C. weakened palmer grasp reflexes.

85. Pneumothoraces are usually caused by one or more of the following EXCEPT:

A. high pressure gradients from mechanical ventilation or continuous positive airway pressure across poorly compliant alveoli.
B. obstructive pulmonary pathology such as ball-valve air trapping.
C. rupture of the entire lung field.

86. Barlow's maneuver test is for:

A. neurologic intactness.
B. clubfoot anomaly.
C. dislocation of the femoral head from the acetabulum.

87. The respiratory system is composed of all of the following EXCEPT:

A. the pumping systems such as the chest wall muscles, diaphragm, and accessory muscles of respiration.
B. the bony rib cage and conducting airways.
C. oxygen supplementation that generates expansion of the lung on inspiration.

88. To palpate the liver and kidneys, the infant's abdominal musculature needs to be relaxed. The best method to obtain this relaxation is to:

A. flex the knees at the hips.
B. wait for the infant to enter the deep sleep state.
C. hold the infant in a sitting position.

89. The condition that occurs when the Pa_{O_2} is 50, Pa_{CO_2} rises above 45, base deficit −4, bicarbonate 22, and with a pH below 7.35 is called:

A. metabolic acidosis.
B. respiratory acidosis.
C. respiratory alkalosis.

90. This condition is the result of alveolar rupture from overdistention, usually with mechanical ventilation or continuous distending airway pressure.

A. BPD.
B. PIE.
C. RDS.

91. When caring for an infant with a suspected diaphragmatic hernia, the nurse should NOT:

A. do bag and mask ventilation.
B. give the infant chest compression for a heart rate below 80.
C. place an orogastric tube when applying ETT ventilation.

92. The mineral essential for bone mineralization, erythrocyte function, cell metabolism, and generation and storage of energy is:

A. calcium.
B. phosphorous.
C. magnesium.

93. A strategy used to reduce the risk of cell injury secondary to tissue hypoxia is to minimize oxygen demand by minimizing the neonate's metabolic rate. One way to do so is by:

A. maintaining a neutral thermal environment.
B. monitoring intermittent blood transfusions.
C. providing increased inspired oxygen concentrations.

94. The future trend in regionalization probably will be:

A. deregionalization–perinatal partnership.
B. more specialization and smaller units.
C. increased levels of care designations.

95. Nurses caring for the infant receiving surfactant need a working knowledge of the treatment modality to assist infants in achieving optimal outcomes. An essential component of nursing care is to suction the infant approximately:

A. 15 minutes before dosing via the ETT.
B. 15 minutes after dosing via the ETT.
C. one hour after dosing via the ETT.

96. The primary benefit of high frequency ventilation in the management of PIE is that:

A. high rates will help to increase cardiac output.
B. airway pressures can be significantly reduced.
C. hyperinflation does not occur with high-frequency ventilation.

97. Atrial natriuretic factor (ANF), peptide hormone, can be important in the regulation of circulating volume and arterial blood pressure. ANF causes natriuresis, diuresis, and vasodilation. The release of ANF is precipitated by:

A. arterial desaturation.
B. atrial distention.
C. pulmonary edema.

98. The function of thiamin (vitamin B_1) is:

A. coenzyme.
B. ATP component.
C. lipid metabolism.

99. The term used to describe the damage done to lung structures by mechanical stress is:

A. BPD.
B. barotrauma.
C. pneumothorax.

100. Antioxidant therapy is a promising new experimental therapy for the purpose of:

A. reducing the time required for infants placed on ECMO.
B. decreasing complications associated with BPD.
C. minimizing ventilator settings in the first 72 hours of life.

101. Recommended dosage for theophylline in the neonate is:

A. 2–4 mg/kg IV every 12 hours.
B. 6–8 mg/kg IV every 12 hours.
C. 6–8 mg/kg IV every six hours.

102. The corpus luteum is the source of:

A. estrogen.
B. progesterone.
C. HCG.

103. Which of the fetal shunts ensures that the fetal brain receives well-oxygenated blood?

A. ductus arteriosus.
B. ductus venosus.
C. foramen ovale.

104. What is the rationale for the administration of glucose/insulin to patients with hyperkalemia?

A. increase cellular uptake of potassium.
B. increase renal secretion of potassium.
C. antagonist effect of potassium on the cell membrane.

105. Hypoxemia in the first 24 hours of extrauterine life can result in:

A. constriction of pulmonary arterioles and dilation of ductus arteriosus.
B. dilation of ductus arteriosus and dilation of pulmonary arterioles.
C. dilation of pulmonary arterioles and constriction of ductus arteriosus.

106. What is responsible for symptoms of hyponatremia?

A. failure of the Na-K cellular pump.
B. influx of water into brain cells.
C. decreased secretion of magnesium secondary to decreased sodium levels.

107. The overall incidence of congenital heart defects (CHD) is about one percent or 8:1000 livebirths, excluding patent ductus arteriosus in preterm infants. What is the incidence of CHDs in newborns if the mother had a congenital heart defect?

A. one percent or 8:1000.
B. approximately 3–4 percent.
C. approximately 8–10 percent.

108. Bounding pulses are associated with cardiac defects that cause "aortic runoff." Cardiac lesions that lead to "aortic runoff" include:

A. atrial septal defects.
B. persistent truncus arteriosus.
C. tetralogy of Fallot.

109. One of the most important risk management tools is:

A. legal counsel.
B. communication.
C. incident reports.

110. Regurgitation systolic murmurs begin with S1, with no interval between S1 and the beginning of the murmur. Regurgitation murmurs are caused by flow of blood from a chamber other than the receiving chamber at higher pressure throughout systole. Regurgitation systolic murmurs are associated with only three conditions:

A. ASD, mitral regurgitation, and pulmonic regurgitation.
B. VSD, mitral regurgitation, and tricuspid regurgitation.
C. tetralogy of Fallot, mitral regurgitation, and tricuspid regurgitation.

111. Metabolic disease of the mother increases the risk for congenital heart defects. Infants of diabetic mothers have a 10 percent risk of having a congenital heart defect. What are the three most common heart defects found in infants of diabetic mothers (IDM)?

A. endocardial cushion defects (ECD), VSD, and pulmonic stenosis.
B. aortic insufficiency, aortic aneurysm, and aortic stenosis.
C. transposition of the great arteries (TGA), VSD, and hypertrophic cardiomyopathy.

112. The amount of flow through a patent ductus arteriosus is determined by:

A. diameter of ductus, length of ductus, and difference between systemic and pulmonary vascular resistance.
B. diameter and length of ductus and difference between left ventricular and right atrial pressures.
C. size of ductus and presence of pulmonary hypertension.

113. Right ventricular hypertrophy can occur in severe cases of VSD but does not generally occur in small or moderate VSD. What prevents development of right ventricular hypertrophy in these cases?

A. with small or moderate size VSD, low pulmonary venous resistance prevents excessive flow to the right ventricle.
B. in small or moderate VSD, there is almost equal pressure in both ventricles so shunting is minimal. There is no excessive workload on the right ventricle.
C. in moderate VSD, the blood is shunted from the left to right ventricle secondary to higher pressure in the left ventricle and higher systemic vascular resistance. The shunt of VSD occurs during systole when the right ventricle is contracted so blood is shunted into the pulmonary artery.

114. A neonate is tentatively diagnosed with "William Elfin facies" with thick lips, short palpebral fissures, and mental retardation. This infant should be evaluated for the presence of which congenital heart defect?

A. idiopathic hypertrophic subaortic stenosis (IHSS).
B. endocardial cushion defects (ECD; VSD is most common).
C. total or partial anomalous pulmonary venous return.

115. In total anomalous pulmonary venous return (TAPVR), the pulmonary veins drain into the right atrium rather than the left atrium directly or through connection with systemic veins. The degree of cyanosis present in TAPVR depends on the amount of

pulmonary blood flow. With increased pulmonary blood flow, there is highly saturated blood in the right atrium and mild cyanosis. With decreased pulmonary blood flow, cyanosis is severe. What is the cause of decreased pulmonary blood flow in infants with TAPVR?

A. obstruction to pulmonary blood flow secondary to TAPVR below the diaphragm.
B. elevated pulmonary vascular resistance secondary to decreased sensitivity to arterial Pa_{O_2}
C. decreased systemic resistance with decreased arterial blood pressure leading to increased systemic flow.

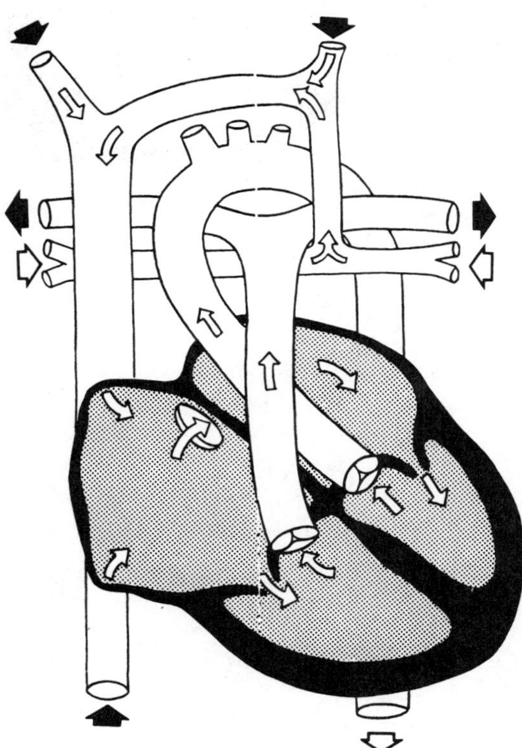

FIGURE 2 Total anomalous pulmonary venous return

116. Diuretics are useful in treatment of CHF to decrease sodium and water retention. Furosemide (Lasix), the most commonly used diuretic, works by:

A. inhibition of sodium and chloride reabsorption along the distal tubules.
B. binding to the cytoplasmic receptor sites and blocking aldosterone action, thus impairing the reabsorption of sodium and the secretion of potassium and hydrogen ions.
C. blocking sodium and chloride reabsorption in the ascending limb of the loop of Henle.

117. Subacute infective endocarditis (SAIE) can be a complication of congenital heart defects. All congenital heart defects that produce turbulent flow or have a significant pressure gradient predispose to bacterial invasion of the cardiac endothelium. Which of the following congenital heart defects does not predispose to SAIE?

A. ASD (secundum).
B. aortic stenosis.
C. VSD.

IN THE NEXT SIX QUESTIONS, IDENTIFY THE CONGENITAL HEART DEFECT DEPICTED IN THE ILLUSTRATION.

118. A. TGA.
B. TOF.
C. COA.

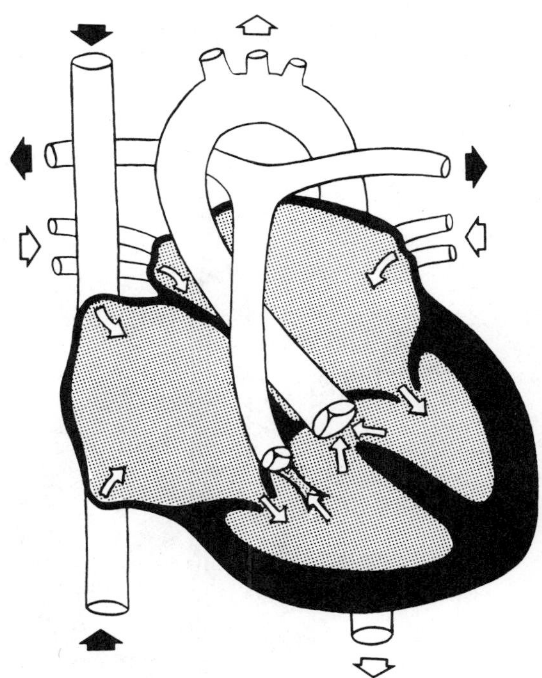

119. A. TGA.
B. VSD.
C. HLHS.

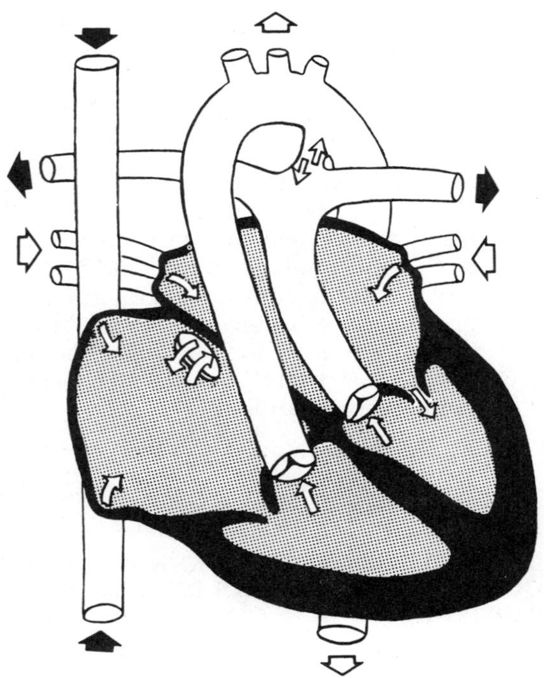

120. A. VSD.
B. ASD.
C. ECD.

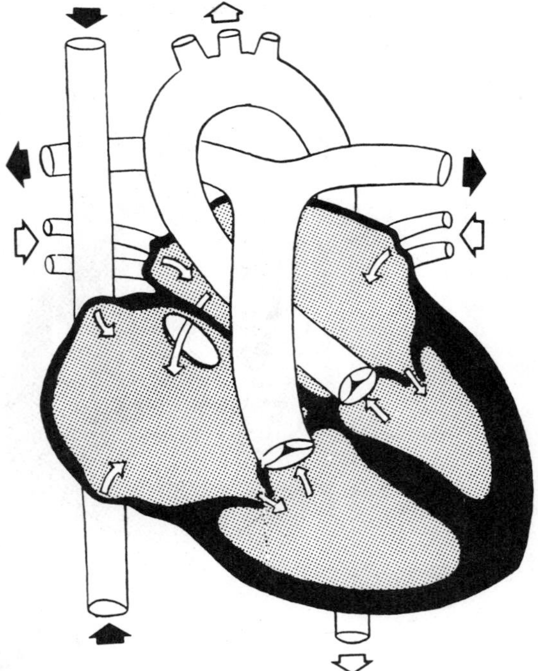

121. A. TAPVR.
B. PS.
C. VSD.

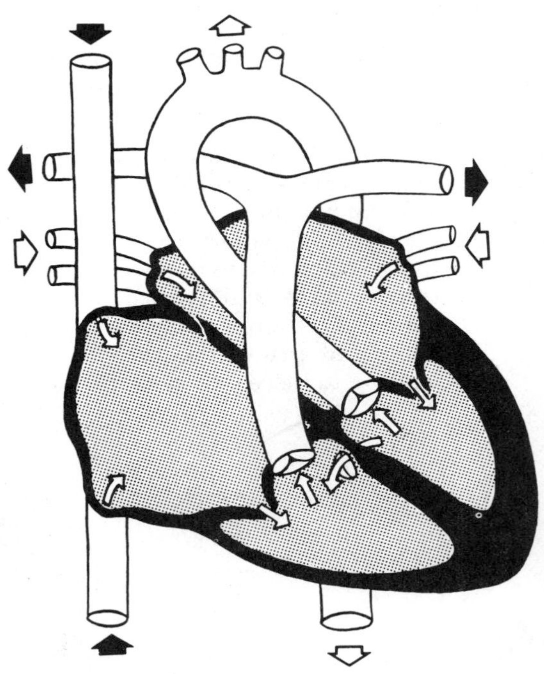

122. A. AV canal.
B. ASD.
C. PDA.

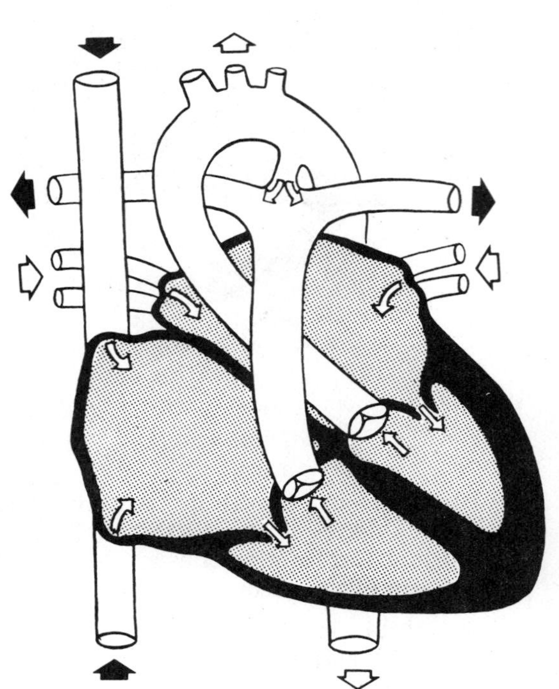

123. A. pulmonic stenosis.
B. COA.
C. HLHS.

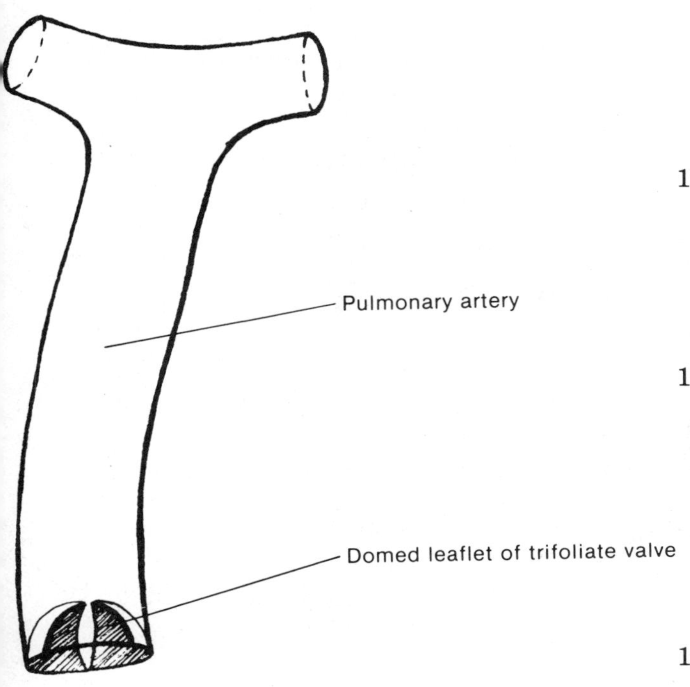

124. There are various developmental stages of neonatal nursing practice. The stage in which independence occurs is seen during which period?

A. beginning practitioner.
B. technician.
C. communicator/translator of neonatal practice.

125. The volume of the ICF is regulated by:

A. Na-K cellular pump.
B. renal adjustment of sodium.
C. colloid osmotic pressure.

126. Transposition of the great arteries (TGA) or transposition of the great vessels (TGV) is the result of inappropriate septation and migration of the truncus arteriosus during fetal cardiac development. What are the hemodynamic consequences of D-TGA?

A. oxygenated blood comes into the left atrium, enters the right ventricle, and goes through the aorta to the systemic circulation.
B. oxygenated blood from the lungs goes to the left atrium, enters the left ventricle, into the pulmonary artery into the lungs.
C. oxygenated blood from the lungs enters the right atrium through the pulmonary valve and is directed into the right ventricle and to the aorta into the systemic circulation.

127. High volumes of parenteral fluids have been associated with which of the following?

A. chronic lung disease.
B. renal tubular acidosis.
C. syndrome of IADH.

128. Which of the following statements about sodium regulation is accurate?

A. sodium is filtered by the tubules and collecting ducts of the kidney.
B. oncotic and hydrostatic pressure in the peritubular capillaries regulate sodium.
C. sodium cannot be absorbed without chloride.

129. What is the most common cause of early (1–2 days postbirth) onset of hyponatremia?

A. perinatal asphyxia.
B. maternal parenteral fluid therapy.
C. insufficient sodium supplementation in parenteral therapy (neonate).

130. Which of the following conditions can be associated with hyponatremia with decreased total body water?

A. renal failure.
B. patent ductus arteriosus.
C. adrenal hemorrhage.

131. When increased volume enters an adult heart, contractility is increased to increase cardiac output to prevent excessive accumulation of blood in the veins. The neonatal response to increased volume is increased heart rate. What is the physiological explanation for this difference in response?

A. venous return is determined by movement of blood through the veins, the thoracic pump, and the venous pump, which adversely affects contractility in the neonate.
B. local factors such as hypoxia, acidosis, hypercarbia, and increased metabolic demand prevent sufficient contractility in the neonatal heart, secondary to decreased glycogen stores for energy.
C. the newborn's heart has fewer fibers and cannot stretch sufficiently to accommodate increased volume.

132. Which of the following ECG changes are associated with hyperkalemia (serum K >5.0 mEq/L)?

A. depression of ST segment, flattened T wave, and increased height of U wave.
B. peaked T waves, disappearance of P waves, and widening of QRS complex.
C. depressed ST segment, narrowed QRS, and fusion with T wave to form a sine wave.

133. What is the most common cause of increased renal loss of chloride?

A. acute tubular necrosis.
B. decreased ADH release.
C. diuretic therapy.

134. What is the characteristic feature of Bartter's syndrome?

A. increased renal loss of chloride.
B. decreased renal secretion of chloride.
C. increased potassium reabsorption and decreased chloride reabsorption in the renal tubules.

135. Increased calcitonin would result in:

A. increased tubular reabsorption of calcium.
B. increased production of 1,25-dihydroxyvitamin D.
C. increased calcium excretion.

136. Why has the prevalence of late hypocalcemia decreased?

A. supplementation of breastfed infants.
B. use of better whey/casein ratio formula.
C. use of formulas with lower phosphate loads.

137. Which of the following conditions is associated with hypercalcemia?

A. subcutaneous fat necrosis.
B. DiGeorge syndrome.
C. IVH.

138. Magnesium is distributed primarily in the:

A. liver, adrenals, and kidneys.
B. skeleton and intracellular spaces.
C. lungs, heart, and thymus.

139. Vitamin B_6 includes pyridoxine, pyridoxal, and pyridoxamine. Which of the following are functions of the B_6 complex vitamins?

A. synthesis of neurotransmitters.
B. metabolism of glucose.
C. electron transport.

140. What other deficiency condition must be considered in the diagnosis/treatment of vitamin B_{12} deficiency?

A. folic acid.
B. vitamin B_6.
C. vitamin C.

141. How is vitamin A transported to the liver for storage?

A. bound to the red blood cell membrane.
B. incorporated into chylomicrons.
C. bound to albumin.

142. What is the purpose of the cardiac sphincter?

A. to prevent reflux of stomach contents into the esophagus.
B. to prevent too rapid transit time in the stomach.
C. to allow for decreased pressure on the esophagus from cardiac blood flow.

143. Vitamin K is necessary for the synthesis of which coagulation factors?

A. I, III, IX, XI.
B. II, VII, IX, X.
C. I, II, VI, X.

144. What is the mechanism responsible for the antibody response to cow's milk protein frequently seen in infants with damaged bowel?

A. relative ineffectiveness of pancreatic digestive phase, resulting in inability to break down polypeptides.
B. direct absorption of macromolecules is impaired.
C. frequent use of gastric or jejunal feedings, which bypasses the mouth, resulting in decreased salivary amylase.

145. Intake of what nutrient can contribute to the development of fluid in the intrapleural space after chest surgery?

A. protein.
B. fat.
C. carbohydrate.

146. How does aldosterone influence sodium regulation?

A. aldosterone controls the Na-K pump.
B. aldosterone increases absorption of sodium in exchange with potassium or hydrogen ions.
C. aldosterone regulates glucose reabsorption that affects sodium reabsorption.

147. The enzymes required for breaking down disaccharides are found in the:

A. pancreas and intestines.
B. endothelium of the ileum.
C. brush border villi of the intestines.

148. What is the action of Wydase in the treatment of IV infiltration?

A. to prevent absorption of the fluid and tissue damage.
B. to break down the cell membrane and dissipate the chemical irritant.
C. to decrease peripheral vascular permeability, allowing absorption of extravascular fluid.

149. Methods used to determine gestational age in utero include all of the following EXCEPT:

A. fetal heart tones.
B. nonstress testing.
C. ultrasound.

150. The philosophical foundation of the collaborative practice model is based on:

A. identification of personal/professional values.
B. avoidance of ethical conflicts as the team's goal.
C. the fact that constancy of caregivers is not always possible.

151. Rickets is caused by:

A. inadequate intake of calcium and phosphorus.
B. inadequate intake of calcium and increased intake of phosphorus.
C. inadequate intake of phosphorus and increased intake of calcium.

152. What is the average daily caloric requirement for enteral feedings for tissue growth and repair in preterm infants?

A. 120 kcal/kg/d.
B. 140 kcal/kg/d.
C. 150 kcal/kg/d.

153. What is the essential function of vitamin D?

A. metabolism of calcium and phosphorus.
B. maintaining the integrity of the red blood cell membrane.
C. synthesis of the parathyroid hormone.

154. The formation of the GI tract is primarily dependent on:

A. proliferation of the dorsal portion of the yolk sac.
B. invagination of the proximal mesodermic cells.
C. folding of the embryo at the end of four weeks.

155. The mouth develops from a surface depression in the ectoderm called the:

A. stomodeum.
B. cloaca.
C. proctodeum.

156. What causes loops of intestines to protrude through the umbilicus out of the abdominal cavity at about seven weeks gestation?

A. rapid growth of intestines and liver.
B. impaired development of abdominal musculature.
C. rotation around superior mesenteric artery.

157. At what point in gestation is the GI tract innervated by the peripheral nervous system?

A. around six weeks.
B. around 12 weeks.
C. around 20 weeks.

158. An inability to establish adequate ventilation at birth with subsequent hypoxemia, respiratory and metabolic acidosis, hypotension, bradycardia, and CNS depression is termed:

A. perinatal asphyxia.
B. fetal demise.
C. neonatal asphyxia.

159. What normally controls the speed of gastric emptying?

A. fundal and antral contractions.
B. chemical composition and amount of chyme.
C. amount of hydrochloric acid secretion.

160. Very low birth weight infants (<1500 g) with respiratory distress and delayed feedings pass their first meconium stool at about:

A. 48 hours after birth.
B. 100–120 hours after birth.
C. 168 hours after birth.

161. What is the process by which lactate and amino acids are converted to glucose?

A. gluconeongenesis.
B. glycolysis.
C. glycogen synthesis.

162. Which parts of the GI tract are more sensitive to distention or irritating stimuli?

A. esophagus, stomach.
B. stomach, duodenum.
C. jejunum, ileum.

163. Why is percussion unreliable in the newborn GI examination?

A. the higher total body water of the newborn causes "muffling" of sounds.
B. the internal abdominal organs are small and close together.
C. the decreased abdominal muscle tone permits increased sound transmission.

164. What is considered the single most significant contribution to screening populations for metabolic disease?

A. detection of phenylpyruvic acid in urine.
B. bacterial inhibition tests.
C. serum phenylalanine tests.

165. What organ is the primary regulator of blood glucose?

A. pancreas.
B. liver.
C. pituitary.

166. Congenital hypothyroidism is characterized by:

A. prematurity.
B. a small posterior fontanelle.
C. delay passing meconium.

167. What is the most sensitive indirect test for the detection of lactose deficiency in term neonates?

A. serum lactic acid levels.
B. breath hydrogen.
C. response to dietary restriction.

168. What is the basis for diagnosis of galactosemia?

A. nuclear cataract development.
B. absence of transferase activity of the red blood cell.
C. presence of glucose reducing substance in the urine.

169. The infant with large, protuberant abdomen and thin chest and extremities is seen in:

A. galactosemia.
B. maple syrup urine disease.
C. glycogen storage disease.

170. Growth hormone deficiency can result in:

A. intrauterine growth retardation.

B. small for gestational age infant.
C. hypoglycemia.

171. Severe acidosis is associated with:

A. glycogen storage disease type I (G-6-PD).
B. glycogen storage disease type II (G-6-PD).
C. glycogen storage disease type IV (G-6-PD).

172. The most frequent cause of SIADH is:

A. prematurity.
B. asphyxia.
C. IVH.

173. An IDM should be monitored during the first few hours of life for:

A. hyperglycemia.
B. seizures.
C. hypoinsulinism.

174. The most common cause of ambiguous genitalia is:

A. congenital adrenal hyperplasia.
B. maternal diabetes.
C. maternal steroid use.

175. Where does ionization of calcium compounds take place?

A. stomach.
B. duodenum.
C. ileum.

176. What is the chief symptom of ABO incompatibility?

A. anemia.
B. jaundice.
C. petechiae.

177. Respiratory syncytial virus is treated with:

A. ampicillin and gentamicin.
B. methicillin.
C. ribovirin.

178. A 32-week AGA male infant is admitted to the NICU with respiratory distress. Maternal history reveals a maternal temperature, PROM × 18 hours, and mild perinatal asphyxia. What antimicrobials should be started on this infant?

A. ampicillin.
B. ampicillin and gentamicin.
C. nafcillin and gentamicin.

179. What is an essential function of vitamin E?

A. antioxidant.
B. antimetabolite.
C. fibrinolysis.

180. A 22-day-old infant was worked up for sepsis and started on ampicillin and gentamicin on Tuesday. On Wednesday, the final sensitivities of the organism are not complete, yet the ID says that it is a penicillinase-producing organism. The antimicrobials should be:

A. nafcillin and gentamicin.
B. methicillin and ticarcillin.
C. vancomycin and clindamycin.

181. What is the major stimulus for RBC production during late fetal development?

A. erythropoietin.
B. prostaglandins.
C. testosterone/estrogen.

182. What is the reason that AO or BO blood type incompatibility occurs more frequently than AB incompatibility?

A. type A blood is not as prevalent as types O and B.
B. type B blood produces anti-A antibodies that are weak and not very effective.
C. in the O mother, antibodies are of IgG and can cross the placenta; A and B type antibodies are of IgM and are too large to cross the placenta.

183. What is the rationale for irradiation of RBC transfusions?

A. reduce risk of HIV transmission from donor blood.
B. reduce risk of graft versus host disease from lymphocytes contained in the transfusion.
C. irradiation removes antibody coating of RBC.

184. What enzyme is necessary for biliary excretion of bilirubin?

A. glucuronide.
B. ligandin.
C. glucuronyl transferase.

185. During a double-volume exchange transfusion, almost 75 percent of the newborn's RBC cell mass is replaced, but only 25 percent of the bilirubin is removed. What is the reason for this difference?

A. the major portion of bilirubin is in the extravascular space and is not affected by the exchange.
B. some hemolysis of the donor blood occurs during the transfusion that decreases the relative effectiveness of the transfusion.
C. the majority of bilirubin is in the arterial system; exchange transfusions are generally performed through the umbilical vein.

186. What is the role of vitamin K in vitamin K-dependent clotting factors?

A. required for synthesis of clotting factors.
B. required for distribution of clotting factors.
C. required for conversion of precursor proteins.

187. The defect in which the spinal cord is open and exposed is:
C. myelomeningocele.
B. meningocele.
C. myeloschisis.

188. As the dietary intake of polyunsaturated fatty acids increases, the requirement of what nutrient also increases?

A. folic acid.
B. iron.
C. vitamin E.

189. Depolarization and repolarization of cells in the nervous system are produced by:

A. movement of sodium and potassium across the cell membrane.
B. transport of calcium into or out of cells.
C. action of acetycholine as a neurotransmitter.

190. Which of the following causes of seizures is associated with the poorest prognosis?

A. hypocalcemia.
B. subarachnoid hemorrhage.
C. birth asphyxia.

191. Which of the following signs is frequently seen early in IVH?

A. fullness of the anterior fontanel.
B. impaired visual tracking.
C. falling hematocrit.

192. What is the initial treatment for linear skull fractures?

A. management for shock and hemorrhage.
B. manual elevation of fracture.
C. observation.

193. Vitamin C deficiency is associated with:

A. decreased vitamin B_{12} absorption.
B. increased iron absorption.
C. transient tyrosinemia.

194. Median nerve injuries are most often caused by:

A. fracture of the humerus.
B. compression of nerve during breech delivery.
C. brachial or radial arterial punctures.

195. What is the most common malformation associated with hydrocephalus?

A. aqueductal (Sylvius) stenosis.
B. Dandy-Walker syndrome.
C. Arnold-Chiari malformation.

196. Achondroplasia is the most common form of dwarfism, having a pattern of inheritance of:

A. multifactorial.
B. autosomal dominant.
C. autosomal recessive.

197. The innermost layer of the GI tract is the:

A. adventitia.
B. submucosa.
C. mucosa.

198. Which of the following families should <u>NOT</u> be referred to a genetics counselor for a calculation of future reproductive risks?

A. a family of an infant with achondroplasia.
B. a family of an infant with distal arthrogryposis.
C. a family of an infant with congenital hip dysplasia.

Case Study

Cindy, a 24-year-old, primpara, gave birth to an 8 lb 7 oz, LGA, 38-week male infant. On examination, the infant, Josh, was found to have syndactyly of the left hand. Other findings revealed an audible hip click, talipes varus, blue sclera, cardiopulmonary status stable. No limitation in movement was found. All other physical parameters were within normal limits. Maternal history: spotting during the first trimester, oliohydramnios; 20 pound weight gain; diagnosed with gestational diabetes one month before delivery.

THE FOLLOWING SIX QUESTIONS ARE BASED ON THIS VIGNETTE.

199. To assess the audible hip click, the NNP or neonatal nurse performed the ______ test. This test is used to determine the dislocation in the hip. It is done by flexing the hip to 90 degrees while bending the knee. The hip is then gently abducted. A positive finding reveals a click or clunk.

A. Barlow's
B. Ortolani's
C. Barlow and Ortolani's

200. ______ test is used to determine the instability of the hip. With this test both hips and knees are flexed, with the hip to be tested in slight adduction. Gentle pressure is exerted by the thumb posteriorly and laterally (down and out). The femoral head can be felt to move out with a clunk.

A. Barlow's
B. Ortolani's
C. Both

201. Josh was found to have congenital dysplasia of the hip (CDH). Treatment for this problem includes:

A. surgical intervention.
B. splinting of the hip.
C. a wait-and-see approach.

202. Clubfoot is referred to as ______.

A. talipes equinovarus.
B. talipes equinovalgus.
C. talipes calcaneous valgus.

203. Hypotheses about the etiology of clubfoot includes:

A. polyhydramnios.
B. multiparity.
C. macrosomia.

204. Surgical correction of syndactyly is necessary to preserve function of the affected digits. This surgical intervention should be done:

A. immediately after birth.
B. within the first six months of life.
C. at 6–12 months of age.

205. Amniotic band syndrome has been associated with all of the following deformities EXCEPT:

A. cleft palate and lip.
B. gastroschisis.
C. congenital hip dislocation.

206. The kidney performs several critical functions for the neonate. These functions include all of the following EXCEPT:

A. secretion.
B. accretion.
C. reabsorption.

207. Tubular ______ is the process by which substances are moved from the epithelial lining of the tubule's capillaries into the interstitial fluid and finally into the lumen.

A. secretion
B. excretion
C. reabsorption

208. Kidney function with production of fetal urine is established by approximately the ______ gestational week.

A. fourth
B. eighth
C. twelfth

209. What is the site of urine formation?

A. nephron.
B. renal tubules.
C. glomeruli.

210. Hydraulic pressure within the renal capillaries depends on:

A. colloid concentration.
B. plasma albumin.
C. renal blood flow.

211. The chief function of the renin-angiotensin cycle is to maintain:

A. arterial blood pressure.
B. renal blood flow.
C. systemic blood flow.

212. How is calcium absorbed?

A. by a carrier-mediated mechanism and passive diffusion.
B. active transport across the mucosal lining.
C. in combination with phosphates.

213. If an abdominal mass is found, which of the following tests is most useful for establishing a diagnosis?

A. abdominal x-ray.
B. computed tomography.
C. abdominal ultrasonography.

214. Which immunoglobulin is readily transferred across the placenta?

A. IgA.
B. IgG.
C. IgM.

215. The most common cause of hydronephrosis is:

A. uretoropelvis junction obstruction.
B. cystic kidneys.
C. Wilms' tumor.

216. The single most significant concern about the skin is:

A. trauma.
B. infection.
C. iatrogenic problems.

217. The tympanic membrane should be examined for thickness, vascularity, and contour. If otitis media is present, the tympanic membrane will appear:

A. mobile.
B. yellow.
C. translucent.

218. Subcutaneous fat begins to be deposited and smooth out the skin's wrinkles by:

A. 26–29 weeks.
B. 30–34 weeks.
C. 35–38 weeks.

219. Photosensitiviy of the full-term newborn's skin is due in part to:

A. reduced melanin production.
B. increased permeability.
C. decreased skin thickness.

220. Rubella most often results in:

A. sensorineural hearing loss.
B. conductive hearing loss.
C. mixed hearing loss.

221. Cutis marmorata is:

A. a normal physiologic vascular response to cool air.
B. a sign of a dermatologic infection.
C. the most common rash of newborns.

222. ______ is a diffuse, generalized edema of the scalp caused by local pressure and trauma during labor. The borders are not well defined, and the swelling crosses suture lines.

A. Caput succedaneum
B. Cephalhematoma
C. Periosteal bleed

223. Epidermolysis bullosa (EB) is a group of congenital blistering disorders that are:

A. always lethal.
B. sex-linked conditions.
C. sometimes responsible for dysphagia.

224. Vibracoustic stimulation to the fetus that results in an impaired fetal response is:

A. not predictive of a compromised fetus.
B. is predictive of a compromised fetus.
C. has less predictive value than a nonstress test.

225. Blueberry muffin syndrome is most often seen with infection from:

A. varicella zoster.
B. cytomegalovirus.
C. toxoplasmosis.

226. Use of Skin Gel or Prep in the care of neonates is generally:

A. encouraged to promote skin integrity.
B. discouraged because absorption is unknown.
C. used only in VLBW infants.

227. The most sensitive period for shaping auditory ability is:

A. one–12 months of life.
B. seven months gestation, 12 months of life.
C. five months gestation, 28 months of life.

228. Endotracheal intubation of longer than ______ days is associated with middle ear effusion.

A. 7
B. 14
C. 21

229. Incidence of ______ hearing loss in infants with severe perinatal asphyxia is about four percent.

A. conductive
B. sensorineural
C. mixed

230. Hearing loss associated with syphilis is:

A. sudden.
B. gradual.
C. mild.

231. Which of the following physical characteristics are associated with auditory problems?

A. absent epicanthic folds.
B. pili torti (twisted hair).
C. long neck.

232. Children requiring hearing aids should be fitted by the age of:

A. three months.
B. 12 months.
C. 18 months.

233. Capillary hemagiomas of the eyelid are tumors that:

A. will cause only a cosmetic problem.
B. can cause both a cosmetic and visual problem.
C. will gradually regress over the first year of life.

234. The term allele refers to:

A. alternative loci on the same gene.
B. two genes from two parents.
C. alternative chromosomes.

235. Cataracts with an oil-drop appearance are indicative of:

A. congenital rubella.
B. galactosemia.
C. infant of a diabetic mother.

236. An infrared thermometer is an example of the ideal biophysical sensor because it:

A. requires only brief patient contact.
B. requires minimal external stimulation for detection.
C. measures directly from emitted electromagnetic energies.

237. An infant receiving phototherapy can have inaccurate biophysical monitor from tranducers due to:

A. signal interference.
B. optical radiation.
C. increase in thermal environment.

238. Which of the following neonates might have more of a chance of inaccurate indirect bilirubin level measured transcutaneously?

A. black male, postmature infant.
B. white male, postmature infant.
C. black female, premature infant.

239. Conditions that have diagnostic benefit from imaging include:

A. cytomegalovirus.
B. Group B *Streptococcus*.
C. rubella.

240. A "burned out" appearance of the lungs on x-ray is indicative of:

A. severe, respiratory distress.
B. overexposed x-ray.
C. inspiratory film.

241. An advantage of MRI over CT scans is:

A. cost and availability.
B. useful for unstable infant.
C. image can be in all planes.

242. Echocardiography is a commonly used diagnostic procedure for the neonate because it can provide information about:

A. blood flow through the heart but cannot measure cardiac output.
B. anatomical structures of the heart.
C. Both.

243. Possible side effects of an upper GI with small bowel follow-through for the neonate are:

A. fluid overload and hypertension.
B. fluid loss and hypotension.
C. fluid loss and hypertension.

244. Fetal surgery should only be done when:

A. neonatal survival is certain with the procedure.
B. neonatal death will result without the procedure.
C. fetal compromise can be reversed.

245. Anesthesia during pregnancy imposes special physiologic considerations for the mother. A physiologic difference between healthy pregnant adults and healthy non-pregnant adult females is:

A. an increase in peripheral vascular resistance.
B. a decrease in functional residual capacity.
C. a decrease in alveolar ventilation.

246. Conditions that are treatable by fetal surgery include all of the following EXCEPT:

A. Arnold-Chiari malformation.
B. bladder outlet obstruction.
C. biliary atresia.

247. In the surgical neonate, acidosis can occur due to all of the following EXCEPT:

A. inadequate ventilatory support.
B. sepsis.
C. sodium acetate administration.

248. Dobutamine achieves organ perfusion by:

A. increasing cardiac output.
B. decreasing acidosis.
C. vasodilatation of renal vessels.

249. What discovery led to a change in the way in which neonatal pain was viewed?

A. the majority of fibers that transmit pain in adults are not myelinated.
B. typical behavioral responses to pain were described.
C. elevated levels of catecholamines were demonstrated after painful stimuli.

250. Which of the following maternal conditions is associated with hypomagnesemia?

A. PIH/pre-eclampsia.
B. placental insufficiency.
C. Graves' disease.

251. What is one of the most challenging tasks of infant pain management?

A. selection of appropriate agents for pain management.
B. differentiation of agitation due to pain or other causes.
C. observation of behavioral responses to painful events.

252. Pain in the infant can be classified as:

A. actual or potential tissue damage.
B. nonexistent.
C. at the level of a semianesthetized adult.

253. Neural plasticity in the development of the CNS is an important factor in pain development. The concept of neural plasticity involves the principles of:

A. environmental interaction.
B. infant interaction.
C. interaction between the infant and the environment.

254. Pain perception for the infant begins:

A. at birth.
B. in utero.
C. not until one month of age.

255. Endorphins are produced in response to asphyxia, acidosis, and maternal drug addiction in the:

A. full-term neonate.
B. fetus.
C. premature neonate.

256. The sympathetic response to pain in newborns is:

A. the same as a pediatric client.
B. less predictable than the adult.
C. the same as an adult.

257. Anand (1990) has done much work with surgical infants and pain. The research findings support that hormonal-metabolic changes are:

A. the same as an adult.
B. greater than an adult.
C. less than an adult.

258. An infant who is cold or vasoconstricted would not be a candidate for IM drug administration. The reasoning behind this includes:

A. all of the drug may not get into the infant because the hub of the syringe will hold about 0.1 ml of solution.
B. absorption of the drug from an IM site is directly related to the blood flow to that site.
C. IM injections can cause drug toxicity in the vasconstricted neonate.

259. Postmaturity syndrome is characterized by:

A. edema.
B. growth failure.
C. decreased alertness.

260. Enteral drug therapy produces unpredictable circulating concentrations for drugs that undergo hepatic first pass elimination. *First pass effect* is the:

A. therapeutic effect created by an initial loading dose of medication.
B. removal of a large portion of a drug dose during the first circulation through an organ.
C. drug level remaining after three-day antibiotic administration.

261. Peak and trough drug concentrations frequently are used in therapeutic drug monitoring. Trough concentration is the:

A. highest concentration one hour after infusion of the drug.
B. lowest concentration just before the administration of the next dose.
C. concentration immediately after the end of the distribution phase.

262. A primary goal of monitoring drug concentrations is to:

A. achieve concentrations that are effective at the site of drug action.
B. give the least amount of drug possible.
C. maintain concentrations in the recommended therapeutic range.

263. A surprisingly small number of drugs are completely contraindicated during nursing. Cocaine and heroin are two such drugs. Another contraindicated drug during nursing would be:

A. aspirin.
B. phenobarbital.
C. bromocriptine.

264. HIV is a ______ that attaches to ______ receptor sites.

A. reovirus, CD^+
B. retrovirus, $CD4^+$
C. reovirus, $CD8^+$

265. HIV exposed infants should be placed in:

A. regular nursery if stable.
B. isolation room of NICU.
C. room with mother.

266. The latency period for perinatally exposed HIV infants is approximately:

A. six months.
B. 12–18 months.
C. 24 months.

267. Early signs and symptoms of HIV include all of the following EXCEPT:

A. inorganic failure to thrive.
B. recurrent infections.
C. thrombocytopenia.

268. Children scheduled to undergo transplantation should:

A. not receive any immunizations, especially hepatitis B.
B. receive all immunizations, especially hepatitis B.
C. receive only the influenza immunization.

269. The ELISA test will tell the practitioner that:

A. neonatal infection is present.
B. HIV antibodies are present.
C. infant is HIV positive.

270. Liver transplantation is offered to:

A. all children with progressive liver failure.
B. only children with inherited metabolic diseases.
C. only children with primary abnormal liver function.

271. Boarder babies is a term used to describe:

A. infants who live in hospital without medical necessity.
B. infants who live in hospital because they are HIV positive.
C. infants who are placed in foster care due to their HIV status.

272. In most cases, pretransplant management includes anticipation of complications from portal hypertension. Signs of portal hypertension include:

A. leukopenia.
B. esophageal strictures.
C. hyposplenism.

273. Rejection of the transplant occurs in approximately ______ of the cases when orthoclone OKT-3 is used in combination with prednisone, and azathioprine initially, later adding cyclosporin.

A. 95 percent
B. 46 percent
C. 25 percent

274. To reduce the number of iatrogenic complications from the bandwagon approach to care, the NNP should initially:

A. review the literature on this new therapy before its initiation.
B. take a wait-and-see approach, watching the patient carefully.
C. design a research study to examine the effects of the therapy.

275. Expected neonatal behavior related to in utero cocaine exposure is described as:

A. a classic withdrawal pattern.
B. a quiet, subdued demeanor.
C. irritability and hypersensitivity to handling.

276. If nurses have the sole responsibility for the introduction of equipment into the NICU, two steps that will smooth the process are:

A. asking standard questions of all sales representatives and creating a critical function list of the equipment.
B. asking standard questions of all sales representatives and requiring on-site technical assistance for the first month.
C. creating a critical function list of the equipment and requiring on-site technical assistance for the first month.

277. Cocaine is metabolized by the esterase-enzymes that are produced in the liver and are present in the plasma. Cholinesterase activity varies for each individual. For the nurse caring for the cocaine exposed neonate this means:

A. cocaine will remain present in the maternal system longer than the neonatal system.
B. cocaine will remain present in the neonatal system longer than the maternal system.
C. both maternal and neonatal systems will metabolize cocaine at the same rate.

278. Which of the following substances is considered teratogenic to the facial development?

A. cocaine.
B. heroin.
C. alcohol.

279. The critical period for alcohol ingestion and fetal alcohol syndrome has been found to be:

A. first trimester.
B. second trimester.
C. immediately before labor.

280. In caring for the family of a drug exposed neonate, it is important to:

A. focus on what damage already may have been sustained.
B. use scare tactics so this does not occur in subsequent pregnancies.
C. focus on the potential good that could occur from detoxification.

281. Computers are used throughout neonatal care units. Data bases hold not only information about the patient but also are useful for:

A. easy storage and retrieval of reference information.
B. calculation of drugs based on the infant's weight.
C. all of the above.

282. Soothing interventions include all the following EXCEPT:

A. swaddling.
B. increasing stimulation.
C. containment.

283. An example of an expert computer system using artificial intelligence would be a system that:

A. provides an algorithm for determining ventilator settings based on ABG data.
B. allows the user to choose nursing diagnoses and applicable interventions.
C. can calculate calories/kg/day.

284. The term CAI refers to:

A. computer access information.
B. computer available interaction.
C. computer assisted instruction.

285. Within the home environment, the ______ was found to be the best predictive factor for later positive development in preterm infants.

A. parent–infant interaction
B. access to stimulating toys
C. feeding interaction

286. To help a mother recognize infant cues for feeding readiness, the nurse might suggest use of:

A. NCAST teaching scale.
B. NCASA records.
C. Fagan Infantest.

287. An infant can be at risk for child abuse because of:

A. lack of social support for mother.
B. behavioral characteristics.
C. prematurity.

288. Contingent interaction depends on:

A. clarity of infant cues.
B. unpredictability of other earlier behaviors.
C. reaction to inappropriate behaviors.

289. Use of protocols for home-based follow-up is important because the protocols:

A. eliminate the need for physician follow-up.
B. complement current agency strategies.
C. preclude need for individualized care plans.

290. State organization can be used to predict:

A. individual infant temperament.
B. developmental outcome.
C. maternal–infant attachment.

291. Parent drop-out syndrome refers to:

A. parents who are unwilling to come to the hospital to learn the infant care needed once at home.
B. parents who are too dependent on home care personnel so they cannot help with their infant's care.
C. parents who are overwhelmed by the prospect of a chronically ill child and opt for foster care.

292. Neonatal Individualized Development Care and Assessment Program (NIDCAP) is based on:

A. naturalistic observation.
B. Brazelton examination.
C. controlled observation.

293. Stress signals include:

A. "Ooh" face.
B. yawning.
C. robust crying.

294. According to Rubin, the second trimester of pregnancy represents the time of beginning all the following EXCEPT:

A. binding in process.
B. claiming process.
C. attachment process.

295. The process of grief:

A. is only applicable to parents whose children die.
B. is applicable to parents who have premature or sick neonates who may or may not die.
C. represents an abnormal coping mechanism.

296. Hospice care for newborns has as its primary goal:

A. to provide an environment that comforts the infant and family.
B. to provide relief or time out for the family.
C. to provide palliative, terminal care.

297. Barriers to hospice care for infants and children include all of the following EXCEPT:

   A. need for a physician's certification of impending death.
   B. lack of or inadequate financial reimbursement for care.
   C. lack of acceptance of hospice as an alternative care approach.

298. The control of the development of advanced practice in neonatal nursing should belong to:

   A. professional organizations.
   B. legislators.
   C. state boards of nursing.

299. Cystic fibrosis is an example of:

   A. autosomal dominant inheritance.
   B. autosomal recessive inheritance.
   C. multifactorial inheritance.

300. What is responsible for the timing of the closure of the aortic and pulmonary valves (S2)?

   A. degree of pulmonary vascular resistance and systemic blood pressure.
   B. volume of blood flow from aorta and pulmonary artery and systemic vascular resistance.
   C. right ventricle filling time and right ventricular ejection time.

REVIEW TEST 2

1. Experienced neonatal nurses act as communicators and translators of neonatal nursing care practices. Nurses at this level of career development:

   A. are informal mentors.
   B. let technical skills lapse.
   C. are not in supervisory roles.

2. How is osteopenia of prematurity different than rickets in older infants or children?

   A. cause is inadequate intake of calcium and phosphorus.
   B. cause is selective demineralization of bones.
   C. occurs with normal serum calcium and phosphorus levels.

3. Signs of abruptio placentae include:

   A. dark red vaginal bleeding.
   B. bright red vaginal bleeding.
   C. no noticeable pain.

4. One role of the level III unit is perinatal outreach education. The focus of this education is on:

   A. orientation of new personnel.
   B. functioning of the perinatal team.
   C. morbidity and mortality rates in the region.

Case History

Kelly, a very pale, thin, unmarried, 16-year-old, who admitted to alcohol use throughout the pregnancy, delivered a 30-week female infant. The infant was noted to be irritable and required ventilatory assistance. On examination, the infant's head circumference and weight were found to be below the 10th percentile. One finger was constricted.

THE FOLLOWING THREE QUESTIONS ARE BASED ON THIS VIGNETTE.

5. From the history, it might be expected that Kelly experienced:

   A. polyhydramnios.
   B. oligohydramnios.
   C. hydramnios.

6. The constriction of the digit can be related to amniotic fluid levels. The constriction is due to a condition called:

   A. amnionitis.
   B. amniotic band syndrome.
   C. polyhydraminos.

7. The intrauterine growth retardation may be directly related to:

   A. prematurity.
   B. maternal age.
   C. alcohol intake.

8. Gametes contain the ______ number of chromosomes.

   A. haploid
   B. diploid
   C. polyploid

9. Abruptio placentae is associated with:

   A. prior abortion.
   B. PIH.
   C. multigestation pregnancy.

10. Which of the following conditions is associated with vitamin A deficiency?

    A. preterm infants on TPN.
    B. infants with BPD.
    C. both A and B.

11. Replication of nursing studies should be:

    A. discouraged because there is no value to repeating studies.
    B. encouraged because repetition helps support first study's findings.
    C. encouraged because a researcher is inexperienced in the process.

12. Which compound is essential for active transport of calcium?

    A. parathyroid hormone.
    B. calcitonin.
    C. 1,25-dihydroxyvitamin D.

13. The legal elements necessary to prove negligence include all of the following EXCEPT:

    A. duty and breach of duty.
    B. injury and causation.
    C. standards of care and evaluation.

14. Niacin deficiency results in:

    A. dermatitis and inflammation of the mucous membranes.
    B. cutaneous vasodilation.
    C. acid gastric secretion.

15. Which of the following infants would be most likely to be hypocalcemic?

    A. preterm 1000-gram infant.
    B. IDM.
    C. birth asphyxiated term infant.

16. Why is digestion of long chain fatty acids difficult for preterm infants?

    A. LCFA require bile acids for absorption and the synthesis of bile acids is slow with a fast turnover.
    B. deficiency of pepsin and hydrochloric acid.
    C. deficiency of maltase, inverlase, and salalinase that are essential for breaking LCFA into short or MC fatty acids.

17. The power of a statistical test is concerned about committing:

    A. type I error.
    B. type II error.
    C. an alpha error.

18. Case management supports the collaborative model of practice. A case manager:

    A. coordinates the formal and informal health services of the neonate.
    B. assumes complete leadership of the neonate's plan of care.
    C. establishes the patient outcomes and conveys these to the team.

19. In addition to its role as a component of the skeleton, calcium also is involved in:

    A. regulation of phosphates.
    B. production of liver enzymes.
    C. blood coagulation.

20. The main purpose of an institution review board is to:

    A. ensure the rights and welfare of subjects.
    B. determine the feasibility of the research design.

C. determine the scientific merit of the design.

21. Employers of advanced practitioners have the right to:

A. set standards of advanced practice.
B. know whether a nurse is qualified.
C. verify advanced practice professional activities.

22. What is the primary enzyme involved in breaking polysaccharides down into mono- and disaccharides?

A. sucrase.
B. lactase.
C. amylase.

23. How is Bartter's syndrome treated?

A. supplementation of chloride.
B. supplementation of potassium and restriction of chloride.
C. indomethacin.

24. The mandate for nurses' participation in ethical deliberations is outlined in:

A. Code for Nurses.
B. Social Policy Statement.
C. Code for Nurses and Social Policy Statement.

25. How can chronic administration of furosemide simulate pulmonary edema?

A. with prolonged administration of lasix, lung receptors demonstrate decreased sensitivity to diuretics and pulmonary fluid can increase.
B. chloride deficiency can lead to metabolic acidosis that can cause hypoventilation and increased $Paco_2$, which also results in pulmonary edema.
C. both low chloride and increased pulmonary fluid cause hyperventilation as compensatory mechanisms leading to a picture of respiratory alkalosis.

26. Activities performed by the neonatal nurse that provide surveillance of physiological variables and comfort for infants are referred to as:

A. generative nursing behaviors.
B. nurturant nursing behaviors.
C. cognitive nursing behaviors.

27. Infants with atrophy of the villi after NEC are usually able to tolerate polycose sooner than infant formulas. What is the reason for this difference?

A. active mucosal transport of monosaccharides.
B. polycose is broken down into disaccharides that are easily absorbed.
C. maltase, isomaltase, invertase, sucrase, and palatinase are present as early as 23 weeks.

28. ______ refers to the obligation to prevent actual or potential harm and to act in a prudent, thoughtful manner.

A. Beneficence
B. Justice
C. Nonmaleficence

29. Zinc is absorbed in the:

A. duodenum.
B. stomach.
C. proximal small intestine.

30. The main purpose of the review of the literature is to:

A. uncover major issues or gaps on specific area of knowledge.
B. formulate a specific research question and research plan.
C. bring together data and theories that pertain to a topic of interest.

31. A Class D diabetic's infant may be:

A. postmature.
B. hyperglycemic.
C. jaundiced.

32. Nurse practitioners and clinical specialists have advanced neonatal nursing to a complex, highly technological enterprise. They have done so in part by:

A. developing a research basis for practice.
B. following physicians' orders without question.
C. maintaining nursing practice at a homogeneous level.

33. What is the main factor that determines the concentration of all other nutrients, based on organ maturity and the disease state?

A. nitrogen balance.
B. total fluid volume.
C. caloric density of nutrients needed.

34. Implications of quality assurance programs for neonatal nursing practice includes all of the following EXCEPT:

    A. to examine interventions to determine if they improve infant functional outcomes.
    B. to provide input for staffs' yearly performance reviews.
    C. to generate new standards of care.

35. The Code for Nurses is an example of the application of:

    A. metaethics.
    B. descriptive ethics.
    C. normative ethics.

36. What are the most common problems associated with TPN administration?

    A. infection (bacterial and/or viral).
    B. liver dysfunction.
    C. hypoglycemia and hyperglycemia.

37. Implantation is completed during the:

    A. first week of gestation.
    B. second week of gestation.
    C. third week of gestation.

38. Standards of care are general guidelines to practice. As the nurse following these standards, it is important to note that:

    A. the nurse must always follow these standards regardless of patient condition.
    B. the nurse must have rationale in addition to knowledge of standards when providing individualized patient care.
    C. if the nurse was not provided this information in orientation, the nurse is not accountable for it in providing patient care.

39. Of the five groups of neonatal nursing care providers, which group is identified as taking research data and relating that information into nursing practice?

    A. translators.
    B. shapers.
    C. generators.

40. Research is a formal, systematic inquiry or examination of a given problem. The goal is all of the following EXCEPT:

    A. to discover new knowledge.
    B. to prove a relationship exists.
    C. to verify existing knowledge.

41. What is the average recommended weight gain per day for preterm infants?

    A. 20 gm/kg/d.
    B. 40 gm/kg/d.
    C. 50 gm/kg/d.

42. Coughing, choking, and cyanosis are common clinical signs of:

    A. tracheoesophageal fistula (TEF).
    B. gastroschisis.
    C. cleft palate.

43. The cephalic portion or foregut gives rise to the:

    A. esophagus, stomach, proximal duodenum, liver, biliary apparatus, and lower respiratory tract.
    B. distal duodenum, small intestine, ascending colon, and most of the transverse colon.
    C. rest of colon, rectum, and genitourinary structures.

Stephanie Amlung, RNC, MSN

Baby Joshua was born prematurely at 28 weeks. His proud parents were thrilled to have a little baby boy but frightened about the aggressive care required to sustain his growth. At birth Joshua was taken to an NICU because he needed ventilatory assistance. He was placed in a warmed incubator with probes monitoring his temperature. Joshua's tiny chest was almost completely covered by the leads connecting him to the cardiopulmonary monitor and the dressing covering the hyperalimentation line. Even to the most loving eyes, the picture of Joshua would seem overwhelming.

This was not the case with Joshua's older sister, Emily. Emily was 4 years old and was anxiously awaiting the birth of her new little brother or sister. She and her parents had just completed the sibling class offered by the local hospital to prepare Emily for being a big sister to a full term, healthy baby. They did not know where to begin to try to explain to Emily about Joshua and his care.

We all agreed that it was important for Emily to come and see Joshua. How do we prepare her for that first visit?

It was ultimately important that Emily feel a part of Joshua's well-being. I thought that if Emily could bring in a doll of her own, that I could begin to basically explain some of the care her brother was receiving before her initial entry into the unit.

Emily had brought her special doll, Anne. I met them at the door, and we all went into a room I had prepared before their arrival. With Emily's permission, we undressed Anne and together we put a diaper on her. We placed her in the warmed incubator. I explained to Emily that Joshua was able to stay warm just like Anne in their own beds. Little by little, we gently placed the various monitor equipment and central line dressing on Anne being careful to speak in language that Emily could understand. The next step was to bring her into the unit and introduce her to her little brother.

As Emily came up to the incubator, we all stood in amazement as we watched a most wonderful sight. Emily was as natural and at ease as if we were in a normal nursery. She did not see tubes and monitors, all she saw was her baby brother. We opened one of the portholes and Emily gently said "Hi Joshua, I'm glad you're my little brother" and then she turned and said "Mommy, look! He opened his eyes to see me."

THE FOLLOWING FIVE QUESTIONS ARE BASED ON THIS VIGNETTE.

44. Emily's parents knew that once Joshua comes home they might expect their 4-year-old to show all of the following EXCEPT:

   A. an increase in aggressive behavior.
   B. regressive behaviors such as thumb-sucking.
   C. a tendency to anger less easily.

45. Emily's visit to the NICU will most likely result in:

   A. providing her with concrete evidence of Joshua's existence.
   B. an increase in regressive behaviors once she is home.
   C. upsetting her and making her fearful of her brother when he comes home.

46. Emily's reaction to the visit was positive. Some negative behaviors that might occur during such a visit are:

   A. clinging excessively to her mother.
   B. asking her mother to play now.
   C. hugging her mother.

47. Emily's parents most likely view the sibling visitation as all of the following EXCEPT:

   A. helping Emily feel a significant part of the family.
   B. a time when they could talk about Joshua with Emily.
   C. a time Emily was more affected by the environment than her brother.

48. Intervention strategies that Joshua's nurses might use with Emily's parents are:

   A. encouraging them to only share a little bit of information with Emily for now.
   B. talking with them about how Joshua's hospitalization can affect Emily.
   C. encouraging them to have Emily visit only this one time until discharge.

49. Normally, human beings have ______ chromosomes in all cells except mature red blood cells and mature sex cells.

   A. 23
   B. 46
   C. 72

50. The organization structure that *best* supports the collaborative practice model is:

   A. centralized.
   B. decentralized.
   C. hierarchical.

51. ______ is the process by which the bilaminar disk is expanded to a trilaminar embryonic disk, and it is the most important event that occurs during early fetal development.

   A. Gastrulation
   B. Neurulation
   C. Primitive streak formation

52. To meet the challenges of intrauterine existence and the transition to extrauterine life, the fetus has numerous adaptations to hypoxia and compensatory mechanisms that provide for what is called:

    A. fetal reserve.
    B. fetal acidosis syndrome.
    C. fetal exchange response.

53. The root principles of ethical decision-making are:

    A. autonomy, nonmaleficence, beneficence, and justice.
    B. autonomy, accountability, integrity, and confidentiality.
    C. autonomy, advocacy, competence, and informed consent.

54. Risk factors in the neonate for bronchopulmonary dysplasia include all of the following EXCEPT:

    A. surfactant deficiency.
    B. pulmonary air leak.
    C. chronic exposure to low levels of inspired oxygen.

55. The main functions of the placenta include all of the following EXCEPT:

    A. temperature control.
    B. respiratory function.
    C. amniotic fluid regulation.

56. The duodenum begins to generate villi between:

    A. 2–3 weeks.
    B. 5–6 weeks.
    C. 9–10 weeks.

57. Statutes of limitations for nurses in neonatal practice is:

    A. a three-year statute of limitation after discharge.
    B. the statute of limitation extends to 18 years of age for the neonate.
    C. statutes of limitation vary from state to state.

58. The biophysical profile is a noninvasive assessment system that allows for the evaluation of fetal status. These parameters include all of the following EXCEPT:

    A. nonstress test and fetal breathing movements.
    B. fetal tone and amniotic fluid volume.
    C. placental grading and chorionic villi sampling.

59. What is responsible for the anatomical location of the transverse colon in front of the duodenum?

    A. the 90 degree rotation of the midgut around the superior mesenteric artery.
    B. the 190 degree counterclockwise rotation.
    C. the 270 degree rotation during herniation and return to the abdominal cavity.

60. The function of the ductus arteriosus in utero is to allow:

    A. blood to flow from the pulmonary artery to the aorta, bypassing the fetal lungs.
    B. the majority of blood from the placenta to bypass the liver and enter the inferior vena cava.
    C. a portion of the blood to flow from the right atrium directly to the left atrium, bypassing the right ventricle.

61. A secondary prevention therapy for BPD would include:

    A. vitamin D administration.
    B. high-frequency ventilation.
    C. prevention of respiratory distress.

62. All of the following are clinical manifestations of perinatal asphyxia EXCEPT:

    A. loss of beat to beat variability.
    B. fetal scalp pH greater than 7.25.
    C. late decelerations.

63. The connective tissue layer making up the outside layer of the esophagus is called

    A. adventitia.
    B. mucosa.
    C. serosa.

64. A pedigree will demonstrate:

    A. a pattern of inheritance.
    B. only affected individuals.
    C. only the proband's genetic risk.

65. Which of the following signs is associated with gastrointestinal obstruction?

A. abdominal distention, either sudden or gradual onset.
B. failure to pass meconium within 24 hours of birth.
C. blood-tinged emesis or frank blood in the stool.

66. Reverse transports are not cost effective for many patients. The costs for these transports are:

A. usually paid for by insurance coverage.
B. often not covered by insurance policies.
C. often ignored by hospitals.

67. Legal evidence of accountability is through:

A. documentation.
B. truth telling.
C. expert witness.

68. In what portion of the gastrointestinal tract are muscular contractions more forceful?

A. esophagus.
B. antrum of stomach.
C. small intestine.

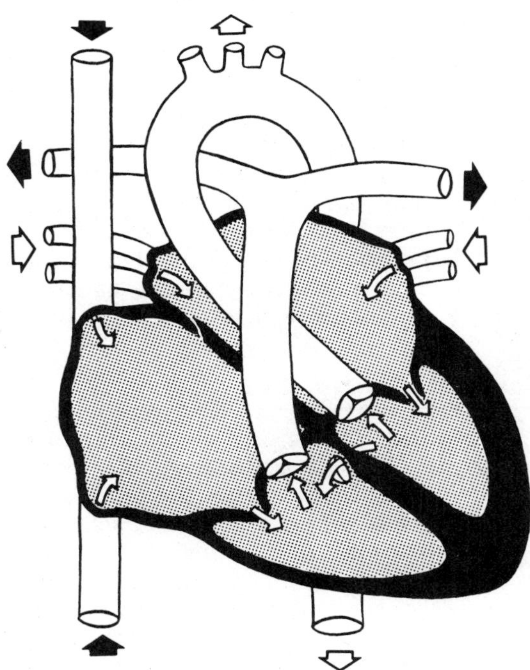

FIGURE 3 Ventricular septal defect

69. A VSD is a defect or opening in the ventricular septum as a result of imperfect ventricular division during early fetal development. The defect can occur anywhere in the muscular or membranous ventricular septum. The severity of the defect is determined by:

A. location of the defect and degree of systemic resistance.
B. size and degree of pulmonary vascular resistance.
C. location and size of defect.

70. The most *common* cause of fetal asphyxia is:

A. cord compression.
B. placental insufficiency.
C. maternal medication.

71. Indications for magnesium sulfate ($MgSO_4$) include all of the following EXCEPT:

A. preeclampsia.
B. preterm labor.
C. hypertension.

72. A trait that affects every generation and is equally distributed between the sexes is:

A. autosomal dominant.
B. autosomal recessive.
C. sex-linked recessive.

73. The major nerve plexus found in the gut wall between the longitudinal and circular layers of muscle that regulates motor function is the:

A. myenteric plexus.
B. mesoteric plexus.
C. submucosal plexus.

74. Clinical assessment of an infant with a pneumothorax include all of the following EXCEPT:

A. asymmetrical chest movements.
B. shifted heart sounds.
C. acrocyanosis.

75. What does the presence of bile-stained emesis mean?

A. obstruction proximal to the ampulla of Vater.
B. obstruction distal to the ampulla of Vater.
C. obstruction secondary to a chronic problem.

76. Use of supportive interventions to help a person through the grief process is most closely associated with:

    A. cognitive models of grief.
    B. attachment models of grief.
    C. holistic models of grief.

77. Transport standards for neonatal nurses are published by:

    A. NANN.
    B. JCAHO.
    C. NAACOG.

78. Gestational age assessments consist of observation of physical characteristics and neuromuscular development. In regard to the accuracy of the exam:

    A. the physical findings remain relatively unchanged in the immediate newborn period.
    B. the neuromuscular component remains stable throughout the entire newborn period.
    C. once the exam is completed, it should not be reevaluated for any reason.

79. A maternal history of polyhydramnios with neonatal excessive oral secretions can indicate:

    A. esophageal atresia.
    B. diaphragmatic hernia.
    C. esophageal duplication.

80. An infant who is cold stressed undergoes multisystem compensatory effects. The system causing the most obvious symptoms is the:

    A. metabolic.
    B. central nervous.
    C. cardiorespiratory.

81. What are the four diseases identified by the International Symposium on Neonatal Screening for inborn errors of metabolism?

    A. PKU, hypothyroidism, galactosemia, and maple syrup urine disease.
    B. PKU, sickle cell anemia, beta thalassemia, and galactosemia.
    C. PKU, tyrosemia, hypothyroidism, and galactosemia.

82. The primary goal of endotracheal suctioning is:

    A. that suctioning be done only when it benefits the patient.
    B. that patency be maintained by suctioning at regular intervals.
    C. that oxygen requirements not increase during the procedure.

83. What is the first effect of an increased blood glucose?

    A. increased insulin production.
    B. increased glycogen synthesis in the liver.
    C. decreased glycogen degradation in the liver.

84. The nurse performing the physical assessment on admission to the nursery must be alert for deviations from the normal. These can include all of the following <u>EXCEPT</u>:

    A. jitteriness.
    B. retractions.
    C. acrocynanosis.

85. Historical research is an example of:

    A. descriptive design.
    B. mixed design.
    C. evaluative design.

86. Indications for surgical correction of VSD include:

    A. development of a grade 2-5/6 regurgitant systolic murmur at the left lower sternal border.
    B. x-ray showing enlarged heart with a prominent main pulmonary artery segment and increased pulmonary vascularity.
    C. presence of significant left-to-right shunting with symptoms of congestive heart failure.

Joyce M. Dohme, RNC, MSN

Mrs. F called for a nurse for the third time in 30 minutes. When I entered the room, I found her in tears because the baby would not nurse. I saw her infant was asleep, and after determining that he had nursed fairly well 5 hours ago, I suggested that she wait until he was more alert. Mrs. F continued to cry. "You're having a rough morning," I said, inviting her to tell me about it.

"Jarrod won't cooperate. My daughter was so easy to nurse. Maybe I'm doing something wrong, or maybe he doesn't like it," she said

ruefully. I answered gently that I thought the likely explanation was that he was still tired from his circumcision. I asked her to tell me about her daughter.

Mrs. F's face brightened. "Chrissie's wonderful. She's 5 years old now. She fit right into our life and family. I thought that would happen all over again with Jarrod." "You know, I love Chrissie so much. How can I possibly love another baby that much? This isn't fair to Jarrod!" Mrs. F began to cry again. I responded, "The love you have for Chrissie has been built over time, as you took care of her and grew to know what makes her special. That will happen with this baby, but it takes time. Jarrod won't be just like Chrissie was because he is a different person. It will be a whole new experience being his mother."

THE FOLLOWING THREE QUESTIONS ARE BASED ON THIS VIGNETTE.

87. The steps to successful role change for Mrs. F includes all the following <u>EXCEPT</u>:

    A. identifying the role of the relevant other.
    B. identifying expectations of new role.
    C. identifying only the role of the person undergoing the change.

88. It appears that Mrs. F may be experiencing a crisis. Crisis is defined as usually being:

    A. an inescapable demand to which the person must respond.
    B. a period of disequilibrium and an upset in steady state.
    C. a development growth-producing event.

89. Roles are:

    A. covert, goal-directed, and static.
    B. overt, goal-directed, and dynamic.
    C. overt, goal-directed, and static.

90. Functional closure of the foramen ovale is caused by:

    A. cord occlusion and the consequent rise in blood pressure.
    B. decreased pulmonary vascular resistance.
    C. increased left atrial pressure and increased systemic resistance.

91. What is the early presenting symptom of carbohydrate intolerance?

    A. hypoglycemia.
    B. lactic acid accumulation.
    C. watery acid stools.

92. The specific mode of transport should be decided by all of the following <u>EXCEPT</u>:

    A. the infant's condition.
    B. local terrain.
    C. individual team member preference.

93. The cardiac valves consist of two sets of one-way valves: the semilunar valves and the atrioventricular (A-V) valves. The semilunar valves consist of the pulmonic and aortic valves. The atrioventricular valves are the tricuspid and the mitral valves. The valve that connects the right atrium and right ventricle is the:

    A. aortic valve.
    B. mitral valve.
    C. tricuspid valve.

94. The infant loses enormous amounts of water through the skin surface. These losses rise dramatically when what type of heating source is used?

    A. convection.
    B. radiation.
    C. conduction.

95. What is a common consequence of untreated galactokinase deficiency?

    A. mental retardation.
    B. cataracts.
    C. failure to thrive.

96. The active neurotransmitter for the parasympathetic/sympathetic nervous system is:

    A. acetylcholine.
    B. epinephrine.
    C. norepinephrine.

97. Mr. and Mrs. Thompson have type O blood. Because the alleles for type O are recessive, Julia, their first child, will have a genotype of ______ .

    A. OO
    B. BO
    C. AO

98. The purpose of the gestational assessment is to:

   A. anticipate problems related to development.
   B. determine approximate length of stay for the newborn.
   C. observe for subtle changes occurring during the transition period.

99. Administration of sorbitol to treat cerebral edema is contraindicated in:

   A. fructose-1, 6-diphosphate deficiency.
   B. essential fructosuria.
   C. sucrose intolerance.

100. Which of the following statements are true about high-frequency oscillatory ventilation (HFOV)?

   A. expiration is passive thus decreasing the risk of air trapping.
   B. HFOV delivers small tidal volumes, less than anatomic dead space at frequencies of 300–3000 breaths per minute.
   C. HFOV must be administered via endotracheal intubation.

101. Cyanosis is the bluish color of the skin, mucous membranes, and nailbeds that occurs when there are at least:

   A. 2 grams/dl of deoxygenated hemoglobin in the circulation.
   B. 5 grams/dl of deoxygenated hemoglobin in the circulation.
   C. 8 grams/dl of deoxygenated hemoglobin in the circulation.

102. As an infant is placed on a weight scale, he or she can lose heat through what mechanism of heat transfer?

   A. evaporative.
   B. convective.
   C. conductive.

103. The term applied to the combination of pulmonary hypertension, subsequent right-to-left shunting through fetal channels away from the pulmonary vascular bed, and a structurally normal heart is:

   A. pneumopericardium.
   B. transient tachypnea of the newborn.
   C. persistent pulmonary hypertension of the newborn.

104. Acyanotic heart defects produce:

   A. decreased pulmonary blood flow.
   B. increased pulmonary blood flow.
   C. normal or slightly decreased pulmonary blood flow.

105. Chloride is an inorganic compound with no buffer effects. Why is it important in acid-base regulation?

   A. serum concentrations of chloride and bicarbonate are inversely correlated, keeping total anion concentration (chloride + bicarbonate) constant. When chloride is retained in the body, serum bicarbonate increases and metabolic alkalosis follows.
   B. chloride acts as an exchange agent for potassium. Low chloride levels would cause increased retention of potassium, which could lead to acidosis.
   C. chloride is one of the principle anions involved in renal tubular reabsorption of sodium, potassium, and calcium.

Marianne McGraw, RN, MSN

The Ms were a young couple in their early 30s. Both were from large families, excited over the thought of having their first baby. Mrs. M sensed she was pregnant very early, and it was confirmed at about six weeks. During the first trimester, she experienced an episode of bleeding that stopped after a few days. Her second trimester was uneventful, until one morning her doctor called with some devastating news. The AFP test done at 16 weeks of gestation was elevated, possibly indicating a neural tube defect. An ultrasound confirmed a myelomeningocele and dilated ventricles. Serial ultrasounds were ordered to monitor the hydrocephalus.

Mary was delivered at 39 weeks gestation by C-section. A low myelomeningocele at the L-5 level was noted. There was active movement of the lower extremities. I promptly assessed the defect to determine size and condition of the sac. The area measured about 4 × 4 cm. Warm, sterile, normal saline dressings were placed over the defect, after the parents had the opportunity to see it. I then bundled Mary to let the parents say "Hi" and take some pictures, before going to the special care nursery. Once in the nursery,

Mary was placed prone in a warmed incubator, with the bed flat. A roll was then placed at the hip level to elevate the lumbosacral region and prevent stress on the sac. I then continued my head-to-toe assessment. Head circumference was 35 cm and appeared normal. Using Ortolani's maneuver, I felt a slight hip click on the right side. She continued to move both legs symmetrically. As I placed a diaper under her, I noted the dribbling of a small amount of urine. No other defects were noted. She was tranferred to a tertiary center.

The next day, Mrs. M and I talked about how Mary was doing. Mary was in surgery. I acknowledged Mrs. M's fears. She stated that it was still difficult for them, but having known about the defect for five months made it a little easier. She then shared some pictures that her husband had taken before the surgery.

At the tertiary center, the closure of the defect was performed without complications. Mary's head circumference remained stable and a V-P shunt was not required. She did require some intermittent catheterizations due to a neurogenic bladder.

She was subsequently discharged on day 14 of life and was breastfeeding well.

THE FOLLOWING FOUR QUESTIONS ARE BASED ON THIS VIGNETTE.

106. Mary's parents should be told that:

A. neural tube defect occurs during the second trimester.
B. neural tube defect occurs during the first 10 weeks of gestation.
C. neural tube defect is an autosomal recessive condition.

107. Mary's parents are told that this problem occurred during the embryonic period. This is the period of time from:

A. weeks 1–4.
B. weeks 2–4.
C. weeks 4–8.

108. Mary's parents are told that she may have some neurologic impairment in her legs. This is due to failure of the:

A. neural crest cells to migrate.
B. neural crest cells to form the sympathetic nervous system.
C. the somites to continue to develop.

109. The hydrocephalus that Mary has is related to:

A. disrupted development of the brain's ventricles.
B. development of back pressure in glial cells.
C. development of an obstruction of the flow of cerebrospinal fluid.

110. A contraindication for the use of extracorporeal membrane oxygenation (ECMO) is:

A. severe respiratory distress.
B. preexisting intracranial hemorrhage.
C. diaphragmatic hernia.

111. Endocardial cushion defects are lesions that result from inappropriate fusion of the endocardial cushions during fetal development. Endocardial cushion defects produce abnormalities of:

A. pulmonary artery, aorta, and pulmonary veins.
B. atrial septum, ventricular septum, and A-V valves.
C. ventricular septum, pulmonic artery, and pulmonary valve.

112. When observing the infant's hands and feet, a simian crease is noted. Simian creases are associated with:

A. Trisomy 21.
B. Trisomy 18.
C. rocker-bottom feet.

113. A common air leak in ventilated VLBW neonates is termed:

A. intrapulmonary interstitial emphysema (IIE).
B. pulmonary interstitial emphysema (PIE).
C. pneumopericardial interstitial emphysema (PPIE).

114. Back transfers benefit regionalization by:

A. optimizing the use of NICU beds.
B. decreasing the accountability of level I or II staff.
C. alleviating the need for the primary physician to become involved.

115. There are four individual heart sounds (S1, S2, S3, S4). S3 and S4 are not generally heard in the neonate. Which statement best describes the cause of the sounds identified as S1 and S2?

A. S1 is the result of closure of the mitral and tricuspid valve after atrial systole; S2 is the result of closure of the aortic and pulmonary valves.
B. S1 is the result of closure of the mitral and tricuspid valves at the end of atrial diastole; S2 is the result of closure of the aortic and pulmonary valves at the end of systole.
C. S1 is the result of closure of the aortic and pulmonary valves after atrial systole; S2 is the closure of the mitral and tricuspid valves at the beginning of ventricular diastole.

116. Mechanisms used to prevent oxygen toxicity injury in the neonate include all of the following EXCEPT:

A. developmental enhancement techniques.
B. limitation of intubation.
C. maximum ventilatory settings.

117. The presence of a single S2 can indicate:

A. atrial septal defect.
B. partial anomalous pulmonary venous return (PAPVR).
C. pulmonic atresia or stenosis.

118. The substance that prevents alveolar collapse and loss of lung volume during expiration is:

A. surfactant.
B. elastin.
C. alveolar fluid.

119. Which of the following is a function of folate?

A. synthesis of DNA nucleotides.
B. carbohydrate and lipid metabolism.
C. synthesis of nucleic acids.

120. Location and transmission patterns of murmurs can be helpful in identification of a cardiac murmur. Diastolic murmurs occur between S1 and S2. Diastolic murmurs are classified according to their timing in relation to heart sounds as early, mid-, or late diastolic (or presystolic). Early diastolic murmurs occur early in diastole after S2. Early diastolic murmurs result from:

A. abnormal ventricular filling or abnormal preload.
B. aortic or pulmonic valve incompetence.
C. flow through AV valves during ventricular diastole as a result of active atrial contraction ejecting blood into the ventricle.

121. The neonate is capable of heat production via the following:

A. shivering and chemical thermogenesis.
B. involuntary muscle activity.
C. decreased metabolic activity.

122. The following are all characteristics of passive high-frequency ventilation EXCEPT:

A. very high rates (greater than 300 breaths per minute) cannot be used with passive high-frequency ventilation because of hyperinflation.
B. passive high-frequency ventilation requires specially designed humidification systems.
C. with passive high-frequency ventilation, expired volume is unlimited.

123. A deficiency of which of the B vitamins is associated with seizures?

A. pyridoxine.
B. pyridoxamine.
C. pyridoxal.

124. What is the most common congenital heart defect (CHD) in term newborns?

A. ASD.
B. PDA.
C. VSD.

125. Jaundice that appears after 24 hours of age and resolves by days 5–7 is considered:

A. physiologic jaundice.
B. pathologic jaundice.
C. breast milk jaundice.

126. Which anion is jointly responsible (with sodium) for maintenance of plasma volume?

A. potassium.
B. chloride.
C. calcium.

Case Study

Baby boy Johnson was born via spontaneous vaginal delivery to a 27-year-old G ii, P i, now ii, mother after an uncomplicated 39 weeks gestation. Prenatal course and maternal history were benign. Apgar scores were 7 (−2 color; −1 respirations) and 8 (−2 color). After stabilization, he was transferred to the NICU in 100% oxygen per hood for diagnosis and management. The differential diagnosis included sepsis, pulmonary disease, cardiac defects, perinatal asphyxia, or neurological defects. The clinical picture points to a complex cyanotic congenital heart defect.

THE FOLLOWING SIX QUESTIONS REFER TO THIS VIGNETTE.

127. Which of the following defects could present with the same clinical picture?
    A. ASD, ECD, VSD.
    B. HLHS, TOF, TGA.
    C. TAPVR, AS, TA.

THE FOLLOWING DATA WAS OBTAINED:

Vital signs:	97.6, 166, 50, 46/28
HEENT:	WNL
Cardiovascular:	Loud grade III/VI harsh systolic murmur; CFT ≈4–5 seconds; Pulses =/decreased/4; Loud single S2
Pulmonary:	BBS =/clear; slightly tachypneic; no retractions, grunting,
GI:	Liver down 2.0 cm RCM; otherwise WNL
Neuro:	Apprehensive; normal reflexes
Lab Data:	CBC: Hemoglobin 15.0, Hematocrit 48.0; 200,000 platelets; 9.0 WBCs, with 28 segs, 1 band, 11 lymphs, 1 eosinophil Lytes: Sodium 140; potassium 5.0; Chloride 110; CO_2 20; BUN 7; Creatinine .1; Glucose 36; Anion Gap 6; Calcium 6.5; Chemstrip 40 ABG: 7.10/25/46/14/−8

128. What management plans should be instituted at this time?

____

____

____

____

____

____

____

FURTHER DIAGNOSTIC TESTS REVEAL:

Chest X-ray: Enlarged heart with narrow base (egg-shaped); increased pulmonary blood flow; no evidence of hyaline membrane disease; ECG: Right axis deviation, Right ventricular hypertrophy; ECHO: Aorta arises from the right ventricle; the pulmonary artery arises from the left ventricle; Large muscular VSD; small PDA.

129. Which CHD produces the reported findings?
    A. TOF with PDA
    B. HLHS with PDA, VSD
    C. TGA with PDA, VSD

130. A continuous infusion of PGE_1 is started to promote ductal patency and increase mixing of oxygenated and deoxygenated blood at the ductal level. What are the adverse effects of PGE_1?
    A. apnea, flush, fever, hypotension, decreased heart rate, and seizure-like activity.
    B. apnea, bradycardia, glucose instability, hypothermia, and rhythm disturbances.
    C. seizures, respiratory failure, renal failure, and decreased platelet aggregation.

131. After infusion of PGE_1, the infant's color improves, and a repeat ABG reveals: 7.30/35/60/24/−3.5. Improvement in color, perfusion, and ABG indicate increased ductal flow has improved mixing of oxygenated and deoxygenated blood. What other procedure can be performed as an emergency procedure without cardiopulmonary bypass to provide improved mixing of oxygenated and deoxygenated blood and to verify the diagnosis?
    A. Blalock-Hanlon procedure.
    B. balloon atrial septostomy.
    C. Mustard procedure.

132. Surgical correction for this infant is planned at about 3–6 months unless signs and symptoms of deterioration are noted. Surgical correction involves switching the right- and left-sided structures at the artery, atrial, or ventricular level. The surgical procedure that involves switching the circulation at the artery level is:

A. Rastelli.
B. Jatene.
C. Senning.

133. Nursing care for infants with respiratory distress syndrome (RDS) is demanding. The risk of pneumothorax is high, and the nurse must carefully assess:

A. quality and symmetry of breath sounds.
B. breath sounds every two hours before and after suctioning.
C. endotracheal tube (ETT) placement.

134. Which of the following statements about body water balance is TRUE?

A. osmolality of the extracellular fluid is normally higher than the intracellular fluid osmolality.
B. osmolality of the ECF is normally equal to the ICF osmolality.
C. osmolality of the ECF is normally lower than the ICF osmolaity.

135. If there are any neonatal abnormalities, these should:

A. not be shown to the parents at the time of transport.
B. be shown to the parents at the time of transport.
C. be discussed but not shown to the parents at the time of transport.

136. A term infant in the newborn nursery was found to have moderate respiratory distress, slight cyanosis, and hypoglycemia. Because of the symptoms, a sepsis workup was done. The Gram stain showed gram-positive cocci in chains. The most likely microorganism causing the infection is:

A. *Listeria monocytogenes.*
B. *Excherichia coli.*
C. Group B streptococcus.

137. Based on the case in the above question, what antimicrobials should be given?

A. ampicillin and vancomycin.
B. ceftazidime and amikacin.
C. ampicillin and gentamicin.

138. A two-month-old, male 32 week AGA infant with BPD who has symptoms indicative of sepsis is "septicized." The Gram stain reveals coagulase-positive cocci in clusters. The most likely microorganism is:

A. Group B streptococcus.
B. *Staphylococcus aureus.*
C. *Neisseria gonorrhea.*

139. Based on the case in the above question, which antimicrobials should be started?

A. vancomycin and gentamicin.
B. nafcillin and gentamicin.
C. amikacin and gentamicin.

140. Approximately how much water is required for each 100 kcal of energy expenditure?

A. 100 ml.
B. 200 ml.
C. 300 ml.

141. What is the chief source of blood cell production in a 36 weeks' gestation fetus?

A. liver.
B. bone marrow.
C. thymus.

142. Transcutaneous Po_2 ($TcPo_2$) is measured by an electrode applied to the skin. The nurse monitoring these readings is aware that the numbers can become unreliable when:

A. there is a change in the local skin perfusion.
B. the neonate's Pao_2 level is over 50.
C. the infant is crying.

143. What is the purpose of "correcting" the WBC count in the first few days after birth?

A. high percentage of fetal hemoglobin cells leads to inaccurate counts.
B. immature RBC with intact nucleus can be incorrectly counted as WBC.
C. leukocytes are sometimes counted initially due to the similar size.

144. A sudden or dramatic change in infant temperature can cause:

A. bradycardia.
B. apnea.
C. tachypnea.

145. Sodium, the main ECF ion, is primarily absorbed in the:

A. stomach.
B. duodenum.
C. jejunum.

146. In the management of neonatal hypoxemia, the perinatal caregiver's first line of defense for the prevention or treatment of hypoxemia is to:

A. increase fluid intake.
B. provide increased inspired oxygen.
C. change positions frequently.

147. Stridor is common in neonates with:

A. upper airway obstruction.
B. lower airway obstruction.
C. decreased functional residual capacity.

148. Congestive heart failure (CHF) is a condition in which the blood supply to the body is insufficient to meet the metabolic requirements of the organs and tissues. The end effects of CHF include:

1. decreased cardiac output.
2. decreased renal perfusion.
3. systemic venous engorgement.
4. Pulmonary venous engorgement.

Which of these effects are responsible for triggering stimulation of the sympathetic nervous system?

A. decreased cardiac output.
B. decreased renal perfusion.
C. pulmonary venous engorgement.

149. Subcutaneous edema of the soft tissues of the scalp is:

A. cephalohematoma.
B. molding.
C. caput succedaneum.

150. How does antidiuretic hormone (ADH) influence sodium regulation?

A. ADH is necessary for the effective function of the Na-K pump.
B. ADH production is stimulated by decreased sodium levels causing increased sodium reabsorption.
C. ADH regulates excretion or reabsorption of free water.

151. *Candida* sepsis is treated with:

A. methicillin.
B. clindamycin.
C. amphotericin B.

152. Inotropic drugs are frequently used in the medical management of CHF to improve cardiac output. Of the three drugs listed below, which has a decreased effect on heart rate and rhythm and causes less peripheral constriction?

A. dopamine.
B. dobutamine.
C. isoproterenol.

153. Magnesium is involved in:

A. red blood cell production.
B. bone marrow stem cell production.
C. mitrochondrial function.

154. The American Academy of Pediatrics (AAP) recommends that under all but emergency situations, surfactant be administered in what type of nurseries?

A. all but level I facilities.
B. level II facilities able to maintain infants on continuous positive airway pressure.
C. level III facilities able to sustain long-term mechanical ventilation.

155. Hypermagnesemia is associated with:

A. hypotonia.
B. hypocalcemia.
C. hypoglycemia.

156. What is the leading cause of death from congenital heart defects in the first month?

A. bacterial infection (subacute bacterial endocarditis).
B. congestive heart failure.
C. complications from hypoplastic left heart syndrome (HLHS).

157. Which of the following is an adverse effect of the use of soy-based formulas?

A. increased phosphorus.
B. decreased phosphorus.
C. hypocalcemia.

158. By day three of life, the IDM is at risk for:
    A. hypocalcemia.
    B. hypermagnesemia.
    C. hyperglycemia.

159. Which phase of lung development is marked by sequential branching of the lung bud?
    A. alveolar.
    B. embryonic.
    C. canalicular.

160. Fanconi syndrome is characterized by:
    A. deficient activity of renal 1-α hydroxylase.
    B. impaired intestinal absorption of phosphorus and increased renal losses of phosphorus.
    C. renal tubular reabsorption disorders.

161. In persistent truncus arteriosus (PTA), both pulmonary and systemic circuits receive blood from the truncus arteriosus. In the immediate newborn period in an infant with PTA, pulmonary and systemic blood flows are about equal. Gradually pulmonary blood flow increases. What is responsible for this change?
    A. constriction of systemic vessels secondary to hypoxia.
    B. right atrial hypertrophy occurs that enables the heart to shunt more blood through the pulmonary circuit.
    C. pulmonary vascular resistance gradually falls, increasing the amount of pulmonary blood flow.

162. Clinical evaluation of adequate cardiac output includes all of the following EXCEPT:
    A. brisk capillary refill.
    B. strong pulse strength.
    C. warm extremities.

163. Potassium is the main intracellular cation. Its most important function is:
    A. regulation of cell membrane potential.
    B. involvement with acid-base balance regulation.
    C. exchange of ion for chloride in renal tubules.

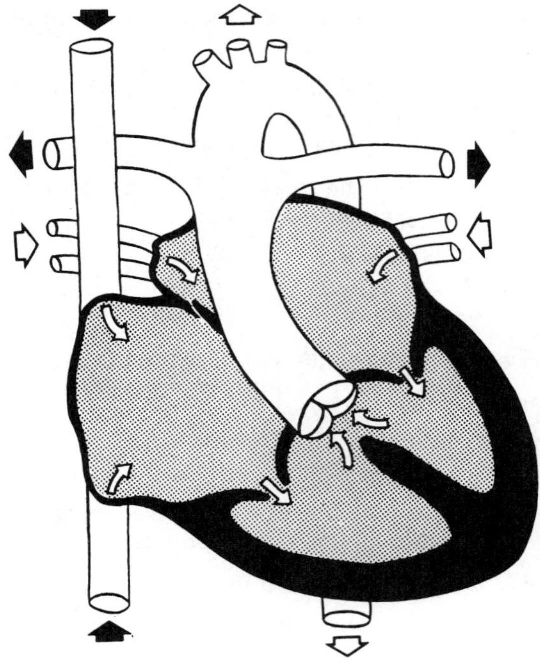

FIGURE 4 Persistent truncus arteriosus

164. An infant requires an exchange transfusion for hyperbilirubinemia. During the exchange transfusion, the CVP is noted to be low. This infant was a breech delivery with Apgars of 3, 4, and has erythroblastosis fetalis (EBF). What condition should be considered in the differential for cause of hyperbilirubinemia?
    A. rupture of the spleen.
    B. adrenal hemorrhage.
    C. hepatic rupture.

165. Seventy-five percent of encephaloceles occur in the:
    A. frontal region.
    B. occipital region.
    C. posterior cranial region.

166. What is the preferred indication for a transfusion of an anemic infant?
    A. impaired tissue oxygenation.
    B. hematocrit less than 40 percent.
    C. failure to gain weight.

167. Tetralogy of Fallot (TOF) consists of a large VSD, pulmonic stenosis (or other right ventricular outflow obstruction), overriding aorta, and hypertrophied

right ventricle. What are the hemodynamic consequences of the VSD in TOF?

A. the VSD causes equalization of pressures in the ventricles. Unsaturated blood flows through the VSD into the aorta because of the obstruction to blood flow from the right ventricle into the artery.
B. blood is shunted from the left to the right ventricle because of higher pressure in the right ventricle and pulmonary artery.

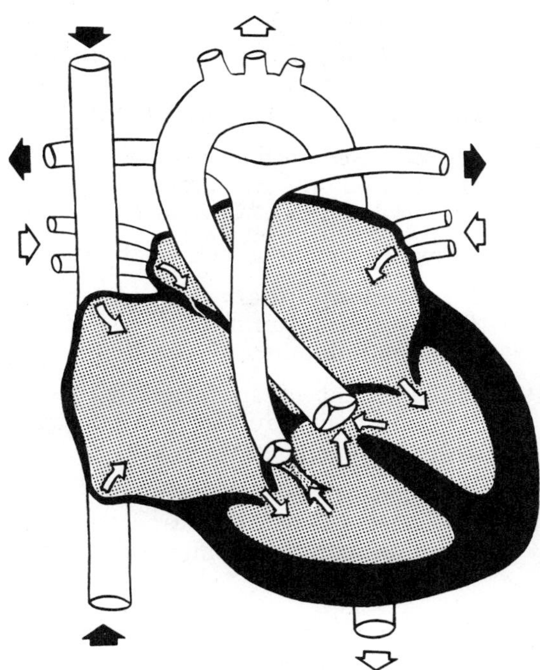

FIGURE 5 Tetralogy of Fallot

C. the VSD results in obstruction to blood flow from the right ventricle to the pulmonary artery. The right ventricle hypertrophies in response to increased pressure caused by obstruction to outflow.

168. What is the electrolyte imbalance that often occurs with prolonged administration of loop diuretics?

A. metabolic acidosis.
B. metabolic alkalosis.
C. hyperchloremia.

169. Treatment of SIADH is:

A. liberalization of fluids.
B. restriction of fluids.
C. IV of hypotonic saline.

170. What is considered normal head growth for a term infant?

A. 0.5 cm/week.
B. 1.0 cm/week.
C. 1.5 cm/week.

171. Why are VLBW infants (<1500 grams) at greater risk for hyponatremia?

A. inability to reabsorb urinary sodium secondary to immature kidneys.
B. relative decreased response to normal sodium levels.
C. inability to provide adequate sodium through parenteral fluids without causing fluid overload.

172. What type of seizure is most commonly seen in neonates?

A. generalized tonic.
B. multifocal clonic.
C. subtle.

173. Treatment of hypothyroidism is:

A. methimazole.
B. propranolol.
C. L-thyroxine.

174. What other deficiency can lead to hypocalcemia?

A. phosphorous.
B. potassium.
C. maternal vitamin D.

175. ______ is an example of home-based protocols of care for preterm infants and their families.

A. NCAST
B. NSTEP-P
C. HOME

176. Signs of SIADH include:

A. edema.
B. hypernatremia.
C. low urine osmolality.

177. The most common location for a PVH/IVH in a preterm infant is the:
    A. subependymal germinal matrix at the head of the caudate nucleus.
    B. choroid plexus.
    C. subarachnoid space in the posterior fossa.

178. What is the most common cause of hyperbilirubinemia?
    A. sepsis.
    B. asphyxia.
    C. prematurity.

179. Which of the following would be appropriate for initial management of hypoxic-ischemic encephalopathy (HIE)?
    A. fluid restriction.
    B. barbiturate therapy.
    C. continuous dopamine therapy.

180. What are the side effects of excessive riboflavin (B_{12}) intake?
    A. epithelial abnormalities.
    B. normocytic anemia.
    C. none reported.

181. What type of renal failure can result from hypoxia?
    A. prerenal failure.
    B. renal failure.
    C. postrenal failure.

182. Which form of bilirubin is able to migrate into brain cells?
    A. unconjugated (indirect).
    B. conjugated (direct).
    C. free.

183. Physical exam findings of a smooth, solid abdominal or flank mass accompanied by hypertension and fever are associated with:
    A. congenital adrenal hyperplasia.
    B. nephroblastoma.
    C. Wilms' tumor.

184. Hypoglycemia is most common and severe in infants with:
    A. glycogen storage disease type I (G-6-PD).
    B. glycogen storage disease type II (G-6-PD).
    C. glycogen storage disease type IV (G-6-PD).

185. Dermatoglyphics is the study of:
    A. the pattern of epidermal ridges.
    B. skin changes.
    C. structural changes in the skin.

186. Careful monitoring of which electrolyte is essential in the presence of renal failure?
    A. sodium.
    B. calcium.
    C. potassium.

187. Conductive hearing loss is most often a result of:
    A. an inner ear problem.
    B. a cochlear ear problem.
    C. a middle ear problem.

188. The NNP managing the care of an infant with achondroplasia should consider all of the following EXCEPT:
    A. increased need for calories.
    B. reduced lung capacity.
    C. increased risk of fractures.

189. Growth hormone is secreted by the:
    A. anterior pituitary.
    B. posterior pituitary.
    C. hypothalamus.

190. Management of an infant with constriction bands due to amniotic band syndrome includes:
    A. frequent vascular checks.
    B. liberal use of diuretics.
    C. minimizing movement of affected part.

191. Otitis media most often results in:
    A. sensorineural hearing loss.
    B. conductive hearing loss.
    C. mixed hearing loss.

192. A measurement of presence of antibody on the RBC surface is the:
    A. direct Coombs.
    B. indirect Coombs.
    C. antibody screen.

193. Overt neonatal reactions to sounds include all of the following EXCEPT:
    A. gross body movements.
    B. pupillary constriction.
    C. crying.

194. Congenital muscular torticollis refers to a primary disorder of the:

A. trapezius muscle.
B. sternocleidomastoid muscle.
C. brachial plexus.

195. The mother admits to the nurse she is still fearful for her infant's life. This fear is a sign of:

A. vulnerable child syndrome.
B. positive coping.
C. adaptive behavior.

Case History

Peter was a 28-week AGA, white male, born to a teen mother who was a known crack cocaine user. There had been no prenatal care, and she presented in active labor with a low grade fever. At 12 hours of age, he began to experience increasing respiratory distress despite surfactant therapy. He appeared ashen and mottled with periods of bradycardia and hypotension. A sepsis workup was done including a lumbar puncture. Urine latex was done, with blood cultures. An ELISA test also was done. When the culture and laboratory reports came back, there was a high IgM level. His blood count showed increased bands and neutrophilia.

THE FOLLOWING EIGHT QUESTIONS ARE BASED ON THIS VIGNETTE.

196. Peter's IgM level reflects:

A. maternally derived antibodies.
B. fetally derived antibodies.
C. antibodies for HIV.

197. The rationale for doing the ELISA test is to determine:

A. HIV status of the infant.
B. exposure to a viral agent.
C. if a bacterial infection is present.

198. The urine latex is used when ______ is suspected.

A. HIV
B. *Escherichia coli* sepsis
C. Group B *Streptococcus*

199. Peter's maternal history would suggest that his diagnosis is probably:

A. HIV.
B. cocaine withdrawal.
C. perinatally acquired infection.

200. Peter's treatment pending culture results should be:

A. broad-spectrum antimicrobials.
B. symptomatic approach.
C. wait-and-see approach.

201. The culture results are gram-positive cocci. The organism most likely responsible for his infection is:

A. *S. aureus*.
B. Group B streptococcus.
C. *Chlamydia*.

202. If Peter had been meconium stained and the organism was a gram-positive rod, the suspected organism might be:

A. *E. coli*.
B. *Listeria*.
C. *Chlamydia*.

203. Op-Site can be used as a second skin EXCEPT:

A. when *Staphylococcus epidermidis* is present.
B. when *Monilia* rash is present.
C. when *Candida albicans* is present.

Case History

Mrs. Smith is a 31-week gestation primipara. She was just admitted for preterm labor and placed on ritodrine hydrochloride.

THE FOLLOWING TWO QUESTIONS ARE BASED ON THIS VIGNETTE.

204. Ritodrine hydrochloride:

A. readily crosses the placenta.
B. does not cross the placenta.
C. slowly crosses the placenta.

205. An effect that Mrs. Smith's fetus may experience from ritodrine hydrochloride is:

A. an increase in fetal glomerular perfusion.
B. a decrease in fetal glomerular perfusion.
C. an increase in fetal glomerular filtration rate.

206. An infant who presents with distended bladder, paradoxical breathing, and relaxed abdominal muscles should be evaluated for:

A. brain injury.
B. meningocele.
C. spinal cord injury.

207. Red scaly skin lesions especially at the groin and perianal areas can be related to:

A. copper deficiency.
B. niacin deficiency.
C. zinc deficiency.

208. A number of factors increase risk of ototoxicity of drug therapy. One such factor is:

A. decreased serum drug levels.
B. increased renal function.
C. concurrent noise.

209. Renal vein thrombosis can be associated with:

A. umbilical artery or vein catheterization.
B. hydronephrosis.
C. renal tubular acidosis.

210. Approximately 15 percent to 20 percent of infants are ABO group incompatible with their mothers, but only about 3 percent exhibit symptoms of incompatibility. What is the rationale for this discrepancy?

A. A and B antigens on fetal RBCs are not well developed, and only a small amount of antibodies will actually attach to the antigen.
B. agglutination or clumping of ABO incompatible reactions cause minimal disruption to circulation so symptoms may not be evident.
C. ABO incompatibilities cause small amounts of IgM in the plasma that do not activate the complement system.

211. Where is cerebrospinal fluid primarily produced?

A. choroid plexus.
B. lateral ventricles.
C. aqueduct of Sylvius.

212. Hearing loss most often associated with cleft palate is:

A. sensorineural.
B. conductive.
C. mixed.

213. Large hemangiomas can:

A. reduce spontaneously.
B. result in heart failure.
C. result from bacterial infection.

214. Palpation of abdominal masses should be omitted if:

A. hematuria is present.
B. Wilms' tumor is suspected.
C. hepatosplenomegaly is present.

215. Scalded skin syndrome is a result of:

A. *Listeria monocytogenes.*
B. *Staphylococcus epidermidis.*
C. *Staphylococcus aureus.*

216. What stimulates the growth of the renal pelvis and calices from the ureteric bud?

A. gonadotropin.
B. testosterone.
C. glucocorticosteroids.

217. Sodium filtration in the renal tubules depends on:

A. chloride concentration.
B. sodium concentration.
C. glomerular filtration rate.

218. Hypopigmentation can be a sign of:

A. Niemann-Pick disease.
B. Marfan's syndrome.
C. PKU.

219. ______ is the most common cause of hearing loss in infants.

A. Otitis media
B. Meningitis
C. Perinatally acquired infection

Case History

Cindy, a 24-year-old primipara, gave birth to an 8 lb 7 oz, LGA, 38-week male infant. On examination, infant Josh was found to have syndactyly of the left hand. Other findings revealed an audible hip click, talipes varus, blue sclera, and stable cardiopulmonary status. No limitation in movement was found. All other physical parameters were within normal limits. Maternal history: spotting during the first trimester, oligohydramnios; 20 pound weight gain; diagnosed with gestational diabetes one month before delivery.

THE FOLLOWING THREE QUESTIONS ARE BASED ON THIS VIGNETTE.

220. The nurse practitioner should explain to the mother that:

A. outward turning of the foot may be due to low levels of amniotic fluid.
B. extra digits are possibly directly related to her diabetes.
C. upper extremities form earlier than the lower extremities.

221. The NNP ordered a series of chest and long bone x-rays to detect:

A. malformations of the long bones.
B. fractures of the chest and long bones.
C. muscular changes.

222. Blue sclera should increase suspicion for a diagnosis of:

A. osteogenesis imperfecta.
B. achondroplasia.
C. muscular dystrophy.

223. Therapeutic success of drug administration is determined by:

A. physiologic changes achieved at the target site for which the drug was used.
B. reaching the therapeutic drug concentration within the neonate by day two of treatment.
C. maintaining a constant drug level within the circulatory system throughout the drug administration period.

224. The skin's normal pH is:

A. 4.
B. 5.
C. 6.

225. Studies have shown close correlations between creatinine clearance and gentamicin clearance as well as gentamicin half-life and birth weight. With this in mind, an adequate dosing schedule for an infant less than 28 weeks would be:

A. gentamicin every 8 hours.
B. gentamicin every 12 hours.
C. gentamicin every 24 hours.

226. Constriction of the vessels leading into the glomerular capillary and increased resistance to blood flow into the capillary would result in:

A. higher filtration rate.
B. higher hydraulic pressure.
C. lower filtration rate.

227. A nursing implication of middle effusion associated the endotracheal intubation is:

A. use of prophylactic antibiotics during intubation time.
B. inclusion of visualization of middle ear during sepsis workup.
C. use of hearing tests during period of intubation.

228. A common problem in neonates that can alter enteral drug absorption is:

A. shortened gastric emptying time increases drug distribution.
B. delayed intestinal peristalsis increases drug absorption.
C. delayed intestinal peristalsis decreases drug absorption.

229. Liberal use of povidone-iodine as a prepping agent has been associated with:

A. hypothyroid goiter.
B. hypothyroidism.
C. low iodine levels.

230. Complications of otitis media include:

A. immobile stapes.
B. brain abscess.
C. white shadows of the ossicles.

231. Premature neonates can have circulating unbound drug concentrations that are higher than their total drug concentrations. This is primarily due to:

A. lower concentrations of serum proteins in the premature neonate.
B. higher concentrations of serum proteins in the premature neonate.
C. decreased availability of tissue receptors in the premature neonate.

232. One side effect of pain is:

A. lack of autoregulation.
B. an increase in blood pressure.
C. a decrease in blood pressure.

233. In neonates, many drugs have prolonged half-lives. This is due to:

A. decreased rate of infusion necessary for the neonate.
B. immaturity of the renal and liver systems.
C. a neonate's NPO status requiring intravenous fluids only.

234. The gonads should be shielded whenever they are within _____ cm of the primary x-ray beam.

A. 5
B. 10
C. 15

235. The term ARC or AIDS-related complex has been replaced by the term:

A. HIV positive.
B. AIDS.
C. HIV complex.

236. Assessment components essential for safe care of the neonate after cardiac catheterization include:

A. evaluation of signs of hypotension.
B. evaluation of signs of hypertension.
C. signs of generalized bleeding.

237. Pain is associated with adverse physiologic effects in:

A. the cardiorespiratory system.
B. the renal system.
C. all major organ systems.

238. Stabilization of the HIV exposed neonate in the delivery room includes:

A. standard protocol, no special considerations.
B. standard protocol, with use of double clothing protection.
C. standard protocol, but increase suction pressure to compensate for thick secretions.

Case History

Jenny is a 30-week AGA infant who was born at 24 weeks' gestation. She received surfactant therapy and was on a ventilator with 80 percent oxygen for five days. Currently, Jenny is in a head hood with 30 percent oxygen. Her blood gases still reflect carbon dioxide retention at times and oxygen levels in the low to moderate range. Jenny is noted to have a whitish-appearing pupil with an active purulent discharge.

THE FOLLOWING SEVEN QUESTIONS ARE BASED ON THIS VIGNETTE.

239. Jenny's eyes can be affected by her immaturity and her need for supplemental oxygen. The ophthalmologist is going to examine her eyes today. This examination should include an evaluation of:

A. the cornea.
B. the pupillary response.
C. visual acuity.

240. Use of dilating eye drops (cycloplegic or mydriatrics) can produce side effects. Jenny's nurse should anticipate this possibility and diminish the complications by:

A. placing pressure over the eyelids for one minute after instillation.
B. placing Jenny in a side-lying position for one minute after instillation.
C. immediately wiping excess medications off the skin surrounding the eye.

241. _____ is the descriptive term for a whitish-appearing pupil.

A. Cataract
B. Leukocoria
C. Toxocariasis

242. In Jenny's case, the most probable cause of this pupillary abnormality is:

A. immaturity.
B. retinopathy of prematurity.
C. rubella.

243. Jenny is believed to be at high risk for retinopathy of prematurity (ROP). Risk factors for ROP include all the following <u>EXCEPT</u>:

A. low birth weight.
B. sepsis.
C. infant of a diabetic mother.

244. Jenny's NNP should arrange follow-up eye examinations after this initial visit:

A. weekly.
B. monthly.
C. every 3–4 months.

245. Jenny's mother is told that Jenny has ROP that will require cryotherapy. The nurse should explain to her that cryotherapy will:

A. create scar tissue that will reverse the disease.
B. reattach the retina and improve visual acuity.

C. break up the fibrinous scar tissue in the vessels.

246. The diagnosis of Hirschsprung's disease can be easily supported by the procedure of:

A. sweat chloride.
B. upper GI series.
C. barium enema.

247. The fight-or-flight stress response is exhibited by:

A. 15–20 days of life.
B. at birth, even in the premature.
C. at birth, in the full-term infant.

248. ______ imaging is a radiologic technique used to evaluate the motion of an organ.

A. Fluroscopic
B. Xeroradioraphic
C. Tomographic

249. A ground wire will:

A. protect the patient from excessive current flow.
B. not protect the patient from excessive current flow.
C. protect the patient from microshocks.

250. ______ is one of the most important indices of a newborn's health status.

A. Skin temperature
B. Core temperature
C. Ratio of skin to core temperature

251. The selection of a particular diagnostic imaging technique should be based on all of the follow EXCEPT:

A. neonatal risks.
B. parental wishes.
C. diagnostic benefits.

252. Cord care for an HIV-exposed infant includes:

A. use of alcohol only.
B. use of antimicrobial ointment.
C. sterile dressing.

253. A major force in the advancement of neonatal pain was:

A. parents.
B. nurses.
C. physicians.

254. An HIV positive infant should:

A. not receive immunization at all.
B. receive standard immunization on a delayed schedule.
C. receive inactivated immunizations on a regular schedule.

255. Mask ventilation is contraindicated when there is a TEF:

A. without esophageal atresia.
B. with esophageal atresia.
C. that is an H-type.

256. The term multiple system organ failure refers to:

A. progression of AIDS.
B. initial sites of AIDS.
C. term used instead of AIDS.

257. Pregnant women are more sensitive to inhalation anesthetics because their:

A. endorphin level is elevated.
B. endorphin level is decreased.
C. epidural veins are decreased.

258. ______ is the most frequent respiratory opportunistic infection for the HIV-positive infant.

A. *Pneumocystis carinii* (PCP)
B. Lymphoid interstitial pneumonia (LIP)
C. *Pseudomonas*

259. A neonatal electroencephalogram is a procedure important in diagnosing:

A. functional areas of the brain.
B. sleep disorders.
C. the focus of seizure activity.

260. In the adult which statement most accurately reflects the role of myelination in transmission of pain stimulus?

A. complete myelination.
B. partial (>50%) myelination.
C. 80 percent of the fibers that transmit pain remain unmyelinated.

261. One important issue concerning the use of *expert* computer systems is:
   A. to have access for use based only on data entry codes.
   B. to understand that expert systems can supplement but never replace a nurse's knowledge and expertise.
   C. that computer down time can cause a backlog of information about the patient.

262. Pharmacologic intervention is indicated for the neonate experiencing neonatal abstinence syndrome. The drug of choice is:
   A. paregoric.
   B. dilantin.
   C. morphine.

263. _____ procedures carry fewer risks to the mother but may be less beneficial to the fetus.
   A. Closed
   B. Open
   C. Later gestational

264. Current technology exists for NICUs to use computerized nursing documentation systems at the "point of care." This refers to:
   A. bedside terminals.
   B. lab retrieval from the computer.
   C. physician orders verified through the computer.

265. Capillary-leak syndrome is a result of:
   A. movement of fluids from the tissue to the vascular space.
   B. generalized ascites in the abdominal region.
   C. a change in membrane permeability.

266. Fetal alcohol syndrome (FAS) is diagnosed by reported alcohol consumption during pregnancy and characteristic neonatal features One such feature is:
   A. large for gestational age (LGA).
   B. facial anomalies.
   C. syndactyly of fingers and toes.

267. Which of the following factors influence neonatal pain management:
   A. fear of addiction and side effects (by practitioners).
   B. lack of ability to evaluate pain objectively.
   C. relative lack of response to existing medications.

268. Glucose metabolism can be altered because of surgery. A Dextrostix should be monitored during the immediate postoperative period every:
   A. 30 minutes to one hour.
   B. one to two hours.
   C. four hours.

269. The VLBW infant who is vulnerable to CNS problems should have an environment that:
   A. is dimly lit if possible.
   B. is close to the nursing station.
   C. offers quiet, continuous music.

270. Postoperative complications after liver transplantation should be suspected if:
   A. hypothermia is present.
   B. leukopenia is present.
   C. leukocytosis is present.

271. Neonatal abstinence syndrome refers to a triad of findings among heroin-exposed infants. The combination of symptoms includes:
   A. SGA, cardiac, and pulmonary symptoms.
   B. SGA, CNS, and GI symptoms.
   C. SGA, CNS, and cardiac symptoms.

272. What essential process of brain growth or maturation is most vulnerable to negative environmental influences?
   A. cerebral blood flow vascularization.
   B. remodeling of the neuronal structure.
   C. proliferation of myelin sheaths.

273. Lactobezoars are an example of an iatrogenic complication. These are due to:
   A. whey predominate formulas.
   B. casein predominate formulas.
   C. use of 27 calorie formulas.

274. Management of portal hypertension centers on:
   A. control of ascites.
   B. control of infection.
   C. restriction of calories.

275. The proper positioning of the premature infant is:

A. neck extended with right-sided head preference.
B. flexion of limbs and trunk and facilitation of midline skills.
C. retracted and abducted shoulders.

276. Heroin exposure in utero creates a condition of:

A. passive fetal addiction.
B. active fetal addiction.
C. fatal withdrawal.

277. Iatrogenic complications due to human error can be reduced through the quality assurance/quality improvement (QA/QI) evaluation process. This process should include all the following EXCEPT:

A. a systematic review of unusual incidents.
B. informing the staff of errors and who was responsible.
C. keeping staff informed of errors.

278. A potential complication of cocaine use during pregnancy includes:

A. placental abruption.
B. increased incidence of postmaturity.
C. decreased fetal heart rate variability.

279. Focus of care for boarder babies should be:

A. normalizing their environment.
B. caring for their intensive medical needs.
C. keeping mother–infant contacts to a minimum.

280. What one fetal hazard has been documented as having a strong association with maternal smoking?

A. dysmorphic features.
B. low birth weight.
C. respiratory distress.

281. Indications for transplantation include all of the following EXCEPT:

A. progressive end-stage liver disease.
B. fatal hepatic-based metabolic disease.
C. premature infant with liver and chronic lung diseases.

282. Cue-based care is based on all the following EXCEPT:

A. observations of infant's state.
B. observations for signs of stress.
C. observations of caregiver's signals.

283. One factor that can help staff to accept the use of computers in the hospital setting includes:

A. immediate, tangible benefits.
B. increased complexity of system use.
C. using standard software applications.

Case History

Baby Gilbert is a 28-week male whose Apgars were 1, 5, and 8. He is now 34 weeks corrected age, just under five pounds, and ready for discharge.

THE FOLLOWING TWO QUESTIONS ARE BASED ON THIS VIGNETTE.

284. His parents should be told:

A. his behavior is well organized and predictable now.
B. his behavior is disorganized and unpredictable now.
C. he will be socially responsive in most situations.

285. His mother has noticed that he tends to drop off to sleep when he first starts to feed. This behavior indicates:

A. a neurologic problem.
B. maternal inability to arouse infant.
C. preterm behavior due to limited energy.

286. Assessing the ______ to home care is perhaps the most critical factor determining the success of failure of home health care.

A. infant's readiness for discharge
B. family's commitment
C. physician's commitment

287. Important components of any follow-up program include:

   A. highly structured, rigid protocols of care.
   B. home visiting by a paraprofessional.
   C. parent involvement in care.

288. Neonatal individualized development care and assessment program (NIDCAP) should be used to assess:

   A. high risk full-term or preterm infants.
   B. high risk preterm infants.
   C. any infant in the NICU.

Marianne McGraw, RN, MSN

Jacob had followed a typical course for a baby born at 32 weeks. He had moderate RDS, which required ventilatory support and transfer to a tertiary center soon after delivery. He weaned quickly and began feeding on day five of life. The next week he was readmitted to the level II referral hospital, where he continued to grow. On Jacob's second day back at the hospital, he began having episodes of apnea with occasional bradycardia. He was closely monitored via cardiac monitor and pulse oximeter. His assessment appeared normal, revealing no lethargy, hypothermia, or cyanosis. Lab studies ruled out sepsis, anemia, hypoxia, and metabolic disturbances. X-rays (chest and abdominal) and a head ultrasound were all within normal limits. The apneic episodes were limited and did not compromise his status.

Jane, his primary nurse, started using Jacob's discharge teaching sheet to assess not only the infant's readiness but the parents' readiness as well.

Mr. and Mrs. W visited often and became involved in Jacob's care. They were initially thrilled to hear about their son's discharge within the week but then feelings of fear and uncertainty hit them.

A home visit, during this first week at home, was made. Mrs. W stated that it had been difficult getting to know Jacob's routines and schedules and that she was still trying to get to know his cues. "How do I know if I'm doing the right thing?" she asked. Mrs. W then stated that she was still afraid that Jacob might stop breathing.

THE FOLLOWING THREE QUESTIONS ARE BASED ON THIS VIGNETTE.

289. Mothers of preterm infants such as the one described above report:

   A. they expect their infants to be similar to full-term infants.
   B. they expect their infants to be different than full-term infants.
   C. they know as much of what to expect from their infants just as full-term mothers do.

290. True to her concerns about the discharge, the transition to home for Jacob and his mother may represent:

   A. a crisis.
   B. an achievement.
   C. a developmental passage.

291. Immediate informational needs for Jacob's mother include all the following <u>EXCEPT</u>:

   A. normal newborn care.
   B. how to keep him healthy.
   C. immunization schedule.

292. Home care may be short- or long-term care. Long-term care is defined as:

   A. care required for longer than one year.
   B. care provided by paraprofessionals for longer than six months.
   C. care required for longer than six months.

293. _____ is most often required by infants with hyperbilirubinemia, respiratory distress, apnea, and alternative feeding needs.

   A. Hospice care
   B. Long-term care
   C. Short-term care

ANSWERS TO REVIEW TEST 1

1. Answer: (**A**) Because the new NICU nurse lacks experience and others on the staff do not know how much they can rely on the new nurse's judgment, direct supervision by a more experienced person is essential. In other words, the newer nurse must begin by helping a more seasoned nurse with an assignment. Early work assignments should be routine. However, it is important for the beginning level neonatal nurse not to be tied only to work that is tedious and detailed. She or he should be expected to show some initiative. Central activities of this role include helping, learning, and following directions. The beginning level neonatal nurse is a dependent practitioner.

REFERENCES

France, M.H. & McDowell, C. (1983). A systematic career development model: An overview. *Canadian Vocational Journal, 19*(1), 31–34.

Harrigan, R.C. & Perez, D. (1993). Neonatal nursing and its role in comprehensive care (pp. 3–8). In C. Kenner, A. Brueggemeyer, & L.P. Gunderson (eds.), *Comprehensive neonatal nursing: A physiologic perspective.* Philadelphia: W.B. Saunders.

Perez, R. (1981). *Protocols for perinatal nursing practice.* St. Louis: C.V. Mosby.

2. Answer: (**A**) A trait can be controlled by a single gene regardless of whether that single gene is dominant or recessive. The single gene transmission follows mendelian laws of inheritance.

REFERENCES

Cohen, F.L. (1984). *Clinical genetics in nursing practice.* Philadelphia: J.B. Lippincott.

Connor, J. & Ferguson-Smith, M. (1987). *Essential medical genetics.* Oxford: Blackwell Scientific.

Cummings, M. (1988). *Human heredity: Principles and issues.* New York: West Publishing.

Thompson, S. & Thompson, M. (1986). *Genetics in medicine* (4th ed.). Philadelphia: W.B. Saunders.

Workman, M.L., Kenner, C., & Hilse, M. (1993). Human genetics (pp. 101–131). In C. Kenner, A. Brueggemeyer, & L.P. Gunderson (eds.), *Comprehensive neonatal nursing: A physiologic perspective.* Philadelphia: W.B. Saunders.

3. Answer: (**B**) There should be a relationship between the certification standards, requirements, and options, and titles and content of curricula used to prepare advanced practitioners of nursing. Students and the public have the right to know whether the certification will be available and under what auspices and whether there is an acceptable level of congruence between program content and certification requirements. State boards of nursing usually do not set standards for advanced nursing practice or have a separate licensure procedure.

REFERENCES

Harrigan, R.C. & Perez, D. (1993). Neonatal nursing and its role in comprehensive care (pp. 3–8). In C. Kenner, A. Brueggemeyer, & L.P. Gunderson (eds.), *Comprehensive neonatal nursing: A physiologic perspective.* Philadelphia: W.B. Saunders.

Harper, R.G., Little, G.A., & Sia, C.G. (1982). The scope of nursing practice in level III neonatal intensive care units. *Pediatrics, 70,* 875–878.

Sherwen, L. (1990). Interdisciplinary collaboration in perinatal/neonatal health care. A worthwhile challenge. *Journal of Perinatology, 10*(1), 1–2.

4. Answer: (**B**) The concept of collaboration does *not* assume the contribution of each member of the group of providers is equal. In fact, the concept of collaboration assumes that each profession has something unique and important to contribute to the well-being of the infant and family. In addition, collaborative practice requires that professionals have mature role competence and highly developed technological expertise.

REFERENCES

Aradine, C.R. & Hansen, M.F. (1970). Interdisciplinary teamwork in family health care. *Nursing Clinics of North America, 5*(2), 211–222.

Leininger, M. (1971). This I believe: About interdisciplinary health education for the future. *Nursing Outlook, 19*(12), 787–791.

Harrigan, R. & Perez, D. (1993). Collaborative practice in the NICU (pp. 9–13). In C. Kenner, A. Brueggemeyer, & L.P. Gunderson (eds.), *Comprehensive neonatal nursing: A physiologic perspective.* Philadelphia: W.B. Saunders.

5. Answer: (**C**) Organizational characteristics that suggest successful collaboration include: (1) low staff turnover, (you must know someone to collaborate); (2) adequate numbers of staff; (3) decentralized decision making; and (4) delegation of authority for caregiving to small groups of staff for a cohort of patients.

REFERENCES

Harrigan, R. & Perez, D. (1993). Collaborative practice in the NICU (pp. 9–13). In C. Kenner, A. Brueggemeyer, & L.P. Gunderson (eds.), *Comprehensive neonatal nursing: A physiologic perspective.* Philadelphia: W.B. Saunders.

Sherwen, L. (1990). Interdisciplinary collaboration in perinatal/neonatal health care. A worthwhile challenge. *Journal of Perinatology, 10* (1), 1–2.

6. Answer: (**C**) Clinical ethics frequently has been equated with medical ethics. This misconception is based on the notion that the nurse–client relationship is secondary to the physician–client relationship. The scope of clinical ethics is larger and incorporates the problems and situations that nurses encounter in the independent and collaborative domains of practice.

REFERENCES

Beauchamp, T.L. & Childress, J.F. (1983). *Principles of biomedical ethics.* New York: Oxford University Press.

Fowler, M.D. (1987). Introduction to ethics and ethical theory (pp. 659–670). In M.D. Fowler & J. Levine-Ariff (eds.), *Ethics at the bedside: A source book for the critical care nurse.* New York: McGraw-Hill.

Southwell, S.M. & Archer-Dusté, H. (1993). Ethical aspects of perinatal care (pp. 14–35). In C. Kenner, A. Brueggemeyer, & L.P. Gunderson (eds.), *Comprehensive neonatal nursing: A physiologic perspective.* Philadelphia: W.B. Saunders.

7. Answer: (**A**) Four key elements to informed consent are: disclosure of accurate information and assurance that the information is comprehended by the receiving party constitute the two information elements. Determination of voluntary participation without coercion and the competence of the individual to make an autonomous decision are the two consent elements.

REFERENCES

Beauchamp, T.L. & Childress, J.F. (1983). *Principles of biomedical ethics.* New York: Oxford University Press.

Cunningham, N. & Hutchinson, S. (1990). Neonatal nurses and issues in research ethics. *Neonatal Network, 8*(5), 29–48.

Fowler, M.D. (1987). Introduction to ethics and ethical theory. In M.D. Fowler & J. Levine-Ariff (eds.), *Ethics at the bedside: A source book for the critical care nurse* (pp. 659–670). New York: McGraw-Hill.

National Commission for the Protection of Human Subjects of Biomedical and Behavioral Research. (1979). *The Belmont report: Ethical principles and guidelines for the protection of human subjects of research* (DHEW Publication No. (OS) 78-0013 and No. (OS) 78-0014). Washington, DC: U.S. Government Printing Office.

Southwell, S.M. & Archer-Dusté, H. (1993). Ethical aspects of perinatal care (pp. 14–35). In C. Kenner, A. Brueggemeyer, & L.P. Gunderson (eds.), *Comprehensive neonatal nursing: A physiologic perspective.* Philadelphia: W.B. Saunders.

8. Answer: (**C**) The hallmark of an expert neonatal nurse is knowing the limits of professional knowledge. Expect neonatal nurses must (1) be able to use appropriate knowledge, (2) have sufficient expertise to evaluate the knowledge for its appropriateness in improving the quality of life, and (3) contribute to the development of a body of knowledge relevant to neonatal health care. This is impossible unless the neonatal nurse is competent both in technically and theoretically sense. Neonatal nurses must be prepared to empirically investigate the adequacy of a statement's plausibility or the relevance of predictive factors associated with treatment approaches. Neonatal nurse researchers are needed to conduct research and further develop the empirical foundation for neonatal nursing practice.

REFERENCES

Harrigan, R.C. & Perez, D. (1993). Neonatal nursing and its role in comprehensive care (pp. 3–8). In C. Kenner, A. Brueggemeyer, & L.P. Gunderson (eds.), *Comprehensive neonatal nursing: A physiologic perspective.* Philadelphia: W.B. Saunders.

Sherwen, L. (1990). Interdisciplinary collaboration in perinatal/neonatal health care. A worthwhile challenge. *Journal of Perinatology, 10*(1), 1–2.

9. Answer: (**C**) Normative ethics explores ethical norms or standards and their application to the human world. Metaethics and descriptive ethics are nonnormative; they do not prescribe behaviors (Fowler, 1987). Teleologists assert that an action can be judged right or wrong by the consequences of the action as measured against a spe-

cific end that is sought. The common illustration of teleologic thought is utilitarianism: "The greatest possible balance of values over disvalue for all persons who would be affected" (Beauchamp & Childress, 1983, p. 20).

REFERENCES

Beauchamp, T.L. & Childress, J.F. (1983). *Principles of biomedical ethics.* New York: Oxford University Press.

Fowler, M.D. (1987). Introduction to ethics and ethical theory. In M.D. Fowler & J. Levine-Ariff (eds.), *Ethics at the bedside: A source book for the critical care nurse* (pp. 659–670). New York: McGraw-Hill.

Southwell, S.M. & Archer-Dusté, H. (1993). Ethical aspects of perinatal care (pp. 14–35). In C. Kenner, A. Brueggemeyer, & L.P. Gunderson (eds.), *Comprehensive neonatal nursing: A physiologic perspective.* Philadelphia: W.B. Saunders.

10. Answer: (**B**) Metaethics and descriptive ethics are nonnormative; they do not prescribe behaviors (Fowler, 1987). Deontological thought affirms that the intrinsic quality of the action determines its rightness or wrongness. Utilitarianism: "The greatest possible balance of values over disvalue for all persons who would be affected" (Beauchamp & Childress, 1983, p. 20). Normative ethics examines norms or standards.

REFERENCES

Beauchamp, T.L. & Childress, J.F. (1983). *Principles of biomedical ethics.* New York: Oxford University Press.

Fowler, M.D. (1987). Introduction to ethics and ethical theory (pp. 659–670). In M.D. Fowler & J. Levine-Ariff (eds.), *Ethics at the bedside: A source book for the critical care nurse.* New York: McGraw-Hill.

Southwell, S.M. & Archer-Dusté, H. (1993). Ethical aspects of perinatal care (pp. 14–35). In C. Kenner, A. Brueggemeyer, & L.P. Gunderson (eds.), *Comprehensive neonatal nursing: A physiologic perspective.* Philadelphia: W.B. Saunders.

11. Answer: (**B**) U.S. Department of Health and Human Services' Baby Doe Regulations (Moreno, 1987) state that treatment should be effective in "reasonable medical judgment" and can be withheld or with drawn only if (1) the infant is chronically and irreversibly comatose; (2) the provision of such treatment would merely prolong dying, not be effective in ameliorating or correcting all the infant's life-threatening conditions, or would otherwise be futile in terms of the survival of the infant; or (3) the provision of such treatment would be virtually futile in terms of the survival of the infant, and the treatment itself under such circumstances would be inhumane.

REFERENCES

Moreno, J.D. (1987). Ethical and legal issues in the care of the impaired newborn. *Clinics in Perinatology 14,* 345–360.

Southwell, S.M. & Archer-Dusté, H. (1993). Ethical aspects of perinatal care (pp. 14–35). In C. Kenner, A. Brueggemeyer, & L.P. Gunderson (eds.), *Comprehensive neonatal nursing: A physiologic perspective.* Philadelphia: W.B. Saunders.

12. Answer: (**B**) Substantive standards of judgment for treatment have to be chosen, against which the strategies are measured (Arras, 1987). The first are sanctity-of-life standards. An extreme form of this type is "vitalism," which views the continuation of life as the greatest good. Another view is the "medical indications" policy. Under this policy, the sanctity of life is upheld, but treatment is medically contraindicated. Quality of life standards are "social worth," in which the quality of life is measured by its degree of benefit or burden to others, primarily parents and society. "Best interests" standard are choices based on what is in the best interest of the infant from the infant's perspective.

REFERENCES

Arras, J.D. (1984). Toward an ethic of ambiguity. *Hastings Center Report, 14*(2), 25–33.

Imperiled newborns. (1987). *Hastings Center Report, 17*(6), 5–32.

Moreno, J.D. (1987). Ethical and legal issues in the care of the impaired newborn. *Clinics in Perinatology 14,* 345–360.

Southwell, S.M. & Archer-Dusté, H. (1993). Ethical aspects of perinatal care (pp. 14–35). In C. Kenner, A. Brueggemeyer, & L.P. Gunderson (eds.), *Comprehensive neonatal nursing: A physiologic perspective.* Philadelphia: W.B. Saunders.

13. Answer: (**A**) Without research, nursing care would be based simply on tradition. Judgments of efficacy based on observation of small numbers of infants or treatments based on the principle of "if a little is good, more is better" have resulted in significant morbidity and mortality for neonates. The use of clinical research trials to scientifically evaluate new therapies before widespread application has become more common in neonatal care.

REFERENCES

Brink, P.J. & Wood, M.J. (eds.). (1989). *Advanced design in nursing research.* Newbury Park, California: Sage Publications.

Franck, L.S., Gunderson, L.P., & Kenner, C. (1993). Collaborative research in neonatal nursing (pp. 52–66). In C. Kenner, A. Brueggemeyer, & L.P. Gunderson (eds.), *Comprehensive neonatal nursing: A physiologic perspective.* Philadelphia: W.B. Saunders.

14. Answer: (**B**) The law uses the term malpractice to describe negligence of individuals who violate a standard of care that can only be known by virtue of education in a field.

REFERENCES

American Nurses' Association. (1984). *Code for nurse with interpretive statements.* Kansas City, MO: Author.

Driscoll, K.M. (1993). Legal aspects of perinatal care (pp. 36–51). In C. Kenner, A. Brueggemeyer, & L.P. Gunderson (eds.), *Comprehensive neonatal nursing: A physiologic perspective.* Philadelphia: W.B. Saunders.

Pegalis, S.E. & Wachsman, H.F. (1990). *American law of medical malpractice.* (Cum. Suppl.). Rochester, NY: Lawyers Co-Operative Publishing.

15. Answer: (**A**) Accountable professionals practice prudently and reasonably based on their education and experience. Knowing and practicing nursing according to current standards help to ensure that a legal challenge to one's practice can be successfully defended. Nursing documentation provides evidence of both professional accountability and legal accountability.

REFERENCES

American Nurses' Association. (1984). *Code for nurse with interpretive statements.* Kansas City, MO: Author.

Driscoll, K.M. (1993). Legal aspects of perinatal care (pp. 36–51). In C. Kenner, A. Brueggemeyer, & L.P. Gunderson (eds.), *Comprehensive neonatal nursing: A physiologic perspective.* Philadelphia: W.B. Saunders.

Pegalis, S.E. & Wachsman, H.F. (1990). *American law of medical malpractice.* (Cum. Suppl.). Rochester, NY: Lawyers Co-Operative Publishing.

16. Answer: (**C**) Incident reports involving neonates should mirror descriptions of the same event found in the medical record. Incident reports should contain *facts* surrounding the event. Conclusory or blaming statements should be absent from the report. The report should reflect the facts of the incident and steps taken to assess for and alleviate any actual injury that occurred. Incident reporting systems should require professionals not only to disclose their own mistakes but also to report those of peers. Ideally, neonatal nurses should view incident reports as an extension of their ethical obligation to safeguard the health and safety of clients.

REFERENCES

American Academy of Pediatrics/American College of Obstetrician and Gynecologists. (1992). *Guidelines for perinatal care.* Elk Grove Village, IL: Author.

American Nurses' Association. (1984). *Code for nurse with interpretive statements.* Kansas City, MO: Author.

Driscoll, K.M. (1993). Legal aspects of perinatal care (pp. 36–51). In C. Kenner, A. Brueggemeyer, & L.P. Gunderson (eds.), *Comprehensive neonatal nursing: A physiologic perspective.* Philadelphia: W.B. Saunders.

Pegalis, S.E. & Wachsman, H.F. (1990). *American law of medical malpractice.* (Cum. Suppl.). Rochester, NY: Lawyers Co-Operative Publishing.

17. Answer: (**A**) The IRBs review research proposals to ensure protection for human subjects under the regulations.

REFERENCES

Driscoll, K.M. (1993). Legal aspects of perinatal care (pp. 36–51). In C. Kenner, A. Brueggemeyer, & L.P. Gunderson (eds.), *Comprehensive neonatal nursing: A physiologic perspective.* Philadelphia: W.B. Saunders.

National Commission for the Protection of Human Subjects of Biomedical and Behavioral Research. (1979). The Belmont Report: Ethical principles and guideline for the protection of human subjects of research (DHEW Publication No. (OS) 78-0013 and No. (OS) 78-0014). Washington, DC: U.S. Government Printing Office.

18. Answer: (**A**) H.E.L.L.P. syndrome is a complex of symptoms described as a severe forerunner of PIH that has a sudden onset and is diagnosed from signs and symptoms of hemolysis, elevated liver enzymes, and low platelets.

REFERENCES

Creasy, R. & Resnick, M. (1989). *Maternal fetal medicine: Principles and practice.* Philadelphia: W.B. Saunders.

Gilbert, E. & Harmon, J. (1986). *High risk pregnancy and delivery.* St. Louis: C.V. Mosby.

Harmon, J.S. (1993). High-risk pregnancy (pp. 157–170). In C. Kenner, A. Brueggemeyer, & L.P. Gunderson (eds.), *Comprehensive neonatal nursing: A physiologic perspective.* Philadelphia: W.B. Saunders.

Moore, K. (1989). *The developing human* (4th ed.). Philadelphia: W.B. Saunders.

19. Answer: (**A**) The level of inquiry is considered by many as occurring on a continuum. Brink and Wood (1989) identify three levels of nursing research: (1) exploratory-descriptive, (2) comparative, and (3) experimental. If the purposes of the research are to become more familiar with phenomena, to gain new insights, to formulate a more specific research problem or hypothesis, the research is *exploratory*. Comparative studies involve more structure than exploratory-descriptive studies, and the samples are usually randomized or stratified. The "gold standard" of experimental research is the randomized clinical trial. In this most rigorous of research designs, carefully controlled prospective, blind trials can definitively establish risks and benefits of new treatments, minimizing bias and error.

REFERENCES

Brink, P.J. & Wood, M.J. (eds.). (1989). *Advanced design in nursing research.* Newbury Park, California: Sage Publications.

Chalmers, T.C. (1990). A belated randomized control trial, *Pediatrics, 85,* 366–369.

Franck, L.S., Gunderson, L.P., & Kenner, C. (1993). Collaborative research in neonatal nursing. (pp. 52–66). In C. Kenner, A. Brueggemeyer, & L.P. Gunderson (eds.), *Comprehensive neonatal nursing: A physiologic perspective.* Philadelphia: W.B. Saunders.

20. Answer: (**C**) Qualitative studies categorize and describe data by patterns, themes and categories of response at a nominal or naming level. Ethnographers, for example, attempt to describe characteristics of certain groups via qualitative methods (Fetterman, 1989). The data are collected through either unstructured or semistructured methods.

REFERENCES

Brink, P.J. & Wood, M.J. (eds.). (1989). *Advanced design in nursing research.* Newbury Park, California: Sage Publications.

Fetterman, D.M. (1989). *Ethnography: Step by step.* Applied social research methods series (Vol. 17). Newbury Park, California: Sage Publications.

Franck, L.S., Gunderson, L.P., & Kenner, C. (1993). Collaborative research in neonatal nursing (pp. 52–66). In C. Kenner, A. Brueggemeyer, & L.P. Gunderson (eds.), *Comprehensive neonatal nursing: A physiologic perspective.* Philadelphia: W.B. Saunders.

21. Answer: (**B**) The data from these qualitative studies are analyzed through content analysis, reporting the categories or themes found.

REFERENCES

Brink, P.J. & Wood, M.J. (eds.). (1989). *Advanced design in nursing research.* Newbury Park, California: Sage Publications.

Franck, L.S., Gunderson, L.P., & Kenner, C. (1993). Collaborative research in neonatal nursing (pp. 52–66). In C. Kenner, A. Brueggemeyer, & L.P. Gunderson (eds.), *Comprehensive neonatal nursing: A physiologic perspective.* Philadelphia: W.B. Saunders.

22. Answer: (**C**) The data are collected through either unstructured or semistructured methods. The sample usually consists of those persons available for interview—a convenience sample.

REFERENCES

Brink, P.J. & Wood, M.J. (eds.). (1989). *Advanced design in nursing research.* Newbury Park, California: Sage Publications.

Franck, L.S., Gunderson, L.P., & Kenner, C. (1993). Collaborative research in neonatal nursing (pp. 52–66). In C. Kenner, A. Brueggemeyer, & L.P. Gunderson (eds.), *Comprehensive neonatal nursing: A physiologic perspective.* Philadelphia: W.B. Saunders.

23. Answer: (**C**) The purpose of the research project will dictate the form of the specific objectives. Not all research investigations will have hypotheses. In descriptive studies, research questions not hypotheses direct the investigation, whereas in experimental studies specific hypothesis are tested.

REFERENCES

Brink, P.J. & Wood, M.J. (eds.). (1989). *Advanced design in nursing research.* Newbury Park, California: Sage Publications.

Franck, L.S., Gunderson, L.P., & Kenner, C. (1993). Collaborative research in neonatal nursing (pp. 52–66). In C. Kenner, A. Brueggemeyer, & L.P. Gunderson (eds.), *Comprehensive neonatal nursing: A physiologic perspective.* Philadelphia: W.B. Saunders.

24. Answer: (**B**) Morality is established by consensus and conveys a sense of a common social tradition or acceptable behaviors. Ethics is the area of intellectual contemplation beyond the simple acceptance of social norms (Fowler, 1987). Normative ethics explores ethical norms or standards and their application to the human world.

REFERENCES

Beauchamp, T.L. & Childress, J.F. (1983). *Principles of biomedical ethics*. New York: Oxford University Press.

Cunningham, N. & Hutchinson, S. (1990). Neonatal nurses and issues in research ethics. *Neonatal Network, 8*(5), 29–48.

Fowler, M.D. (1987). Introduction to ethics and ethical theory (pp. 659–670). In M.D. Fowler & J. Levine-Ariff (eds.), *Ethics at the bedside: A source book for the critical care nurse*. New York: McGraw-Hill.

Southwell, S.M. & Archer-Dusté, H. (1993). Ethical aspects of perinatal care (pp. 14–35). In C. Kenner, A. Brueggemeyer, & L.P. Gunderson (eds.), *Comprehensive neonatal nursing: A physiologic perspective*. Philadelphia: W.B. Saunders.

25. Answer: (**B**) Validity—Does the instrument or technique measure what it purports to measure? Reliability—Does the instrument or technique measure consistently? Suitability—Utility is the instrument appropriate for the setting/subjects.

REFERENCES

Brink, P.J. & Wood, M.J. (eds.). (1989). *Advanced design in nursing research*. Newbury Park, California: Sage Publications.

Franck, L.S., Gunderson, L.P., & Kenner, C. (1993). Collaborative research in neonatal nursing (pp. 52–66). In C. Kenner, A. Brueggemeyer, & L.P. Gunderson (eds.), *Comprehensive neonatal nursing: A physiologic perspective*. Philadelphia: W.B. Saunders.

26. Answer: (**B**) Completion of a research study is not the end of the research process. A key step often neglected is the dissemination of the information obtained in the study. This dissemination serves two purposes: (1) the sharing of information learned so others can benefit and (2) the promotion of critical dialogue among professionals related to the study design, results, and interpretation. Sharing research results can take place through presentation, posters, and abstracts at professional meetings and through publication in peer-reviewed journals.

REFERENCES

Brink, P.J. & Wood, M.J. (eds.). (1989). *Advanced design in nursing research*. Newbury Park, California: Sage Publications.

Franck, L.S., Gunderson, L.P., & Kenner, C. (1993). Collaborative research in neonatal nursing (pp. 52–66). In C. Kenner, A. Brueggemeyer, & L.P. Gunderson (eds.), *Comprehensive neonatal nursing: A physiologic perspective*. Philadelphia: W.B. Saunders.

27. Answer: (**A**) In a large, randomized, controlled trial, CLSE used in a prevention mode (delivery room administration) was compared with CLSE used in the rescue mode (given only to infants with established RDS). More infants less than 30 weeks' gestation survived in the prevention group, 88 percent versus 89 percent. Two different artificial surfactants have been tested in newborn infants with RDS. Artificial surfactants can be distinguished from natural surfactants by the absence of the surfactant associated proteins.

    Two doses of Exosurf® given as rescue therapy to infants with RDS weighing 700 to 1350 grams were evaluated in a multicenter, blinded, placebo-controlled trial. The first dose was given between 2–24 hours of age. The second dose was given 12 hours after the first. Pulmonary function improved with Exosurf® as evidenced by an improvement in the arterial/alveolar oxygen.

REFERENCES

Donovan, E.F. & Spangler, L.L. (1993). New technologies applied to the management of respiratory dysfunction. In C. Kenner, A. Brueggemeyer, & L.P. Gunderson (eds.), *Comprehensive neonatal nursing: A physiologic perspective*. Philadelphia: W.B. Saunders.

Gluck, L. & Nugent, J. (1991). Surfactant replacement (pp. 185–196). In J. Nugent (ed.). *Acute respiratory care of the neonate*. Petaluma, CA: NICU, Ink.

Horbar, J.D., Soll, R.F., Sutherland, J.M., et al. (1989). A multicenter randomized, placebo-controlled trial of surfactant therapy for respiratory distress syndrome. *The New England Journal of Medicine, 320*(15), 959–965.

Miller, E.D. & Armstrong, C.L. (1990). Surfactant replacement therapy: Innovative care for the premature infant. *JOGNN, 19*(1), 14–17.

28. Answer: (**B**) Polycythemia develops as a compensatory mechanism to increase the oxygen-carrying capacity of the blood. In the presence of decreased volume, the increased viscosity of the blood can impede cerebral circulation and increase risks for cerebral infarcts. Volume deficits secondary to nausea, vomiting, and diarrhea are serious threats of gastroenteritis because of the polycythemia.

    Infants with TOF are at no greater risk for calcium imbalances than children with normal cardiac anatomy and function. Volume overload probably will not occur in the presence of gastroenteritis.

REFERENCES

Lott, J.W. (1993). Assessment and management of cardiovascular dysfunction (pp. 355–391). In C. Kenner, A. Brueggemeyer, & L.P. Gunderson (eds.), *Comprehensive neonatal nursing: A physiologic perspective*. Philadelphia: W.B. Saunders.

Mair, D.D., Edwards, W.D., Julsrud, P.R., Sewards, J.B., & Danielson, G.K. (1989). Truncus arteriosus (pp. 504–515). In F.H. Adams, G.C. Emmanouilides, & T.A. Riemenschneider (eds.), *Heart disease in infants, children, and adolescents*. Baltimore: Williams & Wilkins.

Park, M.K. (1984). Cyanotic congenital heart defects (pp. 157–196). *Pediatric cardiology for practitioners*. Chicago: Year Book Medical Publishers.

29. Answer: (**C**) The symbolic interaction theory relates to individuals who create and construct their personal environment as they interact, shape, and adapt to their own social environment. These individual behaviors aid in constructing the meaning of roles.

REFERENCES

Berns, S.P., Geiser, R., & Levi, L.A. (1993). The changing family unit (pp. 69–79). In C. Kenner, A. Brueggemeyer, & L.P. Gunderson (eds.), *Comprehensive neonatal nursing: A physiologic perspective*. Philadelphia: W.B. Saunders.

Edwards, L.D. & Saunders, R.B. (1990). Symbolic interaction: A framework for the care of parents of preterm infants. *Journal of Pediatric Nursing, 5*(2), 123–128.

Thomas, E. & Biddle, B. (1979). Basic concepts for classifying the phenomena of role. In B. Biddle & E. Thomas (eds.), *Role theory: Concepts and research*. New York: Wiley.

30. Answer: (**B**) Role theory identifies seven problems associated with roles: (1) role ambiguity; (2) role conflict; (3) role incongruity; (4) role overload; (5) role underload; (6) role overqualification; and (7) role underqualification. Role ambiguity refers to unclear boundaries or rules about a role.

REFERENCES

Berns, S.P., Geiser, R., & Levi, L.A. (1993). The changing family unit (pp. 69–79). In C. Kenner, A. Brueggemeyer, & L.P. Gunderson (eds.), *Comprehensive neonatal nursing: A physiologic perspective*. Philadelphia: W.B. Saunders.

Hardy, M. & Conway, M.E. (1988). *Role theory: Perspectives for health professionals* (2nd ed.). Norwalk, CT: Appleton & Lange.

Thomas, E. & Biddle, B. (1979). Basic concepts for classifying the phenomena of role. In B. Biddle & E. Thomas (eds.), *Role theory: Concepts and research*. New York: Wiley.

31. Answer: (**B**) A lessening of the intense emotional reactions and increased ability to begin caring for their infant's emotional and physical needs is characteristic of adaptation. Reorganization is the final stage. Here parents come to terms with their infant's problems.

REFERENCES

Berns, S.P., Geiser, R., & Levi, L.A. (1993). The changing family unit (pp. 69–79). In C. Kenner, A. Brueggemeyer, & L.P. Gunderson (eds.), *Comprehensive neonatal nursing: A physiologic perspective*. Philadelphia: W.B. Saunders.

Drotar, D., Baskiewicz, A., Irvin, N., Kennell, J., & Klaus, M. (1975). The adaptation of parents to the birth of an infant with a congenital malformation: A hypothetical model. *Pediatrics, 56*, 710–717.

32. Answer: (**C**) Presenting this information with some optimism allows the family some hope. However, the information should be factual and, ideally, presented to both parents at the same time. Information should be simple with short explanations. The staff's pet names for the infant further reinforces parents' fears. Nursing can help the family by encouraging them to personalize the infant's care. Bringing in clothes, toys, picture of other family members, and making cassette tapes of family voices are ways parents contribute to caretaking.

REFERENCES

Berns, S.P., Geiser, R., & Levi, L.A. (1993). The changing family unit (pp. 69–79). In C. Kenner, A. Brueggemeyer, & L.P. Gunderson (eds.), *Comprehensive neonatal nursing: A physiologic perspective*. Philadelphia: W.B. Saunders.

Goldson, E. (1979). Parents' reaction to the birth of a sick infant. *Children Today, 8*(4), 13.

Hall-Johnson, S.H. (1986). *Nursing assessment and strategies for the family at risk: High-risk parenting*. Philadelphia: J.B. Lippincott Company.

33. Answer: (**C**) Caretaking is a normal part of parenting. However, parents of sick or premature infants have been deprived of time to prepare psychologically and develop their caretaking skills (Goldson, 1979). If the staff never allows the family to become involved in caretaking tasks, parents may feel inadequate or resent the nurse. Positive reinforcement builds self-confidence in parenting abilities. Assessment of readiness to participate in caretaking activities is important.

The nurse can assist parents in identifying additional means of support. Ideally, parents should be permitted to define their "family" as needed to provide support during this crisis, allowing them to visit as unit policy dictates. Grandparents, siblings, extended family, neighbors, and friends comprise this group.

REFERENCES

Berns, S.P., Geiser, R., & Levi, L.A. (1993). The changing family unit (pp. 69–79). In C. Kenner, A. Brueggemeyer, & L.P. Gunderson (eds.), *Comprehensive neonatal nursing: A physiologic perspective.* Philadelphia: W.B. Saunders.

Goldson, E. (1979). Parents' reaction to the birth of a sick infant. *Children Today, 8*(4), 13.

Hall-Johnson, S.H. (1986). *Nursing assessment and strategies for the family at risk: High-risk parenting.* Philadelphia: J.B. Lippincott Company.

34. Answer: (**B**) Adaptive—Mother becomes involved with care when encouraged and supported by staff. Maladaptive—When encouraged by staff to participate in care, mother refuses, terminates visit, or does only minimal care.

REFERENCES

Berns, S.P., Geiser, R., & Levi, L.A. (1993). The changing family unit (pp. 69–79). In C. Kenner, A. Brueggemeyer, & L.P. Gunderson (eds.), *Comprehensive neonatal nursing: A physiologic perspective.* Philadelphia: W.B. Saunders.

Goldson, E. (1979). Parents' reaction to the birth of a sick infant. *Children Today, 8*(4), 13.

Hall-Johnson, S.H. (1986). *Nursing assessment and strategies for the family at risk: High-risk parenting.* St. Louis: J.B. Lippincott Company.

35. Answer: (**C**) Adaptive—Although visits are frequent and last longer than 30 minutes, makes statements about missing infant (e.g. expresses that he or she misses infant at home or that he or she wishes he or she could visit more often and stay longer. Expresses reluctance to terminate visit. Maladaptive—Makes no statements about missing infant, or states he or she misses infant at home and wishes he or she could visit more often, but comments are not validated by frequent or lengthy visits.

REFERENCES

Berns, S.P., Geiser, R., & Levi, L.A. (1993). The changing family unit (pp. 69–79). In C. Kenner, A. Brueggemeyer, & L.P. Gunderson (eds.), *Comprehensive neonatal nursing: A physiologic perspective.* Philadelphia: W.B. Saunders.

Hall-Johnson, S.H. (1986). *Nursing assessment and strategies for the family at risk: High-risk parenting.* Philadelphia: J.B. Lippincott Company.

36. Answer: (**C**) One or more of the major signs of respiratory difficulty (cyanosis, tachypnea, grunting, retractions, and nasal flaring) are usually present in neonates with both pulmonary and nonpulmonary causes of respiratory distress. Tachypnea typically presents in patients with decreased lung compliance such as respiratory distress syndrome, whereas patients with high airway resistance (e.g. airway obstruction) usually have deep but slow breathing. Grunting, which helps maintain lung volume, is more typical of infants with decreased functional residual capacity. Chest wall retractions occur more frequently in the very premature infants because of their highly compliant chest wall.

REFERENCES

Avery, G.B. (1987). *Neonatology: Pathophysiology and management of the newborn* (3rd ed.). Philadelphia: J.B. Lippincott Company.

Haywood, J.L., Coghill III, C.H., Carlo, W.A., & Ross, M. (1993). Assessment and management of respiratory dysfunction (pp. 294–312). In C. Kenner, A. Brueggemeyer, & L.P. Gunderson (eds.), *Comprehensive neonatal nursing: A physiologic perspective.* Philadelphia: W.B. Saunders.

Ryckman, F.C. & Ballisteri, W.F. (1987). The neonatal gastrointestinal tract. In A.A. Fanaroff & R. Martin (eds.), *Neonatal-perinatal medicine: Diseases of the fetus and infant* (14th ed.). St. Louis: C.V. Mosby.

37. Answer: (**A**) Bereavement is the state of having suffered a loss. Grief is an individual's response to the loss.

REFERENCES

Bowlby, J. (1980). Loss, sadness and depression. In J. Bowlby (ed.). *Attachment and loss* (Vol. 3). New York: Basic Books.

Nichols, J.A. (1993). Bereavement: A state of having suffered a loss (pp. 84–98). In C. Kenner, A. Brueggemeyer, & L.P. Gunderson (eds.), *Comprehensive neonatal nursing: A physiologic perspective.* Philadelphia: W.B. Saunders.

Panuthos, C. & Romeo, C. (1984). *Ended beginnings.* South Hadley, MA: Bergin & Garvey.

Parkes, C.M. & Weiss, R. (1983). *Recovery from bereavement.* New York: Basic Books.

Stillion, J.M. (1986). The demise of dualism: Toward a convergence of brain research and therapy. *Death Studies, 10,* 313–329.

38. Answer: (**A**) Alpha, or a type I error, refers to the rejection of the null hypothesis when in fact it is true. Beta,

or type II error refers to accepting a false null hypothesis when in fact it is true.

REFERENCES

Brink, P.J. & Wood, M.J. (eds.). (1989). *Advanced design in nursing research.* Newbury Park, California: Sage Publications.

Franck, L.S., Gunderson, L.P., & Kenner, C. (1993). Collaborative research in neonatal nursing (pp. 52–66). In C. Kenner, A. Brueggemeyer, & L.P. Gunderson (eds.), *Comprehensive neonatal nursing: A physiologic perspective.* Philadelphia: W.B. Saunders.

39. Answer: **(C)** This thermoneutral state is one in which body temperature is maintained within a normal range with the minimization of calorie expenditure and oxygen consumption. The broad range of what constitutes normal body temperature is related more to gestational age than to birth weight because small for gestational age infants can have a better ability to self-regulate than their size indicates.

    Thermoneutrality can be difficult to achieve in the very low birth weight (VLBW) infant and the extremely low birth weight infant (ELBW) in the first few days after delivery. Despite an inability to sweat, premature infants (<37 weeks' gestational age) have high evaporative heat losses because of increased permeability of their skin. The very thin, gelatinous epidermis, typical of the gestationally immature neonate, affords little protection against losses.

REFERENCES

Brueggemeyer, A. (1993). Neonatal thermoregulation (pp. 247–262). In C. Kenner, A. Brueggemeyer, & L.P. Gunderson (eds.), *Comprehensive neonatal nursing: A physiologic perspective.* Philadelphia: W.B. Saunders.

Nalepka, C.D. (1976). Understanding thermoregulation in newborns. *Journal of Obstetrical, Gynecological and Neonatal Nursing, 5*(6), 17–19.

Sauer, P.J.J. & Visser, H.K.A. (1984). The neutral temperature of very low-birth-weight infants. *Pediatrics, 74*(2), 288–289.

40. Answer: **(A)** Grief is a natural human response to any loss, whether the loss is real, perceived, threatened, or anticipated.

REFERENCES

Benfield, D.G., Leib, S.A., & Reuter, J. (1976). Grief response of parents following referral of the critically ill newborn. *New England Journal of Medicine, 294,* 975–978.

Benfield, D.G., Leib, S.A., & Vollman, J.H. (1978). Grief response of parents to neonatal death and parent participation in deciding care. *Pediatrics, 62,* 171–177.

Nichols, J.A. (1993). Bereavement: A state of having suffered a loss (pp. 84–98). In C. Kenner, A. Brueggemeyer, & L.P. Gunderson (eds.), *Comprehensive neonatal nursing: A physiologic perspective.* Philadelphia: W.B. Saunders.

Panuthos, C. & Romeo, C. (1984). *Ended beginnings.* South Hadley, MA: Bergin & Garvey.

Parkes, C.M. (1970a). The first year of bereavement. *Psychiatry, 33,* 444–467.

Parkes, C.M. (1970b). "Seeking" and "finding" a lost object: Evidence from recent studies of the reaction to bereavement. *Social Science and Medicine, 4,* 187–201.

Parkes, C.M. & Weiss, R. (1983). *Recovery from bereavement.* New York: Basic Books.

Schneider, J. (1984). *Stress, loss, and grief.* Baltimore: University Park Press.

Rando, T.A. (1984). *Grief, dying, and death: Clinical interventions for caregivers.* Champaign, IL: Research Press.

Rando, T.A. (ed.). (1986). *Parental loss of a child.* Champaign, IL; Research Press.

Worden, J.W. (1982). *Grief counseling and grief therapy.* New York: Springer.

41. Answer: **(C)** Grief is a natural human response to any loss, whether the loss is real, perceived, threatened, or anticipated. Grief can accompany any loss not just death. Individuals can grieve when a loss is only threatened.

REFERENCES

Bowlby, J. (1980). Loss, sadness and depression. In J. Bowlby (ed.), *Attachment and loss.* (Vol. 3). New York: Basic Books.

Benfield, D.G., Leib, S.A., & Reuter, J. (1976). Grief response of parents following referral of the critically ill newborn. *New England Journal of Medicine, 294,* 975–978.

Benfield, D.G., Leib, S.A., & Vollman, J.H. (1978). Grief response of parents to neonatal death and parent participation in deciding care. *Pediatrics, 62,* 171–177.

Nichols, J.A. (1993). Bereavement: A state of having suffered a loss (pp. 84–98). In C. Kenner, A. Brueggemeyer, & L.P. Gunderson (eds.), *Comprehensive neonatal nursing: A physiologic perspective.* Philadelphia: W.B. Saunders.

Panuthos, C. & Romeo, C. (1984). *Ended beginnings.* South Hadley, MA: Bergin & Garvey.

Parkes, C.M. (1970a). The first year of bereavement. *Psychiatry, 33,* 444–467.

Parkes, C.M. (1970b). "Seeking" and "finding" a lost object: Evidence from recent studies of the reaction to bereavement. *Social Science and Medicine, 4,* 187–201.

Parkes, C.M. & Weiss, R. (1983). *Recovery from bereavement.* New York: Basic Books.

Schneider, J. (1984). *Stress, loss, and grief.* Baltimore: University Park Press.

Rando, T.A. (1984). *Grief, dying, and death: Clinical interventions for caregivers.* Champaign, IL: Research Press.

Rando, T.A. (ed.). (1986). *Parental loss of a child.* Champaign, IL; Research Press.
Worden, J.W. (1982). *Grief counseling and grief therapy.* New York: Springer.

42. Answer: (**A**) Acute grief is the initial phase of mourning. During this time, responses are likely to be intense and the sense of loss all-consuming. The self-centered nature of acute grief is such that the fact of death is at the center of the griever's reality. He or she can barely think of anything else.

REFERENCES

Bowlby, J. (1980). Loss, sadness and depression. In J. Bowlby (ed.). *Attachment and loss* (Vol. 3). New York: Basic Books.
Benfield, D.G., Leib, S.A., & Reuter, J. (1976). Grief response of parents following referral of the critically ill newborn. *New England Journal of Medicine, 294,* 975–978.
Benfield, D.G., Leib, S.A., & Vollman, J.H. (1978). Grief response of parents to neonatal death and parent participation in deciding care. *Pediatrics, 62,* 171–177.
Engel, G.L. (1961). Is grief a disease? A challenge for medical research. *Psychosomatic Medicine, 23,* 18–22.
Nichols, J.A. (1993). Bereavement: A state of having suffered a loss (pp. 84–98). In C. Kenner, A. Brueggemeyer, & L.P. Gunderson (eds.), *Comprehensive neonatal nursing: A physiologic perspective.* Philadelphia: W.B. Saunders.
Panuthos, C. & Romeo, C. (1984). *Ended beginnings.* South Hadley, MA: Bergin & Garvey.
Parkes, C.M. (1970a). The first year of bereavement. *Psychiatry, 33,* 444–467.
Parkes, C.M. (1970b). "Seeking" and "finding" a lost object: Evidence from recent studies of the reaction to bereavement. *Social Science and Medicine, 4,* 187–201.
Parkes, C.M. & Weiss, R. (1983). *Recovery from bereavement.* New York: Basic Books.
Schneider, J. (1984). *Stress, loss, and grief.* Baltimore: University Park Press.
Rando, T.A. (1984). *Grief, dying, and death: Clinical interventions for caregivers.* Champaign, IL: Research Press.
Rando, T.A. (ed.). (1986). *Parental loss of a child.* Champaign, IL; Research Press.
Worden, J.W. (1982). *Grief counseling and grief therapy.* New York: Springer.

43. Answer: (**B**) Cargivers cannot relay on the griever to unselfishly engage in a mutual relationship. Similarly, the parents cannot rely on each other during the acute phase of grief. The myth that "they have each other" tends to be true only in the very early days of bereavement, if at all. For instance, couples may be most supportive of each other immediately after the death. However, soon after the funeral, one can observe the parents grieving separately and unable to offer support to each other. Couples can benefit from being forewarned about this possibility as well as being advised on what to do about it.

REFERENCES

Bowlby, J. (1980). Loss, sadness and depression. In J. Bowlby (ed.), *Attachment and loss* (Vol. 3). New York: Basic Books.
Benfield, D.G., Leib, S.A., & Reuter, J. (1976). Grief response of parents following referral of the critically ill newborn. *New England Journal of Medicine, 294,* 975–978.
Benfield, D.G., Leib, S.A., & Vollman, J.H. (1978). Grief response of parents to neonatal death and parent participation in deciding care. *Pediatrics, 62,* 171–177.
Engel, G.L. (1961). Is grief a disease? A challenge for medical research. *Psychosomatic Medicine, 23,* 18–22.
Kushner, H.S. (1981). *When bad things happen to good people.* New York: Avon Books.
Nichols, J.A. (1993). Bereavement: A state of having suffered a loss (pp. 84–98). In C. Kenner, A. Brueggemeyer, & L.P. Gunderson (eds.), *Comprehensive neonatal nursing: A physiologic perspective.* Philadelphia: W.B. Saunders.
Panuthos, C. & Romeo, C. (1984). *Ended beginnings.* South Hadley, MA: Bergin & Garvey.
Parkes, C.M. (1970a). The first year of bereavement. *Psychiatry, 33,* 444–467.
Parkes, C.M. (1970b). "Seeking" and "finding" a lost object: Evidence from recent studies of the reaction to bereavement. *Social Science and Medicine, 4,* 187–201.
Parkes, C.M. & Weiss, R. (1983). *Recovery from bereavement.* New York: Basic Books.
Schneider, J. (1984). *Stress, loss, and grief.* Baltimore: University Park Press.
Rando, T.A. (1984). *Grief, dying, and death: Clinical interventions for caregivers.* Champaign, IL: Research Press.
Rando, T.A. (ed.). (1986). *Parental loss of a child.* Champaign, IL; Research Press.
Worden, J.W. (1982). *Grief counseling and grief therapy.* New York: Springer.

44. Answer: (**B**) The nature of acute grief also has implications for the surviving children. Parents can be so consumed by grief that their parenting skills become seriously compromised. In this manner, surviving children may temporarily experience the loss of their parents. Special arrangements may be needed—not to remove the children from their parents (for young children need the reassurance of their parents' presence) but to provide in-home child care.

REFERENCES

Katenbaum, R. (1967). The child's understanding of death: How does it develop? In E.A. Grollman (ed.). *Explaining death to children*. Boston: Beacon Press.

Koocher, G.P. (1981). Children's conceptions of death. In R. Bibace & M.E. Walsh (eds.), *Children's conceptions of health, illness, and bodily functions*. San Francisco: Jossey-Bass.

LaTour, K. (1983). *For those who live: Helping children cope with the death of a brother or sister*. Omaha, NE: Centering Corp.

Limbo, R.K. & Wheeler, S.R. (1986). *When a baby dies: A handbook for healing and helping*. LaCrosse, WI: Resolve Through Sharing.

Nichols, J.A. (1993). Bereavement: A state of having suffered a loss (pp. 84–98). In C. Kenner, A. Brueggemeyer, & L.P. Gunderson (eds.), *Comprehensive neonatal nursing: A physiologic perspective*. Philadelphia: W.B. Saunders.

45. Answer: (**A**) Grief is highly individualized. It is unique to each person and to each circumstance. Worden (1982) identified variables that combine to determine how a person might respond to a loss. These variables include the strength of attachment and degree of ambivalence in the relationship; the mode of death; and personality facts such as the sex, age, and coping skills of the survivor. Additionally, Worden cited the kinds of life crises in the survivor's past, how they were handled, and what they meant to the individual as well as a variety of social variables such as the presence of supportive persons and the uses of rituals. Rando (1984) added other determinants, including the individual's level of maturity, cultural and ethnic factors, the circumstances of the death itself, and whether or not death was expected.

REFERENCES

Bowlby, J. (1980). Loss, sadness and depression. In J. Bowlby (ed.), *Attachment and loss* (Vol. 3). New York: Basic Books.

Benfield, D.G., Leib, S.A., & Reuter, J. (1976). Grief response of parents following referral of the critically ill newborn. *New England Journal of Medicine, 294*, 975–978.

Benfield, D.G., Leib, S.A., & Vollman, J.H. (1978). Grief response of parents to neonatal death and parent participation in deciding care. *Pediatrics, 62*, 171–177.

Engel, G.L. (1961). Is grief a disease? A challenge for medical research. *Psychosomatic Medicine, 23*, 18–22.

Hutti, M.H. (1988). A quick reference table of interventions to assist families to cope with pregnancy loss or neonatal death. *Birth, 15*, 33–35.

Kushner, H.S. (1981). *When bad things happen to good people*. New York: Avon Books.

Nichols, J.A. (1993). Bereavement: A state of having suffered a loss (pp. 84–98). In C. Kenner, A. Brueggemeyer, & L.P. Gunderson (eds.), *Comprehensive neonatal nursing: A physiologic perspective*. Philadelphia: W.B. Saunders.

Panuthos, C. & Romeo, C. (1984). *Ended beginnings*. South Hadley, MA: Bergin & Garvey.

Parkes, C.M. (1970a). The first year of bereavement. *Psychiatry, 33*, 444–467.

Parkes, C.M. (1970b). "Seeking" and "finding" a lost object: Evidence from recent studies of the reaction to bereavement. *Social Science and Medicine, 4*, 187–201.

Parkes, C.M. & Weiss, R. (1983). *Recovery from bereavement*. New York: Basic Books.

Schneider, J. (1984). *Stress, loss, and grief*. Baltimore: University Park Press.

Rando, T.A. (1984). *Grief, dying, and death: Clinical interventions for caregivers*. Champaign, IL: Research Press.

Rando, T.A. (ed.). (1986). *Parental loss of a child*. Champaign, IL; Research Press.

Worden, J.W. (1982). *Grief counseling and grief therapy*. New York: Springer.

46. Answer: (**A**) Worden (1982) provides 10 principles a nurse can use to assist people with their grieving:

    1. Help the survivor actualize the loss.
    2. Help the survivor identify and express feelings.
    3. Assist adjustment to living without the deceased.
    4. Facilitate emotional withdrawal from the deceased.
    5. Provide time to grieve.
    6. Interpret "normal" behavior.
    7. Allow for individual differences.
    8. Provide continuing support.
    9. Examine defenses and coping styles.
    10. Recognize one's limitations and know when to refer.

    These principles can be translated into specific interventions such as:

    1. Encourage parents to name the infant. Know the name and use it.
    2. Speak openly and candidly about the infant.
    3. Be supportive of the need to recall memories of the pregnancy, labor, delivery, and events in the nursery, as well as fantasies and expectations revolving around the in-
fant.
    4. Create memories by providing occasions for parents to see, touch,

hold, talk to, give something to, bathe, sing to, or in other ways parent their child before or after death, even if the infant is deformed.

5. Arrange to take the infant to the mother, if she desires to see him or her and cannot come to the NICU.
6. Prepare the family for any change in the infant's appearance since their last visit.
7. Remove the tubes, if possible, and bathe the infant.
8. Dress the infant in clothing that allows parents easy exploration so they can see the infant for themselves. Wrap the infant in a fresh blanket.
9. Provide tangible mementos: a lock of hair, the hospital bracelet, footprints, pictures or videotapes (Johnson et al., 1985), birth and death certificates, a death notice, the infant's blanket.
10. Help grievers clarify the nuances of feeling.
11. Encourage funeral rituals and disposition of the body that are in keeping with family and cultural values and serve as an opportunity to gain closure.

REFERENCES

Borg, S. & Lasker, J. (1981). *When pregnancy fails.* Boston: Beacon Press.

Gardner, S.L. & Merenstein, G.B. (1986). Helping families deal with perinatal loss. *Neonatal Network, 5*(2), 17–33.

Hutti, M.H. (1988). A quick reference table of interventions to assist families to cope with pregnancy loss or neonatal death. *Birth, 15,* 33–35.

Irion, P. (1976). The funeral and the bereaved. In V.R. Pine, A., Kutscher, D. Peretz, R. Salter, R. Bellis, R. Volk, & D. Cherico (eds.), *Acute grief and the funeral.* Springfield, IL: Charles C Thomas.

Johnson, S.M., Johnson, J., Cunningham, J.H., & Weinfeld, I.J. (1985). *A most important picture.* Omaha, NE: Centering Corp.

Nichols, J.A. & Doka, K.J. (1991). No more rosebuds. In K.J. Doka (ed.), *Death and spirituality.* Amityville, NY: Baywood Publishing.

Nichols, J.A. (1993). Bereavement: A state of having suffered a loss (pp. 84–98). In C. Kenner, A. Bruegemeyer, & L.P. Gunderson (eds.), *Comprehensive neonatal nursing: A physiologic perspective.* Philadelphia: W.B. Saunders.

Worden J.W. (1982). *Grief counseling and grief therapy.* New York: Springer.

47. Answer: **(B)** Many parents have reported emotional distress when they have not been given options as to the final disposition of their infant. In particular, many mothers have expressed anger that they were excluded from planning and attending the funeral service. Funerals offer parents many psychological, social, and spiritual benefits, including reinforcement of the reality of death, opportunity for catharsis and receiving comfort, and reaffirmation of one's religious beliefs (Irion, 1976). For the bereaved family of a newborn, the funeral also can provide an opportunity to introduce their beloved infant to the rest of the family so that they, too, can acknowledge the reality of her or his existence. An infant's funeral can be a therapeutic experience for survivors (Nichols & Doka, 1991). As such, the funeral can be thought of as a worthy bereavement tool. Some caregivers, however, have been hesitant to encourage funerals for infants because of their desire to protect parents from additional expenses. Yet, it has long been the custom among funeral directors in the United States to provide infant funerals at a minimal charge.

REFERENCES

Bowlby, J. (1980). Loss, sadness and depression. In J. Bowlby (ed.), *Attachment and loss* (Vol. 3). New York: Basic Books.

Hutti, M.H. (1988). A quick reference table of interventions to assist families to cope with pregnancy loss or neonatal death. *Birth, 15,* 33–35.

Irion, P. (1976). The funeral and the bereaved. In V.R. Pine, A., Kutscher, D. Peretz, R. Salter, R. Bellis, R. Volk, & D. Cherico (eds.), *Acute grief and the funeral.* Springfield, IL: Charles C Thomas.

Johnson, S.M., Johnson, J., Cunningham, J.H., & Weinfeld, I.J. (1985). *A most important picture.* Omaha, NE: Centering Corp.

Nichols, J.A. & Doka, K.J. (1991). No more rosebuds. In K.J. Doka (ed.), *Death and spirituality.* Amityville, NY: Baywood Publishing.

Nichols, J.A. (1993). Bereavement: A state of having suffered a loss (pp. 84–98). In C. Kenner, A. Bruegemeyer, & L.P. Gunderson (eds.), *Comprehensive neonatal nursing: A physiologic perspective.* Philadelphia: W.B. Saunders.

Panuthos, C. & Romeo, C. (1984). *Ended beginnings.* South Hadley, MA: Bergin & Garvey.

Parkes, C.M. & Weiss, R. (1983). *Recovery from bereavement.* New York: Basic Books.

Stillion, J.M. (1986). The demise of dualism: Toward a convergence of brain research and therapy. *Death Studies, 10,* 313–329.

Worden J. W. (1982). *Grief counseling and grief therapy.* New York: Springer.

48. Answer: (**A**) Meiosis is the form of cell division that reduces the genetic complement of the cells by half, an actual reduction division different from the duplication division of mitosis.

REFERENCES

Cohen, F.L. (1984). *Clinical genetics in nursing practice.* Philadelphia: J.B. Lippincott.

Connor, J. & Ferguson-Smith, M. (1987). *Essential medical genetics.* Oxford: Blackwell Scientific Publications.

Cummings, M. (1988). *Human heredity: Principles and issues.* New York: West Publishing.

Thompson, S. & Thompson, M. (1986). *Genetics in medicine.* (4th ed.). Philadelphia: W.B. Saunders.

Workman, M.L., Kenner, C., & Hilse, M. (1993). Human genetics (pp. 101–131). In C. Kenner, A. Brueggemeyer, & L.P. Gunderson (eds.), *Comprehensive neonatal nursing: A physiologic perspective.* Philadelphia: W.B. Saunders.

49. Answer: (**C**) Sex-linked recessive inheritance patterns can be responsible for normal variation of some secondary female sex characteristics. In addition, this pattern of inheritance has been associated with a variety of disorders including hemophilia (A and B), Duchenne's muscular dystrophy, ichthyosis, Lesch-Nyhan syndrome, color blindness, and probably fragile X syndrome.

REFERENCES

Cohen, F.L. (1984). *Clinical genetics in nursing practice.* Philadelphia: J.B. Lippincott.

Connor, J. & Ferguson-Smith, M. (1987). *Essential medical genetics.* Oxford: Blackwell Scientific Publications.

Cummings, M. (1988). *Human heredity: Principles and issues.* New York: West Publishing.

Thompson, S. & Thompson, M. (1986). *Genetics in medicine.* (4th ed.). Philadelphia: W.B. Saunders.

Workman, M.L., Kenner, C., & Hilse, M. (1993). Human genetics (pp. 101–131). In C. Kenner, A. Brueggemeyer, & L.P. Gunderson (eds.), *Comprehensive neonatal nursing: A physiologic perspective.* Philadelphia: W.B. Saunders.

50. Answer: (B) The first change is capacitation, an enzymatic reaction that removes the glycoprotein coating from the spermatozoa and plasma proteins from the seminal fluid.

REFERENCES

Lott, J.W. (1993). Fetal development: Environmental influences and critical periods (pp. 132–156). In C. Kenner, A. Brueggemeyer, & L.P. Gunderson (eds.), *Comprehensive neonatal nursing: A physiologic perspective.* Philadelphia: W.B. Saunders.

Moore, K.L. (1989). *The developing human* (4th ed.). Philadelphia: W.B. Saunders.

Sadler, T.W. (1985). *Langman's medical embryology* (5th ed.). Baltimore: Williams & Wilkins.

51. Answer: (**A**) The placenta is mature and completely functional by 16 weeks of development. If the corpus luteum begins to regress before this 16th week and fails to produce enough progesterone (hormone responsible for readying the uterine cavity for the pregnancy), the pregnancy will be aborted because the placenta cannot solely support the pregnancy until about 16 weeks' gestation.

REFERENCES

Lott, J.W. (1993). Fetal development: Environmental influences and critical periods (pp. 132–156). In C. Kenner, A. Brueggemeyer, & L.P. Gunderson (eds.), *Comprehensive neonatal nursing: A physiologic perspective.* Philadelphia: W.B. Saunders.

Moore, K.L. (1989). *The developing human* (4th ed.). Philadelphia: W.B. Saunders.

Sadler, T.W. (1985). *Langman's medical embryology* (5th ed.). Baltimore: Williams & Wilkins.

52. Answer: (**C**) Documentation is a vital part of any quality assurance program. Throughout the entire transport process, beginning with the first phone contact made by the referral hospital until the infant has been transferred and settled into the receiving hospital, the transport team must meticulously pay attention to time. Recording the exact time that every action or communication occurs is particularly crucial when looking at outcome standards and quality assurance issues such as response times, resuscitation techniques, and problem solving.

REFERENCES

Croop, L.H. & Acree, C.M. (1993). Neonatal transport (pp. 1182–1212). In C. Kenner, A. Brueggemeyer, & L.P. Gunderson (eds.), *Comprehensive neonatal care: A physiologic perspective.* Philadelphia: W.B. Saunders.

Tharp, P. (1985). Patient care in the transport environment: Experience and problem solving (p. 164). In *Proceedings of the Sixth Annual Conference on Critical Care Transport.* San Francisco/Danville, CA: Contemporary Forums.

53. Answer: (**A**) Human chorionic gonadotropin (HCG) is the basis for pregnancy testing. Human placental lactogen (HPL), also a protein hormone produced by the placenta, acts as a fetal growth-promoting hormone by giving the fetus priority for maternal glucose.

REFERENCES

Lott, J.W. (1993). Fetal development: Environmental influences and critical periods (pp. 132–156). In C. Kenner, A. Brueggemeyer, & L.P. Gunderson (eds.), *Comprehensive neonatal nursing: A physiologic perspective*. Philadelphia: W.B. Saunders.

Moore, K.L. (1989). *The developing human* (4th ed.). Philadelphia: W.B. Saunders.

Sadler, T.W. (1985). *Langman's medical embryology* (5th ed.). Baltimore: Williams & Wilkins.

54. Answer: (**A**) Circulation of essential components to and from the fetus depends on several factors. The surface area of the placenta, specifically the integration of the villi, dictates the amounts and rate of diffusion of necessary nutrients and other biochemical components. Depending on gestation from the 20th week on, approximately 400 to 700 ml of maternal blood flow through the uterus. Approximately 80 percent of this blood flow goes into the intervillous space. There, in the "lake" surrounding the "peninsula"-like villi, maternal blood exchanges, through villous tissue, nutrients and oxygen for wastes and carbon dioxide. Nutrients are stored in the placenta and released on the fetus' need independent of blood flow or concentration.

    The umbilical cord, or life-line to the fetus, is made up of two arteries and one vein encased in Wharton's jelly. The umbilical cord delivers biochemical components to and from the fetus. Since the placenta functions as the fetal lung, the arteries carry the relatively unoxygenated blood from the fetus to the placenta, whereas the vein carries reoxygenated blood from the placenta to the fetus. The arteries are firmer walled than the vein, and thus the vein, or the more oxygenated blood flow, constricts more easily. Under healthy circumstances, all blood flow to the uterus and through the placenta is a low-pressure system through widely dilated vessels. Therefore, maternal disease and pregnancy complications that affect the mother's cardiac or vascular systems inevitably have an impact on nutrition and ultimately oxygen and carbon dioxide exchange across the placental membrane to the fetus.

REFERENCES

Creasy, R. & Resnick, M. (1989). *Maternal fetal medicine: Principles and practice*. Philadelphia: W.B. Saunders.

Gilbert, E. & Harmon, J. (1986). *High risk pregnancy and delivery*. St. Louis: C.V. Mosby.

Harmon, J.S. (1993). High-risk pregnancy (pp. 157–170). In C. Kenner, A. Brueggemeyer, & L.P. Gunderson (eds.), *Comprehensive neonatal nursing: A physiologic perspective*. Philadelphia: W.B. Saunders.

Moore, K. (1989). *The developing human* (4th ed.). Philadelphia: W.B. Saunders.

55. Answer: (**C**) The cause of placenta previa is unknown. It is frequently associated with factors that cause uterine scarring or interfere with blood supply to the endometrium. Predisposing factors are (1) abortion, (2) cesarean birth, (3) increased parity, (4) prior previa, (5) uterine infection, (6) closely spaced pregnancies, (7) uterine tumors, (8) multiple pregnancy, and (9) maternal age over 35 years.

REFERENCES

Creasy, R. & Resnick, M. (1989). *Maternal fetal medicine: Principles and practice*. Philadelphia: W.B. Saunders.

Gilbert, E. & Harmon, J. (1986). *High risk pregnancy and delivery*. St. Louis: C.V. Mosby.

Harmon, J.S. (1993). High-risk pregnancy (pp. 157–170). In C. Kenner, A. Brueggemeyer, & L.P. Gunderson (eds.), *Comprehensive neonatal nursing: A physiologic perspective*. Philadelphia: W.B. Saunders.

Moore, K. (1989). *The developing human* (4th ed.). Philadelphia: W.B. Saunders.

56. Answer: (**C**) There is no defined national standard by which to determine the difference between level II and level III care. In some states, individual hospitals classify their level of care; in others, the state sets the perinatal designation (OTA, 1987).

REFERENCES

American Academy of Pediatrics. (1991). *Guidelines for perinatal care* (3rd ed.). Washington, DC: American Academy of Pediatrics and American College of Obstetricians and Gynecologists.

U.S. Congress, Office of Technology Assessment. (1987). *Neonatal intensive care for low birthweight infants: Costs and effectiveness* (OTA-HCS-38). Washington, DC: U.S. Government Printing Office.

Wolfe, L.S. (1993). Regionalization of care (pp. 171–181). In C. Kenner, A. Brueggemeyer, & L.P. Gunderson (eds.), *Comprehensive neonatal care: A physiologic perspective*. Philadelphia: W.B. Saunders.

57. Answer: (**C**) Studies support an improvement in mortality when high-risk mothers are transferred to perina-

tal centers before delivery. There is minimal difference between the survival rates of infants born after antenatal transport and those deliveries schedule at the referral center.

REFERENCES

Jones, D.B. & Modica, M.M. (1989). Assessment strategies for the outreach educator. *The Journal of Perinatal & Neonatal Nursing, 2*(3), 1–9.

National Perinatal Information Center, Inc. (1988). *The Perinatal partnership: An approach to organizing care in the 1990s.* (Project No. 12129). Providence, RI: Cooke, Schwartz, & Gagoron.

Ryan, G.M. (1975). Toward improving the outcome of pregnancy. Recommendations for the regional development of perinatal health services. *Journal of Obstetrics and Gynecology, 46*(4), 375–384.

U.S. Congress, Office of Technology Assessment. (1987). *Neonatal intensive care for low birthweight infants: Costs and effectiveness* (OTA-HCS-38). Washington, DC: U.S. Government Printing Office.

Wolfe, L.S. (1993). Regionalization of care (pp. 171–181). In C. Kenner, A. Brueggemeyer, & L.P. Gunderson (eds.), *Comprehensive neonatal care: A physiologic perspective.* Philadelphia: W.B. Saunders.

58. Answer: (**B**) In general, transport teams typically use ground transport if traveling within a 100-mile radius. Little time is saved by flying within this range because of the arrangements that must be made for loading, unloading, and ground transport from the landing site to the hospital. Helicopter transport have been found to be most advantageous when used for transports between 100 and 250 miles. Because helicopters can typically land in close proximity to the hospital, time is not lost on ground transport at each end of the flight. Any transport greater than 250 miles usually requires the use of some type of fixed-wing aircraft.

REFERENCES

Croop, L.H. & Acree, C.M. (1993). Neonatal transport (pp. 1182–1212). In C. Kenner, A. Brueggemeyer, & L.P. Gunderson (eds.), *Comprehensive neonatal care: A physiologic perspective.* Philadelphia: W.B. Saunders.

Weinger, W. (1987). Setting standards for critical care transport. Fitz-Gibbons' law revisited. *International Anethesiology Clinics, 25*(2), 139–159.

59. Answer: (**B**) A reverse transport (back-transport, back-transfer) is the return of a previously ill neonate from a level III newborn intensive care unit to another level I, II, or III nursery for intermediate or convalescing care or both.

REFERENCES

Croop, L.H. & Acree, C.M. (1993). Neonatal transport (pp. 1182–1212). In C. Kenner, A. Brueggemeyer, & L.P. Gunderson (eds.), *Comprehensive neonatal care: A physiologic perspective.* Philadelphia: W.B. Saunders.

Croop, L. & Kenner, C. (1990). Protocol for reverse neonatal transports. *Neonatal Network, 9*(1), 49–53.

60. Answer: (**C**) The ductus arteriosus normally closes in response to increased arterial oxygen saturation after the onset of pulmonary oxygenation. In preterm neonates, the muscle is less responsive to arterial saturation and closure may be incomplete or intermittent. As the newborn recovers from respiratory distress, decreased pulmonary vascular resistance causes blood to shunt from left to right and re-enter the pulmonary circulation. The increased flow of blood into the pulmonary circulation causes increased pulmonary venous congestion, which decreases lung compliance.

REFERENCES

Avery, G. B. (1987). *Neonatology: Pathophysiology and management of the newborn.* Philadelphia: J.B. Lippincott.

Heymann, M.A. (1989). Fetal and neonatal circulations (pp. 24–35). In F.H. Adams, G.C. Emmanouilides, & T.A. Riemenschneider (eds.), *Heart disease in infants, children, and adolescents.* Baltimore: Williams & Wilkins.

Heymann, M.A. (1989). Patent ductus arteriosus (pp. 209–223). In F.H. Adams, G.C. Emmanouilides, & T.A. Riemenschneider (eds.), *Heart disease in infants, children, and adolescents.* Baltimore, MD.: Williams & Wilkins.

Lott, J.W. (1993). Assessment and management of cardiovascular dysfunction (pp. 355–391). In C. Kenner, A. Brueggemeyer, & L.P. Gunderson (eds.), *Comprehensive neonatal nursing: A physiologic perspective.* Philadelphia: W.B. Saunders.

Park, M.K. (1984). Left-to-right shunts (pp. 125–144). *Pediatric cardiology for practitioners.* Chicago: Year Book Medical Publishers.

61. Answer (**B**) The syncytiotrophoblast forms the primitive uteroplacental circulation through erosion of the maternal blood vessels of the decidua, resulting in the formation of the intervillous space. The intervillous space allows for transfer of oxygen and nutrients from the maternal circulation. The development of the fetal cardiovascular system begins during the third week of gestation in the wall of the yolk sac. Primitive fetal blood is formed in the walls of yolk sac begin-

ning during the third week. Blood vessels from the yolk sac connect with those in the connecting stalk and chorion to form the primitive cardiovascular system. As the development progresses, the blood travels throughout the entire fetus in a unique pattern.

REFERENCES

Creasy, R.K. & Resnik, R. (1989). *Maternal-fetal medicine: Principles and practice* (2nd ed.). Philadelphia: W.B. Saunders.

Weitkamp, T.L. & Felblinger, D.M. (1993). Effects of labor on the fetus and neonate (pp. 215–230). In C. Kenner, A. Brueggemeyer, & L.P. Gunderson (eds.), *Comprehensive neonatal nursing: A physiologic perspective*. Philadelphia: W.B. Saunders.

62. Answer: (**A**) Baseline fetal heart rate (FHR) is defined as the fetal heart rate between contractions for at least a 10-minute time period. This does not include periodic changes. Most fetuses have a baseline FHR of 120 to 160 beats per minute (bpm) at term.

REFERENCES

Creasy, R.K. & Resnik, R. (1989). *Maternal-fetal medicine: Principles and practice* (2nd ed.). Philadelphia: W.B. Saunders.

Weitkamp, T.L. & Felblinger, D.M. (1993). Effects of labor on the fetus and neonate (pp. 215–230). In C. Kenner, A. Brueggemeyer, & L.P. Gunderson (eds.), *Comprehensive neonatal nursing: A physiologic perspective*. Philadelphia: W.B. Saunders.

63. Answer: (**C**) Variability is a result of interaction between the sympathetic and parasympathetic nervous system. For variability to be present, there must be an unimpaired autonomic nervous system, medulla oblongata, and heart. Average and moderate variability are considered indications of a nonacidotic fetus. Periodic changes are changes that occur in the baseline fetal heart rate during a contraction or as a result of a contraction. The two types of periodic changes are accelerations and decelerations. Accelerations are a result of the β-adrenergic sympathetic nervous system and indicate an intact nervous system. Accelerations of the fetal heart occur with stimulation of the sympathetic nervous system. Accelerations are a sign of fetal wellness. Often, accelerations require no intervention because they are seen as a reassuring sign. However, repetitive accelerations during uterine contractions may be the earliest evidence of a partial cord compression and result as an initial response to mild hypoxia.

Early decelerations occur as a result of pressure, usually on the fetal head, that stimulates the vagus nerve resulting in a decrease in fetal heart rate with recovery occurring once the pressure is removed. When visualizing these, they appear to be mirror images of the contraction pattern. Treatment of early decelerations begins with the identification of the pattern and observation of the fetal status.

REFERENCES

Creasy, R.K. & Resnik, R. (1989). *Maternal-fetal medicine: Principles and practice* (2nd ed.). Philadelphia: W.B. Saunders.

May, K.A. & Mahlmeister, L.R. (1990). *Comprehensive maternity nursing: Nursing process and the childbearing family* (3rd ed.). Philadelphia: J.B. Lippincott.

Murray, M. (1988). Essentials of electronic fetal monitoring: Antepartal and intrapartal fetal monitoring. Washington DC: NAACOG.

Weitkamp, T.L. & Felblinger, D.M. (1993). Effects of labor on the fetus and neonate (pp. 215–230). In C. Kenner, A. Brueggemeyer, & L.P. Gunderson (eds.), *Comprehensive neonatal nursing: A physiologic perspective*. Philadelphia: W.B. Saunders.

64. Answer: (**A**) Late decelerations are a result of uteroplacental insufficiency. Uteroplacental insufficiency occurs when gas exchange is restricted anywhere between the uterus, placenta, and fetus resulting in fetal hypoxia.

Although late decelerations indicate a decrease in placental perfusion, the presence of short-term variability, long-term variability, spontaneous accelerations, and a baseline FHT between 120 to 160 bpm are reassuring signs.

REFERENCES

May, K.A. & Mahlmeister, L.R. (1990). *Comprehensive maternity nursing: Nursing process and the childbearing family* (3rd ed.). Philadelphia: J.B. Lippincott.

Tournaire, M., Sturbois, G., Zorn, J., Breart, G., & Sureau, C. (1980). Clinical monitoring before and during labor (pp. 331–361). In S. Adajern, A.K. Brown, & C. Sureau (eds.), *Clinical perinatology*. St. Louis: C.V. Mosby.

Weitkamp, T.L. & Felblinger, D.M. (1993). Effects of labor on the fetus and neonate (pp. 215–230). In C. Kenner, A. Brueggemeyer, & L.P. Gunderson (eds.), *Comprehensive neonatal nursing: A physiologic perspective*. Philadelphia: W.B. Saunders.

65. Answer: (**C**) Treatment of late decelerations does not include decreasing IV fluids to correct maternal hypotension. Treatment of late decelerations involves increasing the uterine blood flow and gas exchange. Methods to accomplish this depend on etiology and current maternal status, correcting maternal hypotension (increasing IV fluids), decreasing uterine stimulation (stopping or decreasing oxytocic medication or the administration of tocolytic agents), administration of five or more liters of 100 percent oxygen by tight face mask. Variable decelerations are usually a result of umbilical cord compression and result in patterns of FHR decrease that differ is size, duration, and shape from contraction to contraction.

REFERENCES

Knapp, R.M. & Knapp, C.M.W. (1986). Obstetric anesthesia (pp. 283–302). In D.J. Angelini, C.M.W. Knapp, & R. Gibes (eds.), *Perinatal/neonatal nursing: A clinical handbook*. Boston: Blackwell Scientific Publication.

Pedersen, H. (1990) Analgesia and anesthesia during pregnancy and labor (pp. 425–431). In K. Buckley & N. Kulb (eds.), *High risk maternity nursing manual*. Baltimore: Williams & Wilkins.

Weitkamp, T.L. & Felblinger, D.M. (1993). Effects of labor on the fetus and neonate (pp. 215–230). In C. Kenner, A. Brueggemeyer, & L.P. Gunderson (eds.), *Comprehensive neonatal nursing: A physiologic perspective*. Philadelphia: W.B. Saunders.

66. Answer: (**C**) Overshoots of fetal heart rate can be caused by decreased chemoreceptor stimulation. Overshoots are smooth accelerations after a variable deceleration lasting 20 to 30 seconds. The overshoots are thought to be a result of catecholamine release by the fetal adrenal glands. Treatment of variable decelerations involves changing the maternal position to try to relieve the pressure on the umbilical cord. One hundred percent oxygen at a flow rate of five liters or more is administered by a tight face mask if the pattern continues or becomes more severe.

REFERENCES

May, K.A. & Mahlmeister, L.R. (1990). *Comprehensive maternity nursing: Nursing process and the childbearing family* (3rd ed.). Philadelphia: J.B. Lippincott.

Tournaire, M., Sturbois, G., Zorn, J., Breart, G., & Sureau, C. (1980). Clinical monitoring before and during labor (pp. 331–361). In S. Adajern, A.K. Brown, & C. Sureau (eds.), *Clinical perinatology*. St. Louis: C.V. Mosby.

Weitkamp, T.L. & Felblinger, D.M. (1993). Effects of labor on the fetus and neonate (pp. 215–230). In C. Kenner, A. Brueggemeyer, & L.P. Gunderson (eds.), *Comprehensive neonatal nursing: A physiologic perspective*. Philadelphia: W.B. Saunders.

67. Answer: (**A**) The primary goal is immediate restoration of the blood volume and the oxygen-carrying capacity. Decreased maternal perfusion of the placenta includes factors such as hypotension, hypertension, abruptio placentae, and hypotonic contractions.

Maternal *blood loss* or obstetric hemorrhage has been documented as one of the leading causes of maternal mortality. Conditions that can manifest themselves in relation to obstetric hemorrhage include cesarean section, obstetric lacerations, uterine atony, retained placenta, uterine inversion, and the more rare placenta accreta.

The primary goal is the immediate restoration of the blood volume and the oxygen-carrying capacity. The second goal is to be aware of the specific nursing care needs of the patient that are related to the condition causing the hemorrhage. Stabilization of the patient is of paramount importance (Creasy & Resnik, 1989). Without the stabilization of the mother, the effects of blood loss on the fetus have the potential to be ominous. Uteroplacental insufficiency can result in the inability of the fetus to exhibit a physiological response compatible with life-sustaining outcomes. The fetal response to acute blood loss is similar to the maternal reaction. Hypoxemia and acidosis result in bradycardia, vasospasm, and the initial shunting of blood to vital organs. As the maternal condition progresses and these compensatory mechanisms are no longer adequate, brain damage and fetal demise can occur (May & Mahlmeister, 1990). Medications known to have hypotensive effects include ritodrine, magnesium sulfate (has a depressant effect on myometrial contractility), and narcotic substances.

REFERENCES

Creasy, R.K. & Resnik, R. (1989). *Maternal-fetal medicine: Principles and practice* (2nd ed.). Philadelphia: W.B. Saunders.

Pedersen, H. (1990). Analgesia and anesthesia during pregnancy and labor (pp. 425–431). In K. Buckley & N. Kulb (eds.), *High risk maternity nursing manual.* Baltimore: Williams & Wilkins.
Robertson, W.B., Brosen, I., & Dixon, H.G. (1967). The pathological response of the vessels of the placental bed to hypertensive pregnancy. *Journal of Pathology and Bacteriology, 93,* 581.
May, K.A. & Mahlmeister, L.R. (1990). *Comprehensive maternity nursing: Nursing process and the childbearing family* (3rd ed.). Philadelphia: J.B. Lippincott.
Weitkamp, T.L. & Felblinger, D.M. (1993). Effects of labor on the fetus and neonate (pp. 215–230). In C. Kenner, A. Brueggemeyer, & L.P. Gunderson (eds.), *Comprehensive neonatal nursing: A physiologic perspective.* Philadelphia: W.B. Saunders.

68. Answer: (**B**) To treat the patient with pregnancy-induced hypertension (PIH), the nurse must first be aware of the classic triad of symptoms associated with the physiologic changes that accompany PIH. These symptoms include hypertension that is defined as blood pressure of 140/90 or an increase in systolic pressure of 30 mm Hg over baseline nonpregnant levels, or an increase in diastolic pressure of 15 mm Hg above baseline nonpregnant levels; sudden weight gain of greater than two pounds per week accompanied by fluid retention and increasing generalized edema; and proteinuria, 0.5 g/liter in a 24-hour period or a dipstick reading of +1 or +2. Proteinuria is usually the last symptom to occur.

REFERENCES

Creasy, R.K. & Resnik, R. (1989). *Maternal-fetal medicine: Principles and practice* (2nd ed.). Philadelphia: W.B. Saunders.
Cunningham, F.G., MacDonald, P.C., & Gant, N.F. (1989). *Williams obstetrics* (18th ed.). Norwalk, Connecticut: Appleton & Lange.
Lin, C.C., Lindheimer, M.D., River, P., & Moawad, A.H. (1982). Fetal outcome in hypertensive disorders of pregnancy. *American Journal of Obstetrics and Gynecology, 142,* 255.
May, K.A. & Mahlmeister, L.R. (1990). *Comprehensive maternity nursing: Nursing process and the childbearing family* (3rd ed.). Philadelphia: J.B. Lippincott.
Weitkamp, T.L. & Felblinger, D.M. (1993). Effects of labor on the fetus and neonate (pp. 215–230). In C. Kenner, A. Brueggemeyer, & L.P. Gunderson (eds.), *Comprehensive neonatal nursing: A physiologic perspective.* Philadelphia: W.B. Saunders.

69. Answer: (**A**) To keep oxygen consumption to a minimum during rewarming, the incubator should be adjusted to 1 to 1.5 degrees higher than the infant's temperature. Hourly, the incubator temperature may be adjusted upwardly by one degree until infant temperature has been stabilized.

REFERENCES

Dodman, N. (1987). Newborn temperature control. *Neonatal Network, 5*(6), 19–23.
Brueggemeyer, A. (1990). Thermoregulation (pp. 23–38). In L.P. Gunderson & C. Kenner (eds.), *Care of the 24–25 week gestational age infant: Small baby protocol.* Petaluma, CA: Neonatal Network.
Brueggemeyer, A. (1993). Neonatal thermoregulation (pp. 247–262). In C. Kenner, A. Brueggemeyer, & L.P. Gunderson (eds.), *Comprehensive neonatal nursing: A physiologic perspective.* Philadelphia: W.B. Saunders.

70. Answer: (**B**) Oxygen causes the pulmonary arterioles to dilate, whereas the same increase in blood oxygen content causes the ductus arteriosus to close. Circulating and tissue prostaglandin E_2 maintain the ductus vasodilatation in utero. The increase in Po_2 initially affects the ductus by constricting it. Prostaglandin E_2 levels and other vasoactive mediator substances such as serotonin and bradykinin drop with the loss of the placenta (Eden & Boehm, 1990). There is an increase in pulmonary metabolism and degradation of PGE_2 with the increase in pulmonary blood flow. Lower PGE_2 levels and the effects of the other biochemical changes occurring within the cardiopulmonary system allow the ductus to further constrict in response to rising Po_2.

REFERENCES

Eden, R.D. & Boehm, F.H. (1990). *Assessment and care of the fetus.* Norwalk, CT: Appleton & Lange.
London, M.L. (1993). Resuscitation and stabilization of the neonate (pp. 231–246). In C. Kenner, A. Brueggemeyer, & L.P. Gunderson (eds.). *Comprehensive neonatal nursing: A physiologic perspective.* Philadelphia: W.B. Saunders.

71. Answer: (**C**) *Primary apnea* lasts almost 60 seconds. A series of spontaneous deep gasps develop for four to five minutes that then become weaker and stop after about eight minutes of total anoxia. Primary apnea is accompanied by an increase in blood pressure and a decrease in heart rate. The infant is deeply cyanotic but usually well perfused and responds to stimulation with the initiation of respiration. *Secondary apnea* or terminal apnea begins after the last gasp and will result in death if the asphyxia is

not reversed within several minutes. Secondary apnea resists induction of spontaneous respiration by any sensory stimuli and will require assisted ventilation to establish respirations. It is nearly impossible to differentiate whether the newborn is in primary or secondary apnea initially. It is critical to remember that asphyxia can first occur in utero as a result of fetal hypoxia, and the newborn already may have gone through primary apnea and progressed into secondary apnea at the time of birth.

REFERENCES

Banagale, R.C. & Donn, S.M. (1986). Asphyxia neonatorium. *The Journal of Family Practice. 22*(6), 539–545.

London, M.L. (1993). Resuscitation and stabilization of the neonate (pp. 231–246). In C. Kenner, A. Brueggemeyer, & L.P. Gunderson (eds.), *Comprehensive neonatal nursing: A physiologic perspective.* Philadelphia: W.B. Saunders.

Woods, J. (1983). Birth asphyxia: Pathophysiologic events and fetal adaptive changes. *Clinics in Perinatology, 10*(2), 473.

72. Answer: (**B**) A one second assessment of gestational age should be carried out. Remember Apgar scores are in part related to the newborn's level of maturity. Therefore, low Apgar scores can relate more to developmental immaturity rather than fetal distress. The order of importance is pulse, respiratory effort, tone (activity), reflex irritability (grimace), and color. Apgars of three or less at one minute, or five or less at five minutes will require resuscitation and usually reflect severe hypoxic insult and acidosis (Lamb & Rosner, 1987).

REFERENCES

Bloom, R.S. & Cropley, C., & Peckham, G.J. (1983). Principles of neonatal resuscitation (pp. 1–24). *In* R.A. Polin & F.D. Berg (eds.), *Workbook in practical neonatology*. Philadelphia: W.B. Saunders.

Edwards, M.C. (1988). Delivery room resuscitation of the neonate. *Pediatric Annals, 17*(7), 458–464, 466.

Lamb, F.S. & Rosner, M.S. (1987). Neonatal resuscitation. *Emergency Medicine Clinics of North America, 5*(3), 541–557.

London, M.L. (1993). Resuscitation and stabilization of the neonate (pp. 231–246). In C. Kenner, A. Brueggemeyer, & L.P. Gunderson (eds.), *Comprehensive neonatal nursing: A physiologic perspective.* Philadelphia: W.B. Saunders.

Talner, N.S., Lister, G., & Fahey, J.T. (1992). Effects of asphyxia on the myocardium of the fetus and newborn (pp. 759–769). In R.A. Polin & W.W. Fox (eds.), *Fetal and neonatal physiology.* Philadelphia: W.B. Saunders.

73. Answer: (**B**) Cyanosis, early onset respiratory distress, and the scaphoid abdomen are the *classic triad* of symptoms with diaphragmatic hernia. DO NOT attempt to bag and mask ventilate this infant. Intubation is required.

REFERENCES

London, M.L. (1993). Resuscitation and stabilization of the neonate (pp. 231–246). In C. Kenner, A. Brueggemeyer, & L.P. Gunderson (eds.), *Comprehensive neonatal nursing: A physiologic perspective.* Philadelphia: W.B. Saunders.

Ringer, S.A. & Stark, A.R. (1989). Management of neonatal emergencies in the delivery room. *Clinics in Perinatology, 16*(1), 23–42.

74. Answer: (**B**) Infants who have previously been stressed have a depleted reserve of brown fat stores. Premature, small for gestational age and growth retarded neonates have insufficient brown fat stores. They are less able to produce sufficient heat for thermal self-regulation. The last trimester is the period of highest transfer of nutrients across the placenta to the fetus for energy use. The infant born before this time has fewer nutrient stores to produce heat. During the course of a normal delivery, the wet infant can lose as much as 200 calories of heat for every one kilogram of body weight during each minute that the heat loss is allowed to continue. Thus, one of the most important points of neonatal stabilization in the delivery room is rapid drying to decrease the chance of iatrogenic hypothermia.

REFERENCES

Brueggemeyer, A. (1993). Neonatal thermoregulation (pp. 247–262). In C. Kenner, A. Brueggemeyer, & L.P. Gunderson (eds.), *Comprehensive neonatal nursing: A physiologic perspective.* Philadelphia: W.B. Saunders.

Nalepka, C.D. (1976). Understanding thermoregulation in newborns. *Journal of Obstetrical, Gynecological and Neonatal Nursing, 5*(6), 17–19.

Ringer, S.A. & Stark, A.R. (1990). Management of neonatal emergencies in the delivery room. *Clinics in Perinatology, 16*(1), 23–41.

75. Answer: (**A**) The infant can display subtle signs of distress. Heart rate may rise. Tachypnea can present in an infant with temperature instability. In the cold-stressed infant, tachypnea results from an increased need for oxygen due to an increase in metabolism. The heat-stressed infant becomes

tachypneic to increase expiratory heat losses. In the short-term response, the infant can exhibit changes in behavior and response. Long-term responses include poor growth patterns and behavioral changes.

The infant responds to thermal stress and energy demands by hyperventilation. The healthy infant who is cold stressed can double or triple the consumption of oxygen.

The infant can exhibit behavioral signs that indicate poor temperature control. These signs can be subtle at first, but as the infant's temperature continues to change, the signs can become more recognizable.

Body positioning is one of the first signs that the infant is attempting to respond to internal or environmental temperature changes. The term infant is able to assume a flexed body position to generate and retain body heat. The premature infant has a very limited ability to assume a flexed position and can be incapable of changing position.

Skin changes can occur in infants when thermoregulation has been disturbed. In the infant who is cool, skin color can range from pale to cyanotic. Mottling also can occur as peripheral response to cooling attempts to retain core body temperature. The overheated infant can become slightly plethoric. Although the sweating mechanism is poorly developed in the infant, diaphoresis can occur.

REFERENCES

Brueggemeyer, A. (1993). Neonatal thermoregulation (pp. 247–262). In C. Kenner, A. Brueggemeyer, & L.P. Gunderson (eds.), *Comprehensive neonatal nursing: A physiologic perspective*. Philadelphia: W.B. Saunders.

James, L.S. (1973). Acid-base changes in the perinatal period (pp. 185–206). In R.W. Winters (ed.), *The Body Fluids in Pediatrics*. Boston: Little, Brown & Co.

Marks, K.H., Gunther, R.C., Rossi, J.A., & Maisels, M.J. (1980). Oxygen consumption and insensible water loss in premature infants under radiant heaters. *Pediatrics, 66*(2), 228–232.

LeBlanc, M.H. (1982). Relative efficacy of an incubator and an open warmer in producing thermoneutrality for the small premature infant. *Pediatrics, 69*(4), 439–445.

76. Answer: (**A**) Symptoms of ASD occur when pulmonary vascular resistance begins to fall and right ventricular end-diastolic and right atrial pressures fall. In ASD, blood shunts from left to right across the defect because the right ventricle offers less resistance to filling because it is more compliant than the left ventricle. (Answer C describes the hemodynamics of pulmonary atresia with VSD.)

REFERENCES

Feldt, R.H., Porter, C.J., Edwards, W.D., Puga, F.J., & Seward, J.B. (1989). Defects of the atrial septum and the atrioventricular canal (pp. 170–188). In F.H. Adams, G.C. Emmanouilides, & T.A. Riemenschneider (eds.), *Heart disease in infants, children, and adolescents*. Baltimore: Williams & Wilkins.

Hazinski, M.F. (1983). Congenital heart disease in the neonate (Part III): Congestive heart failure. *Neonatal Network, 1*(6), 8–17.

Hazinski, M.F. (1984). Cardiovascular disorders (pp. 63–252). *Nursing care of the critically ill child*. St. Louis: C.V. Mosby.

Lott, J.W. (1993). Assessment and management of cardiovascular dysfunction (pp. 355–391). In C. Kenner, A. Brueggemeyer, & L.P. Gunderson (eds.), *Comprehensive neonatal nursing: A physiologic perspective*. Philadelphia: W.B. Saunders.

Mair, D.D., Edwards, W.D., Julsrud, P.R., Hagler, D.J., & Puga, F.J. (1989). Pulmonary atresia and ventricular septal defects (pp. 289–301). In F.H. Adams, G.C. Emmanouilides, & T.A. Riemenschneider (eds.), *Heart disease in infants, children, and adolescents*. Baltimore: Williams & Wilkins.

Mair, D.D., Edwards, W.D., Julsrud, P.R., Sewards, J.B., & Danielson, G. K. (1989). Truncus arteriosus (pp. 504–515). In F.H. Adams, G.C. Emmanouilides, & T.A. Riemenschneider (eds.), *Heart disease in infants, children, and adolescents*. Baltimore: Williams & Wilkins.

77. Answer: (**C**) Term healthy babies (AGA), when clothed and fed, are able to produce heat to self-thermoregulate. In the presence of a cold environment, these infants are able to increase basal heat production by two to three times the normal rate within one or two days of birth.

LGA can be expected to be able to generate sufficient heat to maintain self-thermoregulation. In reality, these infants can lack sufficient brown fat stores and also may be poor feeders and lack sufficient oral intake to generate heat.

The infant, however, can be limited in its ability to thermally self-regulate. The presence of hypoxia or hypoglycemia can prevent the infant from generating sufficient heat through metabolism.

Oral feedings have shown an increase in neonatal heat production that is not present when protein hydrolysate is administered parenterally. It is not clear as to why heat is produced with oral feedings but it may be due to increased metabolism during digestion or heat gain that can be generated when sufficient energy is provided via ingestion.

REFERENCES

Brueggemeyer, A. (1993). Neonatal thermoregulation (pp. 247–262). In C. Kenner, A. Brueggemeyer, & L.P. Gunderson (eds.), *Comprehensive neonatal nursing: A physiologic perspective.* Philadelphia: W.B. Saunders.

Laburn, D.M. & Laburn, H.P. (1985). Pathophysiology of temperature regulation. *The Physiologist, 28*(6), 507–517.

Mestyán, J. (1978). Energy metabolism and substrate utilization in the newborn (pp. 39–74). In J. Sinclair (ed.), *Temperature regulation and energy metabolism in the newborn.* New York : Grune & Stratton.

78. Answer: (**B**) There are three major assessments in the neonatal period: in the delivery room, on admission to the nursery, and a complete physical assessment before discharge. The assessment at birth is primarily a physical assessment with the objective of evaluating adaptation to extrauterine life. Apgar score values from 7 to 10 reflect a generally vigorous infant with little need for resuscitation. Scores that remain low on a repeat scoring at 10–15 minutes after birth can be predictive of a poor outcome. The second major assessment is performed in the nursery, generally 1 to 4 hours after birth. For the well neonate, this consists of a short physical exam to confirm a stable condition, and a gestational assessment.

REFERENCES

Apgar, V. (1953). A proposal for a new method of evaluation of the newborn infant. *Current Researches in Anesthesia and Analgesia, 32,* 260–267.

Endo, A.S. & Nishioka, E. (1993). Neonatal assessment (pp. 265–293). In C. Kenner, A. Brueggemeyer, & L.P. Gunderson (eds.), *Comprehensive neonatal nursing: A physiologic perspective.* Philadelphia: W.B. Saunders.

Fanaroff, A.A., Martin, R.J., & Miller, M.J. (1989). Identification and management of high risk problems in the neonate (pp. 1150–1193). In R. Creasy & R. Resnick (eds.), *Maternal-fetal medicine: Principles and practice* (2nd ed.). Philadelphia: W.B. Saunders.

Olds, S.B., London, M.L., & Ladewig, P.A. (1988). *Maternal-newborn nursing: A family centered approach* (3rd ed.). Menlo Park: Addison-Wesley.

79. Answer: (**C**) It is accepted that 38 weeks is the dividing line for preterm/term births. Graphs of the distribution of birth weights at given gestational age (LGA; weight >90th percentile) or small for gestational age (SGA; weight <10th percentile)

REFERENCES

Battaglia, F.C., & Lubchenco, L.O. (1967). A practical classification of newborn infants by weight and gestational age. *Journal of Pediatrics, 71*(2), 159–163.

Endo, A.S. & Nishioka, E. (1993). Neonatal assessment (pp. 265–293). In C. Kenner, A. Brueggemeyer, & L.P. Gunderson (eds.), *Comprehensive neonatal nursing: A physiologic perspective.* Philadelphia: W.B. Saunders.

80. Answer: (**C**) Acrocyanosis (blue hands and feet) is common and generally insignificant in the transition period immediately after birth and reflects poor peripheral perfusion. It is also seen with cold stress. Color is best interpreted in the context of the overall clinical assessment.

REFERENCES

Battaglia, F.C., & Lubchenco, L.O. (1967). A practical classification of newborn infants by weight and gestational age. *Journal of Pediatrics, 71*(2), 159–163.

Endo, A.S. & Nishioka, E. (1993). Neonatal assessment (pp. 265–293). In C. Kenner, A. Brueggemeyer, & L.P. Gunderson (eds.), *Comprehensive neonatal nursing: A physiologic perspective.* Philadelphia: W.B. Saunders.

Petrucha, R. (1989). Fetal maturity/gestational age evaluation. *Journal of Perinatology, 9*(1), 100–101.

81. Answer: (**B**) Periodic respiration (intermittent cessation of respiration for up to 10 seconds) is a normal finding, especially among premature infants. Apneic episodes, on the other hand, are of longer duration, >15 seconds, and are accompanied by duskiness or cyanosis. Diagnosis of pathological conditions such as atelectasis, effusion, and pneumothorax are made based on diminished or congested breath sounds or radiographic studies. Rhonchi and rales often can be heard together. The PMI is usually found at the fourth or fifth intercostal space.

REFERENCES

Battaglia, F.C., & Lubchenco, L.O. (1967). A practical classification of newborn infants by weight and gestational age. *Journal of Pediatrics, 71*(2), 159–163.

Endo, A.S. & Nishioka, E. (1993). Neonatal assessment (pp. 265–293). In C. Kenner, A. Brueggemeyer, & L.P. Gunderson (eds.), *Comprehensive neonatal nursing: A physiologic perspective.* Philadelphia: W.B. Saunders.

Petrucha, R. (1989). Fetal maturity/gestational age evaluation. *Journal of Perinatology, 9*(1), 100–101.

82. Answer: (**B**) Nurses and other health professionals should be able to interpret the data obtained from the pulse oximeter, transcutaneous carbon dioxide monitor, and hemodynamic monitor. HFV neonates may require arterial waveform tracings to monitor their heart rate because the ventilator's vibrations can interfere with the ECG tracings. Saline can be used with suctioning because of the tendency of HFV to be less humidified than conventional mechanical ventilation, but no research found mandated this technique with HFV.

REFERENCES

Carlo, W.A. & Chatburn, R.L. (1988). *Neonatal respiratory care*. Chicago: Year Book Medical Publishers, Inc.

Donovan, E.F. & Spangler, L.L. (1993). New technologies applied to the management of respiratory dysfunction. In C. Kenner, A. Brueggemeyer, & L.P. Gunderson (eds.), *Comprehensive neonatal nursing: A physiologic perspective*. Philadelphia: W.B. Saunders.

Gordin, P. (1989). High-frequency jet ventilation for severe respiratory failure. *Pediatric Nursing, 15*(6), 625–629.

HIFI Study Group. (1989). High-frequency oscillatory ventilation compared with conventional mechanical ventilation in the treatment of respiratory failure in preterm infants. *New England Journal of Medicine, 320*(2), 88–93.

Roberts, P.M. & Jones, M.B. (1990). Extracorporeal membrane oxygenation and indications for cardiopulmonary bypass in the neonate. *JOGNN, 19*(6), 391–399.

Wetzel, R.C. & Gioia, F.R. (1987). Extracorporeal membrane oxygenation: Its use in neonatal respiratory failure. *AORN Journal, 45*(3), 725–739.

83. Answer: (**C**) Asymmetrical limbs are associated with maternal diabetes, drug use, and congenital syndromes.

REFERENCES

Battaglia, F.C., & Lubchenco, L.O. (1967). A practical classification of newborn infants by weight and gestational age. *Journal of Pediatrics, 71*(2), 159–163.

Endo, A.S. & Nishioka, E. (1993). Neonatal assessment (pp. 265–293). In C. Kenner, A. Brueggemeyer, & L.P. Gunderson (eds.), *Comprehensive neonatal nursing: A physiologic perspective*. Philadelphia: W.B. Saunders.

Petrucha, R. (1989). Fetal maturity/gestational age evaluation. *Journal of Perinatology, 9*(1), 100–101.

84. Answer: (**B**) There should be full range of joint motion in all extremities. Birth trauma resulting in damage to the firth or sixth cervical nerves results in a paralysis of the upper portion of the arm called Erb-Duchenne paralysis.

REFERENCES

Battaglia, F.C., & Lubchenco, L.O. (1967). A practical classification of newborn infants by weight and gestational age. *Journal of Pediatrics, 71*(2), 159–163.

Endo, A.S. & Nishioka, E. (1993). Neonatal assessment (pp. 265–293). In C. Kenner, A. Brueggemeyer, & L.P. Gunderson (eds.), *Comprehensive neonatal nursing: A physiologic perspective*. Philadelphia: W.B. Saunders.

Petrucha, R. (1989). Fetal maturity/gestational age evaluation. *Journal of Perinatology, 9*(1), 100–101.

85. Answer: (**C**) A pneumothorax is preceded by rupture of the alveoli with interstitial air traveling via fascial planes to the mediastinum, where it breaks through the mediastinal pleura to form collections of air outside the lung. Pneumonthoraxes are usually caused by one or more of the following:

1. High pressure gradients from mechanical ventilation or continuous positive airway pressure across poorly compliant alveoli.
2. Obstructive pulmonary pathology such as ball-valve air trapping associated with meconium aspiration syndrome.
3. Rupture of subpleural blebs from IIE or BPD.

Occasionally a pneumothorax is benign and asymptomatic. More serious leaks needing treatment are usually larger, occur in neonates with preexisting serious lung disease, are under tension, and compress the heart and lungs compromising their function. Serious pneumothoraxes are accompanied by acute, profound respiratory and cardiac decompensation and often require cardiopulmonary resuscitation with evacuation of the air by needle aspiration and chest tube placement.

A pneumopericardium is a rare complication of mechanical ventilation caused by lung overdistention with high peak inspiratory and positive end-expiratory pressures.

REFERENCES

Southwell, S.M. (1993). Complications of respiratory management (pp. 337–354). In C. Kenner, A. Brueggemeyer, & L.P. Gunderson (eds.), *Comprehensive neonatal nursing: A physiologic perspective*. Philadelphia: W.B. Saunders.

Thiebeault, D.W. (1986). Pulmonary barotrauma: Interstitial emphysema, pneumomediastinum, and pneumothorax (pp. 499–517). In D.W. Thibeault & G.A. Gregory (eds.), *Neonatal pulmonary care* (2nd ed.). Norwalk, CT: Appleton-Century-Crofts.

86. Answer: (**C**) Ortolani's maneuver is performed by placing the fingers on both trocanters while the thumbs grip the medial aspects of the femur. Both legs are flexed and abducted to nearly touch the examining table. If dislocation is present, a click may be felt or heard, as the femoral head is reduced into the acetabulum. Conversely, Barlow's maneuver tests for ready dislocation of the femoral head from the acetabulum. With the examiner's hands placed as above, the infant's legs are adducted and pressed down gently. Dislocation, if present, will be palpable. Both Ortolani's and Barlow's tests should be performed to confirm pressure or absence of abnormality.

REFERENCES

Battaglia, F.C., & Lubchenco, L.O. (1967). A practical classification of newborn infants by weight and gestational age. *Journal of Pediatrics, 71*(2), 159–163.

Endo, A.S. & Nishioka, E. (1993). Neonatal assessment (pp. 265–293). In C. Kenner, A. Brueggemeyer, & L.P. Gunderson (eds.), *Comprehensive neonatal nursing: A physiologic perspective.* Philadelphia: W.B. Saunders.

Petrucha, R. (1989). Fetal maturity/gestational age evaluation. *Journal of Perinatology, 9*(1), 100–101.

87. Answer: (**C**) The respiratory system is composed of: (1) pumping systems (the chest wall muscles, diaphragm, accessory muscles of respiration) that move fresh gas into the lungs; (2) the bony rib cage that provides structural support for the respiratory muscles and limits lung deflation; (3) the conducting airways that connect gas-exchanging units with the outside but offer resistance to gas flow; (4) the elastic element of the system that offers some resistance to gas flow but provides pumping force for moving stale air out of the system; (5) air-liquid interfaces that generate surface tension opposing lung expansion on inspiration but supporting lung deflation on expiration; and finally (6) abdominal muscles that aid exhalation by active contraction.

Forces that oppose lung expansion are elastic and resistive forces of the thorax, lungs, abdomen, and airways. Elastic recoil is the natural tendency of the stretched objects to return to their resting state—the stretched chest wall musculature, diaphragm, airways, and lungs. Surface tension at the air-liquid interface in the alveoli acts to decrease the surface area of the interface, favoring collapse of the airway. Opposing these forces is the elastic recoil of the chest wall in the opposite direction and the surface tension-reducing properties of the surfactant film coating normal alveoli. The point where these opposing forces balance at end expiration is the functional residual capacity (FRC). The newborn has a relatively low FRC because his or her comparatively floppy chest wall offers little resistance to collapse, even when there is a normal amount of functional surfactant present.

REFERENCES

Harris, T.R. (1988). Physiologic principles. In J.P. Goldsmith & E.H. Karotkin (eds.), *Assisted ventilation of the neonate* (2nd ed.). Philadelphia: W.B. Saunders.

Haywood, J.L., Coghill III, C.H., Carlo, W.A., & Ross, M. (1993). Assessment and management of respiratory dysfunction (pp. 294–312). In C. Kenner, A. Brueggemeyer, & L.P. Gunderson (eds.), *Comprehensive neonatal nursing: A physiologic perspective.* Philadelphia: W.B. Saunders.

88. Answer: (**A**) Flexing the knees at the hips allows the abdominal muscles to relax. The liver margin is palpated inferior to the right costal margin, and the spleen tip frequently can be felt at the left costal margin. Both kidneys can be palpated as well as the descending colon in the left lower quadrant.

REFERENCES

Battaglia, F.C., & Lubchenco, L.O. (1967). A practical classification of newborn infants by weight and gestational age. *Journal of Pediatrics, 71*(2), 159–163.

Endo, A.S. & Nishioka, E. (1993). Neonatal assessment (pp. 265–293). In C. Kenner, A. Brueggemeyer, & L.P. Gunderson (eds.), *Comprehensive neonatal nursing: A physiologic perspective.* Philadelphia: W.B. Saunders.

Petrucha, R. (1989). Fetal maturity/gestational age evaluation. *Journal of Perinatology, 9*(1), 100–101.

89. Answer: (**B**) The generally accepted normal range of $Paco_2$ is 35 to 45 torr. If $Paco_2$ rises as in hypoventilation, the pH falls and the patient suffers from respiratory acidosis. The patient with a chronic respiratory acidosis may retain bicarbonate, inducing in himself or herself a compensatory metabolic alkalosis. A patient who is hyperventilated with subnormal

Pa_{CO_2} has a respiratory alkalosis. Depressed bicarbonate ion concentration (below approximately 20 mM/L in plasma) is called metabolic acidosis, and can be associated with any cause for anaerobic metabolism, such as poor cardiac output from patent ductus arteriosus or shock from bacterial sepsis. Extremely immature infants can develop metabolic acidosis due to renal bicarbonate wasting.

When presented with an abnormal pH, the clinician rapidly determines whether acidosis or alkalosis exists. An examination of the Pa_{CO_2} and HCO_3^- will determine whether the process is respiratory, metabolic, or mixed. One then tries to determine which derangement came first. For example, an acidotic, acutely ill hypoxemic infant with a high Pa_{CO_2} and depressed HCO_3^- is usually hypoventilating and suffering metabolic acidosis secondary to anerobic metabolism.

With the advent and widespread use of transcutaneous monitoring of Pa_{O_2} and Pa_{CO_2} since the late 1970s, neonatal care has changed dramatically. Continuous monitoring has led to an appreciation of the liability of tissue oxygenation, particularly in ventilatory-dependent patients or those with chronic lung disease. Transcutaneous monitoring also allows for management of less ill neonates without invasive catheters.

REFERENCES

Haywood, J.L., Coghill III, C.H., Carlo, W.A., & Ross, M. (1993). Assessment and management of respiratory dysfunction (pp. 294–312). In C. Kenner, A. Brueggemeyer, & L.P. Gunderson (eds.), *Comprehensive neonatal nursing: A physiologic perspective.* Philadelphia: W.B. Saunders.

Long, L.G., Phillip, A.G.S., & Lucey, J.F. (1980). Excessive handling as a cause of hypoxemia. *Pediatrics, 65,* 203.

90. Answer: (**B**) Many air leak syndromes begin with at least some degree of pulmonary interstitial emphysema (PIE). PIE is the result of alveolar rupture from overdistention, usually concomitant with mechanical ventilation or continuous distending airway pressure. It occurs most commonly in preterm infants but can be seen infants of any gestational age. Lung compliance is nonuniform because there are areas of poor aeration and alveolar collapse. Interspersed are alveoli of normal or near-normal compliance that become overdistended. The more normal lung units (those with better compliance) become overdistended and eventually rupture. Air is forced from the alveolus into the loose tissue of the interstitial space and dissects toward the hilum of the lung, where it may track into the mediastinum and cause a pneumomediastinum, or into pericardium and cause a pneumopericardium.

The astute nurse may notice an infant's chest becoming barrel-shaped with overdistention and notes breath sounds become distant on the affected side. Typically, the infant who suffers a pneumothorax will become unstable, developing cyanosis, oxygen desaturation, and carbon dioxide retention. The infant can become hypotensive and bradycardic as high intrathoracic pressure impedes cardiac output. A tension pneumothorax, in which free pleural air compresses the lung, is a medical emergency, and prompt relief by thoracentesis or tube thoracostomy is indicated.

Transient tachypnea of the newborn occurs typically in infants born by cesarean section, particularly in the absence of labor. The etiology of the disorder is thought to be a transient pulmonary edema, which makes sense when we know that the infant has "missed" the chance during labor to absorb pulmonary alveolar fluid. Pneumonias can be of bacterial, viral, or other infectious etiologies. Pneumonias may be transmitted transplacentally, as has been shown with Group B streptococcus, or via an ascending bacterial invasion associated with maternal amnionitis and prolonged rupture of the fetal membranes.

There is a strong association of bacterial pneumonias with premature birth, which may be due to a developmental deficiency of bacteriostatic factors in the amniotic fluid or the infection as a precipitating factor in preterm labor.

REFERENCES

Avery, M.E., Gatewood, O.B., & Brumley, G. (1966). Transient tachypnea of the newborn: Possible de-

layed resorption of fluid at birth. *American Journal of Diseases in Children, 111,* 380.
Haywood, J.L., Coghill III, C.H., Carlo, W.A., & Ross, M. (1993). Assessment and management of respiratory dysfunction (pp. 294–312). In C. Kenner, A. Brueggemeyer, & L.P. Gunderson (eds.), *Comprehensive neonatal nursing: A physiologic perspective.* Philadelphia: W.B. Saunders.
Naeye, R.L. & Peters, E.C. (1978). Amniotic fluid infections with intact membranes leading to perinatal death: A prospective study. *Pediatrics, 61,* 171.

91. Answer: (**A**) As soon as the diagnosis is suspected, bag and mask ventilation should be avoided as this fills the hernia contents with air and can compress the lungs and worsen ventilation. An orogastric tube should be placed to aid in decompression of the herniated abdominal viscera. The trachea should be intubated promptly and mechanical ventilation begun. Ventilation should be attempted with rapid rate and low inflation pressure. Dopamine infusion should be given.

REFERENCES

Cassani, V.L. (1984). Hypoxemia secondary to suctioning in the neonate. *Neonatal Network, 2,* 8–16.
Hall, B.D. (1979). Choanal atresia and associated multiple anomalies. *Journal of Pediatrics, 95,* 395–398.
Haywood, J.L., Coghill III, C.H., Carlo, W.A., & Ross, M. (1993). Assessment and management of respiratory dysfunction (pp. 294–312). In C. Kenner, A. Brueggemeyer, & L.P. Gunderson (eds.), *Comprehensive neonatal nursing: A physiologic perspective.* Philadelphia: W.B. Saunders.

92. Answer: (**B**) Calcium is the most abundant mineral in the human body. It is an essential component of the skeleton and plays an important role in muscle contraction, neural transmission, and blood coagulation. Phosphorus is essential for bone mineralization, erythrocyte function, cell metabolism, and the generation and storage of energy.

REFERENCES

Costarino, A. & Baumgart, S. (1986). Modern fluid and electrolyte management of the critically ill premature infant. *Pediatric Clinics of North America, 33,* 153–158.
DeMarini, S., Tsang, R.C., & Rath, L.L. (1993). Fluids, electrolytes, vitamins, and trace minerals: Basis of ingestion, digestion, elimination, and metabolism (pp. 393–413). In C. Kenner, A. Brueggemeyer, & L.P. Gunderson (eds.), *Comprehensive neonatal nursing: A physiologic perspective.* Philadelphia: W.B. Saunders.
Tsang, R.C., Chen, I., Hayes, W., Atkinson, W., Atherton, H., & Edwards, N. (1974). Neonatal hypocalcemia in infants with birth asphyxia. *Journal of Pediatrics, 84,* 428–433.
Tsang, R.C. & Oh, W. (1970). Neonatal hypocalcemia in low birthweight infants. *Pediatrics, 45,* 773–781.

93. Answer: (**A**) A third strategy used to reduce the risk of cell injury secondary to tissue hypoxia is to minimize oxygen demand by minimizing the newborn's metabolic rate. Depending on the specific thermal environment, the neonatal energy (and oxygen) expenditure necessary to keep warm can be very great or quite small.

REFERENCES

Carlo, W.A. & Chatburn, R.L. (1988). *Neonatal respiratory care.* Chicago: Year Book Medical Publishers, Inc.
Donovan, E.F. & Spangler, L.L. (1993). New technologies applied to the management of respiratory dysfunction. In C. Kenner, A. Brueggemeyer, & L.P. Gunderson (eds.), *Comprehensive neonatal nursing: A physiologic perspective.* Philadelphia: W.B. Saunders.
Merenstein, G.B. & Gardner, S.L. (1989). *Handbook of neonatal intensive care.* St. Louis: C.V. Mosby.

94. Answer: (**A**) The National Perinatal Information Center's study (1988) recommended the formation of a "perinatal partnership" to replace the regionalization concept outlined by the Committee on Perinatal Health. In the perinatal partnership, hospitals would identify the patient groups for whom they are able to provide services. In the original regional concept, hospital characteristics were defined and patients were directed to an appropriate facility. With perinatal partnership, there is an opportunity for more than one tertiary center to serve the needs of the region. Hospitals would not be restricted to the type of services offered but would have to maintain a determined patient volume and a standard quality of care.

REFERENCES

Burkett, M.E. (1989). The tertiary center and health department in cooperation: The Duke University experience. *The Journal of Perinatal & Neonatal Nursing, 2*(3), 11–13.
National Perinatal Information Center, Inc. (1988). *The Perinatal partnership: An approach to organizing care in the 1990s.* (Project No. 12129). Providence, RI: Cooke, Schwartz, & Gagoron.
Wolfe, L.S. (1993). Regionalization of care (pp. 171–181). In C. Kenner, A. Brueggemeyer, & L.P. Gunderson (eds.), *Comprehensive neonatal care: A physiologic perspective.* Philadelphia: W.B. Saunders.

95. Answer: (**A**) An essential component of nursing care with these infants is to

suction the infant approximately 15 minutes before dosing. This suctioning is important to help prevent endotracheal tube plugging, because suctioning is delayed as long as possible after surfactant dosing. Most drug companies suggest at least 4–6 hours should be left between dose and suctioning. The nurse is to assist with positioning of infants during surfactant instillation. Infants receive some surfactant such as Survanta in four aliquots, each in a different body position. During dosing, the infant is held in each position 30 seconds after doing, while the bed is maintained at a 45-degree angle. When repositioning, the nurses and physicians should be careful not to jar the infant or move the infant quickly because this will increase intracranial pressure. Infants should be reconnected to the ventilator immediately after receiving each aliquot of surfactant. If the infant becomes dusky or bradycardic, surfactant administration should be stopped to allow the infant to recover. Containment (providing barriers such as rolls so infant is given boundaries) should be used to calm the infant and prevent agitation.

REFERENCES

Carlo, W.A. & Chatburn, R.L. (1988). *Neonatal respiratory care.* Chicago: Year Book Medical Publishers, Inc.

Donovan, E.F. & Spangler, L.L. (1993). New technologies applied to the management of respiratory dysfunction. In C. Kenner, A. Brueggemeyer, & L.P. Gunderson (eds.), *Comprehensive neonatal nursing: A physiologic perspective.* Philadelphia: W.B. Saunders.

Horbar, J.D., Soll, RF., Sutherland, J.M., et al. (1989). A multicenter randomized, placebo-controlled trial of surfactant therapy for respiratory distress syndrome. *The New England Journal of Medicine, 320*(15), 959–965.

Miller, E.D. & Armstrong, C.L. (1990). Surfactant replacement therapy: Innovative care for the premature infant. *JOGNN, 19*(1), 14–17.

96. Answer: (**B**) It is generally accepted that HFV has been useful in the management of newborns with severe pulmonary interstitial emphysema (PIE). The primary benefit of HFV in the management of PIE is that airway pressures can be significantly reduced, thus, theoretically decreasing the risk of further air leak and other pressure related airway injury and decreased cardiac output. These experiences suggest that HFV is helpful in the management of newborns with meconium aspiration syndrome, congenital diaphragmatic hernia, and neonatal pulmonary hypertension without primary lung disease. High frequency positive pressure ventilation (HFPPV) can be called conventional ventilation with increased frequencies of 60–150 breaths per minute. In HFPPV, the tidal volume is greater than anatomic dead space but is less than conventional ventilation, and is delivered with very short inspiratory times. HFPPV comes from the Sjostrand technique and employs passive expiration.

High-frequency flow interruption ventilation (HFFI) delivers tidal volumes that can be less than or greater than anatomic dead space, at frequencies of 300 to 900 breaths per minute. This is sometimes classified as a type of high-frequency oscillatory ventilation.

REFERENCES

Boros, S.J., Mammel, M.C., Coleman, J.M., et. al. (1985). Neonatal high-frequency jet ventilation: Four years' experience. *Pediatrics, 75,* 657–663.

Carlo, W.A. & Chatburn, R.L. (1988). *Neonatal respiratory care.* Chicago: Year Book Medical Publishers, Inc.

Donovan, E.F. & Spangler, L.L. (1993). New technologies applied to the management of respiratory dysfunction. In C. Kenner, A. Brueggemeyer, & L.P. Gunderson (eds.), *Comprehensive neonatal nursing: A physiologic perspective.* Philadelphia: W.B. Saunders.

Gordin, P. (1989). High-frequency jet ventilation for severe respiratory failure. *Pediatric Nursing, 15*(6), 625–629.

HIFI Study Group. (1989). High-frequency oscillatory ventilation compared with conventional mechanical ventilation in the treatment of respiratory failure in preterm infants. *New England Journal of Medicine, 320*(2), 88–93.

Nugent, J. (1991). *Acute respiratory care of the neonate.* Petaluma, CA: NICU, INK.

97. Answer: (**B**) The stretching of the atria by increased volume triggers the release of ANF, which causes elimination of sodium and water and causes dilation of veins, to allow for greater volume as a compensatory mechanism. The role of ANF is being studied. ANF release is not related to arterial desaturation or pulmonary edema.

REFERENCES

Lees, M.H. & King, D.H. (1989). Heart disease in the newborn (pp. 842–855). In F.H. Adams, G.C. Emmanouilides, & T.A. Riemenschneider (eds.), *Heart disease in infants, children, and adolescents*. Baltimore: Williams & Wilkins.

Lott, J.W. (1993). Assessment and management of cardiovascular dysfunction (pp. 355–391). In C. Kenner, A. Brueggemeyer, & L.P. Gunderson (eds.), *Comprehensive neonatal nursing: A physiologic perspective*. Philadelphia: W.B. Saunders.

Talner, N.S. (1989). Heart failure (pp. 890–911). In F.H. Adams, G.C. Emmanouilides, & T.A. Riemenschneider (eds.), *Heart disease in infants, children, and adolescents*. Baltimore: Williams & Wilkins.

98. Answer: (**A**) Thiamin is a necessary coenzyme in carbohydrate and amino acid metabolism.

REFERENCES

DeMarini, S., Tsang, R.C., & Rath, L.L. (1993). Fluids, electrolytes, vitamins, and trace minerals: Basis of ingestion, digestion, elimination, and metabolism (pp. 393–413). In C. Kenner, A. Brueggemeyer, & L.P. Gunderson (eds.), *Comprehensive neonatal nursing: A physiologic perspective*. Philadelphia: W.B. Saunders.

Moran, J.R. & Greene, H.L. (1979). The B vitamins and vitamin C in human nutrition. I. General considerations and "obligatory" B vitamins. *American Journal of Diseases of Childhood, 133*, 192–199.

Schanler, R.J. (1988). Water-soluble vitamins: C, B_1, B_2, B_6, niacin, biotin, and pantothenic acid (pp. 236–252). In R.C. Tsang & B.L. Nichols (eds.), *Nutrition during infancy*. St. Louis: C.V. Mosby.

99. Answer: (**B**) Barotrauma, the damage done to lung structures (primarily small airways and alveoli) by mechanical stress, has been implicated as a major contributor to the incidence of BPD. Barotrauma occurs when lung volume exceeds physiologic limits, especially when tissue structures are "stiff" or noncompliant. Overdistention of the airways and alveoli in the premature infant is most often caused by the large and frequently oscillating pressure differences associated with mechanical ventilation. Premature infants are especially susceptible to barotrauma because not only are they likely to need assisted ventilation but also their lungs are noncompliant because of increased surface tension from surfactant deficiency and increased interstitial fluid. Mechanical stresses occur in all planes of the alveolar wall, but the strain is especially significant at the junction of the alveolus and the related bronchioles where large excursions in diameter occur during ventilation. Tissue breakdown, epithelial necrosis, and alveolar rupture occur as a consequence of these large, unbalanced stresses.

REFERENCES

Bonikos, D.S. & Bensch, K.G. (1988). Pathogenesis of bronchopulmonary dysplasia (pp. 33–58). In T.A. Merritt, W.H. Northway, Jr., & B.R. Boynton (eds.), *Bronchopulmonary dysplasia*. Boston: Blackwell Scientific.

Boynton, B.R. (1988). Epidemiology of BPD (pp. 19–32). In T. A Merritt, W.H. Northway, Jr., & B.R. Boynton (eds.), *Bronchopulmonary dysplasia*. Boston: Blackwell Scientific.

Monin, P. & Vert, P. (1987). The management of bronchopulmonary dysplasia. *Clinics in Perinatology, 14*, 531–549.

Obladen, M. (1988). Alterations in surfactant composition (pp. 131–142). In T.A. Merritt, W.H. Northway, Jr., & B.R. Boynton (eds.), *Bronchopulmonary dysplasia*. Boston: Blackwell Scientific.

Southwell, S.M. (1993). Complications of respiratory management (pp. 337–354). In C. Kenner, A. Brueggemeyer, & L.P. Gunderson (eds.), *Comprehensive neonatal nursing: A physiologic perspective*. Philadelphia: W.B. Saunders.

Wispé, J.R. & Roberts, R.J. (1987). Molecular basis of pulmonary oxygen toxicity. *Clinics in Perinatology, 14*, 61–666.

100. Answer: (**B**) A promising experimental therapy is the use of antioxidant therapy to neutralize and clear free oxygen radicals. Both prematures and infants with BPD have immature or poorly functioning antiproteolytic enzymes. In a double-blind study, infants experimentally treated with superoxide dismutase (SOD) had decreased radiologic and clinical signs of BPD and required fewer days on continuous positive airway pressure (CPAP) than control infants but had no difference in survival or amount of oxygen or mechanical ventilation needed. The activity of natural protease inhibitors also can be increased in SOD-treated infants, another protection from tissue damage in the cycle of BPD. Further studies are needed to establish whether SOD therapy is safe and efficacious in the newborn.

REFERENCES

Rosenfeld, W. & Concepcion, L. (1988). Pharmacologic intervention: Use of the antioxidant superoxide dismutase (pp. 365–374). In T.A. Merritt, W.H. Northway, Jr., & B.R. Boynton (eds.), *Bronchopulmonary dysplasia*. Boston: Blackwell Scientific.

Rosenfeld, W., Evans, H., Concepcion, L., Jhaveri, R.,

Schaeffer, H., & Friedman, A. (1984). Prevention of bronchopulmonary dysplasia by administration of bovine superoxide dismutase in preterm infants with respiration distress syndrome. *The Journal of Pediatrics, 105,* 781–785.

Southwell, S.M. (1993). Complications of respiratory management (pp. 337–354). In C. Kenner, A. Brueggemeyer, & L.P. Gunderson (eds.), *Comprehensive neonatal nursing: A physiologic perspective.* Philadelphia: W.B. Saunders.

101. Answer: (**A**) Recommended dosage of theophylline is 5 mg/kg IV for loading dose, and maintenance dose is 2 mg/kg IV every 12 hours (first dose is given 12 hours after loading dose).

REFERENCES

Roberts, R.J. (1984). Methylxanthine therapy: Caffeine and theophylline (pp. 226–249). In R.J. Roberts. *Drug therapy in infants.* Philadelphia: W.B. Saunders.

Southwell, S.M. (1993). Complications of respiratory management (pp. 337–354). In C. Kenner, A. Brueggemeyer, & L.P. Gunderson (eds.), *Comprehensive neonatal nursing: A physiologic perspective.* Philadelphia: W.B. Saunders.

102. Answer: (**B**) The placenta is mature and completely functional by 16 weeks of development. If the corpus luteum begins to regress before this 16th week and fails to produce enough progesterone (hormone responsible for readying the uterine cavity for pregnancy), the pregnancy will be aborted because the placenta cannot solely support the pregnancy until about 16 weeks' gestation.

REFERENCES

Lott, J.W. (1993). Fetal development: Environmental influences and critical periods (pp. 132–156). In C. Kenner, A. Brueggemyer, & L.P. Gunderson (eds.), *Comprehensive neonatal nursing: A physiologic perspective.* Philadelphia: W.B. Saunders.

Moore, K.L. (1989). *The developing human* (4th ed.). Philadelphia: W.B. Saunders.

Sadler, T.W. (1985). *Langman's medical embryology* (5th ed.). Baltimore: Williams & Wilkins.

103. Answer: (**C**) The foramen ovale allows well-oxygenated blood from the right atrium to enter the left atrium, through the left ventricle, and then to the head and neck. The ductus arteriosus allows the majority of fetal blood to bypass the fetal pulmonary circulation. The ductus venosus permits the majority of blood from the placenta to bypass the liver and enter the inferior vena cava.

REFERENCES

Hazinski, M.F. (1984). Cardiovascular disorders (pp. 63–252). *Nursing care of the critically ill child.* St. Louis: C.V. Mosby.

Lott, J.W. (1993). Assessment and management of cardiovascular dysfunction (pp. 355–391). In C. Kenner, A. Brueggemeyer, & L.P. Gunderson (eds.), *Comprehensive neonatal nursing: A physiologic perspective.* Philadelphia: W.B. Saunders.

Moller, J.H. (1987). *Congenital heart anomalies. Clinical education aid.* Columbus OH: Ross Laboratories.

Sacksteder, S. (1978). Embryology and fetal circulation. *American Journal of Nursing,* (Feb), 262–265.

104. Answer: (**A**) An infusion of glucose and insulin at a ratio of 4 g of glucose to 1 unit of insulin (to increase cellular uptake of potassium) is given to decrease the serum potassium level.

REFERENCES

Arieff, A. & Guisado, R. (1976). Effects on the central nervous system of hypernatremic and hyponatremic states. *Kidney International, 10,* 104–116.

Bell, E.F., Warburton, D., Stonestreet, B.S., & Oh, W. (1980). Effect of fluid administration on the development of symptomatic patent ductus arteriosus and congestive heart failure in premature infants. *New England Journal of Medicine, 302,* 598–604.

Costarino, A. & Baumgart, S. (1986). Modern fluid and electrolyte management of the critically ill premature infant. *Pediatric Clinics of North America, 33,* 153–158.

DeMarini, S., Tsang, R.C., & Rath, L.L. (1993). Fluids, electrolytes, vitamins, and trace minerals: Basis of ingestion, digestion, elimination, and metabolism (pp. 393–413). In C. Kenner, A. Brueggemeyer, & L.P. Gunderson (eds.), *Comprehensive neonatal nursing: A physiologic perspective.* Philadelphia: W.B. Saunders.

Gruskay, J.A., Costarino, A.T., Polin, R.A., & Baumgart, S. (1988). Non-oliguric hyperkalemia in the premature infant less than 1000 grams. *Journal of Pediatrics, 113,* 381–386.

105. Answer: (**A**) Hypoxemia can cause a constricted ductus to reopen and may reestablish increased pulmonary vascular resistance leading to persistent pulmonary hypertension of the newborn (PPHN). The ductus arteriosus responds to hypoxemia by opening; the pulmonary arterioles respond by constriction.

REFERENCES

Heymann, M.A. (1989). Patent ductus arteriosus (pp. 209-223). In F.H. Adams, G.C. Emmanouilides, & T.A. Riemenschneider (eds.), *Heart disease in infants, children, and adolescents.* Baltimore: Williams & Wilkins.

Huhta, J.C. (1990). Patent ductus arteriosus in the preterm neonate (pp. 389–400). In W.A. Long (ed.). *Fetal and neonatal cardiology.* Philadelphia: W.B. Saunders.

Lott, J.W. (1993). Assessment and management of cardiovascular dysfunction (pp. 355–391). In C. Kenner, A. Brueggemeyer, & L.P. Gunderson (eds.), *Comprehensive neonatal nursing: A physiologic perspective*. Philadelphia: W.B. Saunders.
Sacksteder, S. (1978). Embryology and fetal circulation. *American Journal of Nursing*, (Feb), 262–265.

106. Answer: (**B**) The increased water content in the brain causes the symptoms and signs of hyponatremia. Vomiting, lethargy, and apnea can occur with various degrees of hyponatremia, but seizures and coma usually do not occur unless serum sodium concentration is less than 115 mEq/L (<115 mmol/L).

REFERENCES

Arieff, A., & Guisado, R. (1976). Effects on the central nervous system of hypernatremic and hyponatremic states. *Kidney International, 10,* 104–116.
Bell, E.F., Warburton, D., Stonestreet, B.S., & Oh, W. (1980). Effect of fluid administration on the development of symptomatic patent ductus arteriosus and congestive heart failure in premature infants. *New England Journal of Medicine, 302,* 598–604.
DeMarini, S., Tsang, R.C., & Rath, L.L. (1993). Fluids, electrolytes, vitamins, and trace minerals: Basis of ingestion, digestion, elimination, and metabolism (pp. 393–413). In C. Kenner, A. Brueggemeyer, & L.P. Gunderson (eds.), *Comprehensive neonatal nursing: A physiologic perspective*. Philadelphia: W.B. Saunders.

107. Answer: (**B**) For the general population 1 percent is the risk. The incidence is higher if the mother had a congenital heart defect.

REFERENCES

Hazinski, M.F. (1983). Congenital heart disease in the neonate (Part III): Congestive heart failure. *Neonatal Network, 1*(6), 8–17.
Hazinski, M.F. (1984). Cardiovascular disorders (pp. 63–252). *Nursing care of the critically ill child*. St. Louis: C.V. Mosby.
Heymann, M.A. (1989). Fetal and neonatal circulations (pp. 24–35). In F.H. Adams, G.C. Emmanouilides, & T.A. Riemenschneider (eds.), *Heart disease in infants, children, and adolescents*. Baltimore: Williams & Wilkins.
Heymann, M.A. (1989). Patent ductus arteriosus (pp. 209–223). In F.H. Adams, G.C. Emmanouilides, & T.A. Riemenschneider (eds.), *Heart disease in infants, children, and adolescents*. Baltimore: Williams & Wilkins.
Lott, J.W. (1993). Assessment and management of cardiovascular dysfunction (pp. 355–391). In C. Kenner, A. Brueggemeyer, & L.P. Gunderson (eds.), *Comprehensive neonatal nursing: A physiologic perspective*. Philadelphia: W.B. Saunders.
Neill, C.A. (1990). Genetics and recurrence risks of congenital heart disease (pp. 125–133). In W.A. Long (ed.), *Fetal and neonatal cardiology*. Philadelphia: W.B. Saunders.

108. Answer: (**B**) In persistent truncus arteriosus, a single large vessel arises from the ventricles and gives rise to the systemic, pulmonary, and coronary circulations. Symptoms include bounding arterial pulses and a widened pulse pressure. In ASD, blood is shunted from left to right, which increases right ventricular volume, but does not cause bounding pulses associated with aortic runoff. Tetralogy of Fallot consists of a large VSD, pulmonic stenosis, over-riding aorta, and hypertrophied right ventricle. Hemodynamic symptoms do not include bounding pulses.

REFERENCES

Avery, G.B. (1987). *Neonatology: Pathophysiology and management of the newborn*. Philadelphia: J.B. Lippincott.
Lott, J.W. (1993). Assessment and management of cardiovascular dysfunction (pp. 355–391). In C. Kenner, A. Brueggemeyer, & L.P. Gunderson (eds.), *Comprehensive neonatal nursing: A physiologic perspective*. Philadelphia: W.B. Saunders.
Park, M.K. (1984). Pathophysiology of cyanotic congenital heart defects (pp. 108–123). *Pediatric cardiology for practitioners*. Chicago: Year Book Medical Publishers.

109. Answer: (**B**) Communication and documentation are the linchpins of professional practice. Nurses' notes should reflect the nurse's discussion with the physician and other nurses and the subsequent treatment decisions and nursing interventions.

REFERENCES

American Academy of Pediatrics/American College of Obstetrician and Gynecologists. (1992). *Guidelines for perinatal care*. Elk Grove Village, IL: Author.
American Nurses' Association. (1984). *Code for nurse with interpretive statements*. Kansas City, MO: Author.
Driscoll, K.M. (1993). Legal aspects of perinatal care (pp. 36–51). In C. Kenner, A. Brueggemeyer, & L.P. Gunderson (eds.), *Comprehensive neonatal nursing: A physiologic perspective*. Philadelphia: W.B. Saunders.
Pegalis, S.E. & Wachsman, H.F. (1990). *American law of medical malpractice*. (Cum. Suppl.). Rochester, NY: Lawyers Co-Operative Publishing.

110. Answer: (**B**) Only VSD, mitral valve regurgitation, and tricuspid regurgitation create a systolic regurgitation murmur. ASD is not associated with a regurgitation murmur; ASD can produce a grade 2-3/6 systolic ejection murmur. Tetralogy of Fallot is associ-

ated with a loud grade 3-5/6 systolic ejection murmur.

REFERENCES

Johnson, G.L. (1990). Clinical examination (pp. 223–235). In W.A. Long (ed.), *Fetal and neonatal cardiology*. Philadelphia: W.B. Saunders.

Lott, J.W. (1993). Assessment and management of cardiovascular dysfunction (pp. 355–391). In C. Kenner, A. Brueggemeyer, & L.P. Gunderson (eds.), *Comprehensive neonatal nursing: A physiologic perspective*. Philadelphia: W.B. Saunders.

Park, M.K. (1984). Physical examination (pp. 9–33). *Pediatric cardiology for practitioners*. Chicago: Year Book Medical Publishers.

111. Answer: (**C**) TGA, VSD, and hypertrophic cardiomyopathy are the three most frequent defects associated with IDMs. Endocardial cushion defects and/or VSD are the most common heart defects associated with Down syndrome (Trisomy 21). Aortic insufficiency and aortic aneurysm are commonly associated with Marfan syndrome.

REFERENCES

Hazinski, M.F. (1983). Congenital heart disease in the neonate (Part III): Congestive heart failure. *Neonatal Network, 1*(6), 8–17.

Hazinski, M.F. (1984). Cardiovascular disorders (pp. 63–252). *Nursing care of the critically ill child*. St. Louis: C.V. Mosby.

Heymann, M.A. (1989). Fetal and neonatal circulations (pp. 24–35). In F.H. Adams, G.C. Emmanouilides, & T.A. Riemenschneider (eds.), *Heart disease in infants, children, and adolescents*. Baltimore: Williams & Wilkins.

Heymann, M.A. (1989). Patent ductus arteriosus (pp. 209–223). In F.H. Adams, G.C. Emmanouilides, & T.A. Riemenschneider (eds.), *Heart disease in infants, children, and adolescents*. Baltimore: Williams & Wilkins.

Lott, J.W. (1993). Assessment and management of cardiovascular dysfunction (pp. 355–391). In C. Kenner, A. Brueggemeyer, & L.P. Gunderson (eds.), *Comprehensive neonatal nursing: A physiologic perspective*. Philadelphia: W.B. Saunders.

112. Answer: (**A**) The amount of blood flow through the PDA and the effects of the ductal flow depend on:

    1. difference between systemic and pulmonary vascular resistance
    2. diameter of ductus
    3. length of ductus

    Blood normally enters the pulmonary artery, into the lungs, through the pulmonary veins and into the right atrium, so the pulmonary artery pressure would be directly involved. High pulmonary blood flow causes increased pulmonary vascular resistance, pulmonary hypertension, and right ventricular hypertrophy.

REFERENCES

Heymann, M.A. (1989). Patent ductus arteriosus (pp. 209–223). In F.H. Adams, G.C. Emmanouilides, & T.A. Riemenschneider (eds.), *Heart disease in infants, children, and adolescents*. Baltimore: Williams & Wilkins.

Huhta, J.C. (1990). Patent ductus arteriosus in the preterm neonate (pp. 389–400). In W.A. Long (ed.), *Fetal and neonatal cardiology*. Philadelphia: W.B. Saunders.

Kirklin, J.K. (1990). Neonatal patent ductus surgery (pp. 754–759). In W.A. Long (ed.), *Fetal and neonatal cardiology*. Philadelphia: W.B. Saunders.

Lott, J.W. (1993). Assessment and management of cardiovascular dysfunction (pp. 355–391). In C. Kenner, A. Brueggemeyer, & L.P. Gunderson (eds.), *Comprehensive neonatal nursing: A physiologic perspective*. Philadelphia: W.B. Saunders.

Park, M.K. (1984). Left-to-right shunts (pp. 125–144). *Pediatric cardiology for practitioners*. Chicago: Year Book Medical Publishers.

113. Answer: (**C**) In moderate VSD, blood is shunted from left to right ventricle secondary to higher pressure in the left ventricle and higher systemic vascular resistance. From the right ventricle, the blood enters the pulmonary artery. The shunt is not affected by pulmonary venous pressure. The pressure is higher in the left ventricle than in the right ventricle; there is a significant amount of blood shunted.

REFERENCES

Graham, T.P., Bender, H.W., & Spach, M.S. (1989) (pp. 189–209). In F.H. Adams, G.C. Emmanouilides, & T.A. Riemenschneider (eds.), *Heart disease in infants, children, and adolescents*. Baltimore: Williams & Wilkins.

Lott, J.W. (1993). Assessment and management of cardiovascular dysfunction (pp. 355–391). In C. Kenner, A. Brueggemeyer, & L.P. Gunderson (eds.), *Comprehensive neonatal nursing: A physiologic perspective*. Philadelphia: W.B. Saunders.

Moller, J.H. (1987). *Congenital heart anomalies. Clinical education aid. Columbus, OH: Ross Laboratories.*

114. Answer: (**A**) William Elfin facies have an association with idiopathic hypertrophic subaortic stenosis (IHSS). Endocardial cushion defects are most commonly found in IDMs. TAPVR has no association with William Elfin facies.

REFERENCES

Avery, G.B. (1987). *Neonatology: Pathophysiology and management of the newborn*. Philadelphia: J.B. Lippincott.

Friedman, W.F. (1988). Congenital heart disease in infancy and childhood (pp. 896–975). In E. Braunwald (ed.), *Heart disease: A textbook of cardiovascular medicine*. Philadelphia: W.B. Saunders.
Friedman, W.F. (1989). Aortic stenosis (pp. 224–243). In F.H. Adams, G.C. Emmanouilides, & T.A. Riemenschneider (eds.), *Heart disease in infants, children, and adolescents*. Baltimore: Williams & Wilkins.
Lott, J.W. (1993). Assessment and management of cardiovascular dysfunction (pp. 355–391). In C. Kenner, A. Brueggemeyer, & L.P. Gunderson (eds.), *Comprehensive neonatal nursing: A physiologic perspective*. Philadelphia: W.B. Saunders.

115. Answer: (**A**) Decreased pulmonary blood flow in infants with TAPVR is secondary to obstruction to pulmonary blood flow with the TAPVR below the diaphragm. Elevated pulmonary venous pressure is present secondary to the obstruction that causes pulmonary edema. The decreased pulmonary blood flow is caused by obstruction to pulmonary flow, not increased systemic flow.

REFERENCES

Bull, C. (1990). Total anomalous pulmonary venous drainage (pp. 439–451). In W.A. Long (ed.), *Fetal and neonatal cardiology*. Philadelphia: W.B. Saunders: Philadelphia.
Lott, J.W. (1993). Assessment and management of cardiovascular dysfunction (pp. 355–391). In C. Kenner, A. Brueggemeyer, & L.P. Gunderson (eds.), *Comprehensive neonatal nursing: A physiologic perspective*. Philadelphia: W.B. Saunders.
Lucas, R.V. & Krabill, K.A. (1990). Anomalous venous connections, pulmonary and systemic. *Pediatric Clinics of North America, 37,* 580–616.

116. Answer: (**C**) Furosemide works by blocking sodium and chloride reabsorption in the ascending loop of Henle. Thiazide diuretics work by inhibition of sodium and chloride reabsorption along the distal tubules. Spironalactone works by binding to the cytoplasmic receptor sites and blocking aldosterone action, thus impairing the reabsorption of sodium and the secretion of potassium and hydrogen ions.

REFERENCES

Lott, J.W. (1993). Assessment and management of cardiovascular dysfunction (pp. 355–391). In C. Kenner, A. Brueggemeyer, & L.P. Gunderson (eds.), *Comprehensive neonatal nursing: A physiologic perspective*. Philadelphia: W.B. Saunders.
Oh, W. (1985). Diuretic therapy (pp. 299–304). In T.F. Yeh (ed.), *Drug therapy in the neonate and small infant*. Chicago: Year Book Medical Publishers.
Schneeweiss, A. (1990). Neonatal cardiovascular pharmacology (pp. 667–681). In W.A. Long (ed.), *Fetal and neonatal cardiology*. Philadelphia: W.B. Saunders.

117. Answer: (**A**) All congenital heart defects EXCEPT secundum type ASD predispose to SAIE. Aortic stenosis, VSD, and TOF are the three defects most commonly associated with development of SAIE.

REFERENCES

Dajani, A.S., Bisno, A.L., Chung, K.J., Durack, D.T., Freed, M., Gerber, M.A., Karchmer, A.W., Millard, D., Rahimtoola, S., Shulman, S.T., Watanakunakorn, C. & Taubert, K.A. (1990). Prevention of bacterial endocarditis: Recommendations by the American Heart Association. *Journal of the American Medical Association, 264*(22), 2919–2922.
Kaplan, E.L. & Shulman, S.T. (1989). Endocarditis (pp. 718–730). In F.H. Adams, G.C. Emmanouilides, & T.A. Riemenschneider (eds.), *Heart disease in infants, children, and adolescents*. Baltimore: Williams & Wilkins.
Lott, J.W. (1993). Assessment and management of cardiovascular dysfunction (pp. 355–391). In C. Kenner, A. Brueggemeyer, & L.P. Gunderson (eds.), *Comprehensive neonatal nursing: A physiologic perspective*. Philadelphia: W.B. Saunders.
Park, M.K. (1984). Cardiovascular infections (pp. 226–237). *Pediatric cardiology for practitioners*. Chicago: Year Book Medical Publishers.

118. Answer: (**B**) Tetralogy of Fallot (TOF)

REFERENCES

Creasy, R.K. & Resnik, R. (1989). *Maternal-fetal medicine: Principles and practice* (2nd ed.). Philadelphia: W.B. Saunders.
Lott, J.W. (1993). Assessment and management of cardiovascular dysfunction (pp. 355–391). In C. Kenner, A. Brueggemeyer, & L.P. Gunderson (eds.), *Comprehensive neonatal nursing: A physiologic perspective*. Philadelphia: W.B. Saunders.
Ross Laboratories. (1985). *Clinical education aid*. Columbus, OH: Ross Laboratories.

119. Answer: (**A**) Transposition of great arteries (TGA)

REFERENCES

Creasy, R.K. & Resnik, R. (1989). *Maternal-fetal medicine: Principles and practice* (2nd ed.). Philadelphia: W.B. Saunders.
Lott, J.W. (1993). Assessment and management of cardiovascular dysfunction (pp. 355–391). In C. Kenner, A. Brueggemeyer, & L.P. Gunderson (eds.). *Comprehensive neonatal nursing: A physiologic perspective*. Philadelphia: W.B. Saunders.
Ross Laboratories. (1985). *Clinical education aid*. Columbus, OH: Ross Laboratories.

120. Answer: (**B**) Atrial septal defect (ASD)

REFERENCES

Creasy, R.K. & Resnik, R. (1989). *Maternal-fetal medicine: Principles and practice* (2nd ed.). Philadelphia: W.B. Saunders.
Lott, J.W. (1993). Assessment and management of cardiovascular dysfunction (pp. 355–391). In C. Kenner, A. Brueggemeyer, & L.P. Gunderson (eds.), *Comprehensive neonatal nursing: A physiologic perspective*. Philadelphia: W.B. Saunders.
Ross Laboratories. (1985). *Clinical education aid*. Columbus, OH: Ross Laboratories.

121. Answer: (**C**) Ventricular septal defect

REFERENCES

Creasy, R.K. & Resnik, R. (1989). *Maternal-fetal medicine: Principles and practice* (2nd ed.). Philadelphia: W.B. Saunders.
Lott, J.W. (1993). Assessment and management of cardiovascular dysfunction (pp. 355–391). In C. Kenner, A. Brueggemeyer, & L.P. Gunderson (eds.), *Comprehensive neonatal nursing: A physiologic perspective*. Philadelphia: W.B. Saunders.
Ross Laboratories. (1985). *Clinical education aid*. Columbus, OH: Ross Laboratories.

122. Answer: (**C**) Patent ductus arteriosus

REFERENCES

Creasy, R.K. & Resnik, R. (1989). *Maternal-fetal medicine: Principles and practice* (2nd ed.). Philadelphia: W.B. Saunders.
Lott, J.W. (1993). Assessment and management of cardiovascular dysfunction (pp. 355–391). In C. Kenner, A. Brueggemeyer, & L.P. Gunderson (eds.), *Comprehensive neonatal nursing: A physiologic perspective*. Philadelphia: W.B. Saunders.
Ross Laboratories. (1985). *Clinical education aid*. Columbus, OH: Ross Laboratories.

123. Answer: (**A**) Pulmonic stenosis

REFERENCES

Creasy, R.K. & Resnik, R. (1989). *Maternal-fetal medicine: Principles and practice* (2nd ed.). Philadelphia: W.B. Saunders.
Lott, J.W. (1993). Assessment and management of cardiovascular dysfunction (pp. 355–391). In C. Kenner, A. Brueggemeyer, & L.P. Gunderson (eds.), *Comprehensive neonatal nursing: A physiologic perspective*. Philadelphia: W.B. Saunders.
May, K.A. & Mahlmeister, L.R. (1990). *Comprehensive maternity nursing: Nursing process and the childbearing family* (3rd ed.). Philadelphia: J.B. Lippincott.
Murray, M. (1988). Essentials of electronic fetal monitoring: Antepartal and intrapartal fetal monitoring. Washington, DC: NAACOG.
Ross Laboratories. (1985). *Clinical education aid*. Columbus, OH: Ross Laboratories.

124. Answer: (**B**) The primary theme in the second developmental stage for neonatal nurses is independence. Transition is accomplished by establishing a reputation as technically competent professional who can work independently to produce designated patient outcomes. This nurse looks forward to having primary responsibility for a small number of patients. At this level, the nurse is expected to evolve his or her technical skills to a high level.

First-line managers never can be effective if they cannot understand the technical aspects of the work that they supervise. Lack of technological expertise will undermine the manager's self-confidence and the trust and confidence of his or her staff. Successful achievement of the developmental tasks associated with this stage is extremely important in the process of long-term career development.

REFERENCES

Bates, B. (1970). Doctor and nurse: Changing roles and relations. *New England Journal of Medicine, 283,* 129.
Harrigan, R.C. & Perez, D. (1993). Neonatal nursing and its role in comprehensive care (pp. 3–8). In C. Kenner, A. Brueggemeyer, & L.P. Gunderson (eds.), *Comprehensive neonatal nursing: A physiologic perspective*. Philadelphia: W.B. Saunders.

125. Answer: (**A**) The volume of the intracellular compartment is maintained mainly by potassium salts and regulated by the Na-K cellular pump.

REFERENCES

Costarino, A.T. & Baumgart, S. (1988). Controversies in fluid and electrolyte therapy for the premature infant. *Clinics in Perinatology, 15,* 863–878.
DeMarini, S., Tsang, R.C., & Rath, L.L. (1993). Fluids, electrolytes, vitamins, and trace minerals: Basis of ingestion, digestion, elimination, and metabolism (pp. 393–413). In C. Kenner, A. Brueggemeyer, & L.P. Gunderson (eds.), *Comprehensive neonatal nursing: A physiologic perspective*. Philadelphia: W.B. Saunders.
Spitzer, A. (1982). The role of the kidney in sodium homeostasis during maturation. *Kidney International, 21,* 539–545.

126. Answer: (**B**) In D-TGA, two separate parallel circulations exist. Oxygenated blood is returned to the pulmonary circulation. The aorta receives unoxygenated systemic venous blood and returns it to the systemic arterial circuit. The end result is that heart and brain and other vital tissues are perfused with desaturated blood. This defect is incompatible with life. A communication between the two circulations must exist to allow mixing of oxygenated and deoxygenated blood.

The communication can be at the ductal, atrial, or ventricular level. Answer A describes the typical blood flow pattern of "corrected" or levotransposition (L-TGA). Circulation in L-TGA with no other defects is functionally normal.

REFERENCES

Kirklin, J.W., Colvin, E.V., McConnell, M.E., & Bargeron, L.M. (1990). Complete transposition of the great arteries: Treatment in the current era. *Pediatric Clinics of North America, 37,* 171–178.

Lott, J.W. (1993). Assessment and management of cardiovascular dysfunction (pp. 355–391). In C. Kenner, A. Brueggemeyer, & L.P. Gunderson (eds.), *Comprehensive neonatal nursing: A physiologic perspective.* Philadelphia: W.B. Saunders.

Paul, M.H. (1989). Complete transposition of the great arteries (pp. 371–423). In F.H. Adams, G.C. Emmanouilides, & T.A. Riemenschneider (eds.), *Heart disease in infants, children, and adolescents.* Baltimore: Williams & Wilkins.

127. Answer: (**A**) In preterm infants, high volumes of parenteral fluids have been associated with increased incidence of BPD, patent ductus arteriosus, and intraventricular hemorrhage.

REFERENCES

Bell, E.F., Warburton, D., Stonestreet, B.S., & Oh, W. (1980). Effect of fluid administration on the development of symptomatic patent ductus arteriosus and congestive heart failure in premature infants. *New England Journal of Medicine, 302,* 598–604.

DeMarini, S., Tsang, R.C., & Rath, L.L. (1993). Fluids, electrolytes, vitamins, and trace minerals: Basis of ingestion, digestion, elimination, and metabolism (pp. 393–413). In C. Kenner, A. Brueggemeyer, & L.P. Gunderson (eds.), *Comprehensive neonatal nursing: A physiologic perspective.* Philadelphia: W.B. Saunders.

Papile, L., Burstein, J., Burstein, R., Koffler, H., & Koops, B. (1978). Relationship of intravenous sodium bicarbonate infusions and cerebral intraventricular hemorrhage. *Journal of Pediatrics, 93,* 834–836.

Spahr, R.C., Klein, A.M., Brown, D.R., Holzman, I.R., & MacDonald, H.M. (1980). Fluid administration and bronchopulmonary dysplasia. *American Journal of Diseases of Childhood, 134,* 958–960.

128. Answer: (**B**) The main factors involved in the regulation of sodium reabsorption are the oncotic and hydrostatic pressure in the peritubular capillaries and the action of the hormone aldosterone, which increases the absorption of sodium in exchange with potassium or hydrogen.

REFERENCES

Bell, E.F., Warburton, D., Stonestreet, B.S., & Oh, W. (1980). Effect of fluid administration on the development of symptomatic patent ductus arteriosus and congestive heart failure in premature infants. *New England Journal of Medicine, 302,* 598–604.

DeMarini, S., Tsang, R.C., & Rath, L.L. (1993). Fluids, electrolytes, vitamins, and trace minerals: Basis of ingestion, digestion, elimination, and metabolism (pp. 393–413). In C. Kenner, A. Brueggemeyer, & L.P. Gunderson (eds.), *Comprehensive neonatal nursing: A physiologic perspective.* Philadelphia: W.B. Saunders.

Spitzer, A. (1982). The role of the kidney in sodium homeostasis during maturation. *Kidney International, 21,* 539–545.

Turnberg, L.A. (1971a). Abnormalities in intestinal electrolyte transport in congenital chloridorrhea. *Gut, 12,* 544–551.

Turnberg, L.A. (1971b). Potassium transport in the human small bowel. *Gut, 12,* 811–818.

Turnberg, L.A., Bieberdort, F.A., Mordowsky, S.G., & Gordtran, J.S. (1970). Interrelations of choloride, bicarbonate, sodium and hydrogen transport in human ileum. *Journal of Clinical Investigation, 49,* 557–567.

129. Answer: (**A**) Infants with early hyponatremia are usually in a state of excess water, and fluid restriction is the appropriate treatment.

REFERENCES

Arieff, A., & Guisado, R. (1976). Effects on the central nervous system of hypernatremic and hyponatremic states. *Kidney International, 10,* 104–116.

Bell, E.F., Warburton, D., Stonestreet, B.S., & Oh, W. (1980). Effect of fluid administration on the development of symptomatic patent ductus arteriosus and congestive heart failure in premature infants. *New England Journal of Medicine, 302,* 598–604.

Costarino, A. & Baumgart, S. (1986). Modern fluid and electrolyte management of the critically ill premature infant. *Pediatric Clinics of North America, 33,* 153–158.

DeMarini, S., Tsang, R.C., & Rath, L.L. (1993). Fluids, electrolytes, vitamins, and trace minerals: Basis of ingestion, digestion, elimination, and metabolism (pp. 393–413). In C. Kenner, A. Brueggemeyer, & L.P. Gunderson (eds.), *Comprehensive neonatal nursing: A physiologic perspective.* Philadelphia: W.B. Saunders.

130. Answer: (**C**) Hyponatremia with dehydration can be caused by either renal or extrarenal sodium and water losses. Renal losses usually are due to adrenal insufficiency (congenital adrenal hyperplasia, adrenal hemorrhage). Cardiopulmonary resuscitation, acidosis, and RDS are causes of hypernatremia in the newborn.

REFERENCES

Arieff, A., & Guisado, R. (1976). Effects on the central nervous system of hypernatremic and hyponatremic states. *Kidney International, 10,* 104–116.

Bell, E.F., Warburton, D., Stonestreet, B.S., & Oh, W. (1980). Effect of fluid administration on the development of symptomatic patent ductus arteriosus and congestive heart failure in premature infants. *New England Journal of Medicine, 302,* 598–604.

Costarino, A. & Baumgart, S. (1986). Modern fluid and

electrolyte management of the critically ill premature infant. *Pediatric Clinics of North America, 33,* 153–158.

DeMarini, S., Tsang, R.C., & Rath, L.L. (1993). Fluids, electrolytes, vitamins, and trace minerals: Basis of ingestion, digestion, elimination, and metabolism (pp. 393–413). In C. Kenner, A. Brueggemeyer, & L.P. Gunderson (eds.), *Comprehensive neonatal nursing: A physiologic perspective.* Philadelphia: W.B. Saunders.

Papile, L., Burstein, J., Burstein, R., Koffler, H., & Koops, B. (1978). Relationship of intravenous sodium bicarbonate infusions and cerebral intraventricular hemorrhage. *Journal of Pediatrics, 93,* 834–836.

Spahr, R.C., Klein, A.M., Brown, D.R., Holzman, I.R., & MacDonald, H.M. (1980). Fluid administration and bronchopulmonary dysplasia. *American Journal of Diseases of Childhood, 134,* 958–960.

131. Answer: (**C**) In adults, contractility is increased in response to stimulation of stretch receptors in the heart muscle. The newborn's heart has fewer fibers and cannot stretch sufficiently to accommodate increased volume, thus, increasing rate is the only effective mechanism to respond to increased volume. Venous return is the amount of blood volume returned to the heart. Local factors that affect venous return to the heart include hypoxia, acidosis, hypercarbia, hyperthermia, increased metabolic demand, and increased metabolites (potassium, ATP, and lactic acid). These factors also would adversely affect an adult heart.

REFERENCES

Braunwald, E., Sonnenblick, E.H., & Ross, J. (1988). Mechanisms of cardiac contraction and relaxation (pp. 383–425). In E. Braunwald (ed.), *Heart disease: A textbook of cardiovascular medicine.* Philadelphia: W.B. Saunders.

Conover, M.B. (1988). Anatomy and physiology of the heart (pp. 1–14). *Understanding electrocardiography: Arrhythmias and the 12-lead EKG.* St. Louis: C.V. Mosby.

Lott, J.W. (1993). Assessment and management of cardiovascular dysfunction (pp. 355–391). In C. Kenner, A. Brueggemeyer, & L.P. Gunderson (eds.), *Comprehensive neonatal nursing: A physiologic perspective.* Philadelphia: W.B. Saunders.

Smith, J.J. & Kampine, J.P. (1984). *Circulatory physiology.* Baltimore: Williams & Wilkins.

132. Answer: (**B**) ECG may be a better measure of serious toxicity than is serum potassium concentration. ECG changes include depression of the ST segment, flattening of the T wave, and increased height of the U wave. Prolongation of the P-R interval, widening of the QRS complex, and various arrhythmias can follow, particularly in newborns treated with digoxin. These ECG changes are indicative of hypokalemia. Hyperkalemia may be identified by ECG changes also. The typical sequence is peaked T waves, disappearance of P waves, and widening of QRS complex and its fusion with the T wave to form sine wave. Ventricular fibrillation may follow.

REFERENCES

DeMarini, S., Tsang, R.C., & Rath, L.L. (1993). Fluids, electrolytes, vitamins, and trace minerals: Basis of ingestion, digestion, elimination, and metabolism (pp. 393–413). In C. Kenner, A. Brueggemeyer, & L.P. Gunderson (eds.), *Comprehensive neonatal nursing: A physiologic perspective.* Philadelphia: W.B. Saunders.

Turnberg, L.A. (1971b). Potassium transport in the human small bowel. *Gut, 12,* 811–818.

Turnberg, L.A., Bieberdort, F.A., Mordowsky, S.G., & Gordtran, J.S. (1970). Interrelations of choloride, bicarbonate, sodium and hydrogen transport in human ileum. *Journal of Clinical Investigation, 49,* 557–567.

Surawicz, B. (1967). Relationship between electrocardiogram and electrolytes. *American Heart Journal, 73,* 814–834.

133. Answer: (**C**) The most common cause of increased renal losses of chloride is diuretic therapy.

REFERENCES

Costarino, A. & Baumgart, S. (1986). Modern fluid and electrolyte management of the critically ill premature infant. *Pediatric Clinics of North America, 33,* 153–158.

DeMarini, S., Tsang, R.C., & Rath, L.L. (1993). Fluids, electrolytes, vitamins, and trace minerals: Basis of ingestion, digestion, elimination, and metabolism (pp. 393–413). In C. Kenner, A. Brueggemeyer, & L.P. Gunderson (eds.), *Comprehensive neonatal nursing: A physiologic perspective.* Philadelphia: W.B. Saunders.

Perkin, R.M. & Levin, D.L. (1980). Common fluid and electrolyte problems in the pediatric intensive care unit. *Pediatric Clinics of North America, 27,* 558–567.

134. Answer: (**A**) The proximal type of Bartter's syndrome is usually diagnosed in the neonatal period and occurs mainly in male infants. A decreased renal threshold for bicarbonate and a failure to decrease the acid level of the urine occur in this condition and result in a hyperchloremic metabolic acidosis.

REFERENCES

Costarino, A. & Baumgart, S. (1986). Modern fluid and electrolyte management of the critically ill premature infant. *Pediatric Clinics of North America, 33,* 153–158.

DeMarini, S., Tsang, R.C., & Rath, L.L. (1993). Fluids, electrolytes, vitamins, and trace minerals: Basis of ingestion, digestion, elimination, and metabolism (pp. 393–413). In C. Kenner, A. Brueggemeyer, & L.P. Gunderson (eds.), *Comprehensive neonatal nursing: A physiologic perspective*. Philadelphia: W.B. Saunders.

Perkin, R.M. & Levin, D.L. (1980). Common fluid and electrolyte problems in the pediatric intensive care unit. *Pediatric Clinics of North America, 27,* 558–567.

Spitzer, A., Berstein, J., Edelman, C.M., & Boichis, H. (1987). The kidney and urinary tract (pp. 981–1015). In A.A. Fanaroff & R.J. Martin (eds.), *Neonatal-perinatal medicine*. St. Louis: C.V. Mosby.

135. Answer: (**C**) Corticosteroids decrease calcium absorption by inhibiting its transfer in the intestinal mucosa. Anticonvulsants can directly inhibit intestinal transfer of calcium (phenytoin) or can interfere with vitamin D metabolism (phenobarbital and phenytoin). Serum calcium concentration is maintained within narrow limits by the action of parathyroid hormone and 1,25-dihydroxyvitamin D, which increase serum calcium, and of calcitonin, which decreases serum calcium. Calcium is excreted by the kidneys; filtered calcium is reabsorbed in most segments of the tubules. Parathyroid hormone increases tubular reabsorption of calcium, whereas calcitonin is thought to increase calcium excretion.

REFERENCES

DeMarini, S., Tsang, R.C., & Rath, L.L. (1993). Fluids, electrolytes, vitamins, and trace minerals: Basis of ingestion, digestion, elimination, and metabolism (pp. 393–413). In C. Kenner, A. Brueggemeyer, & L.P. Gunderson (eds.), *Comprehensive neonatal nursing: A physiologic perspective*. Philadelphia: W.B. Saunders.

Hahn, T.J. (1980). Drug induced disorders of vitamin D and mineral metabolism. *Clinics in Endocrinology and Metabolism, 9,* 107–129.

Kimberg, D.V. (1969). Effects of vitamin D. and steroid hormones on intestinal calcium transport. *New England Journal of Medicine, 280,* 1396–1405.

136. Answer: (**C**) Late hypocalcemia typically occurs by the end of the first week of life and is caused by increased dietary phosphate load. It was common with the use of evaporated cow's milk formulas, which have a phosphate content greatly exceeding that of human milk. With modern "adapted" formulas, whose P content is closer to that of human milk, late neonatal hypocalcemia has become less frequent but has not disappeared. Maternal vitamin D deficiency can represent a predisposing factor.

REFERENCES

DeMarini, S., Tsang, R.C., & Rath, L.L. (1993). Fluids, electrolytes, vitamins, and trace minerals: Basis of ingestion, digestion, elimination, and metabolism (pp. 393–413). In C. Kenner, A. Brueggemeyer, & L.P. Gunderson (eds.), *Comprehensive neonatal nursing: A physiologic perspective*. Philadelphia: W.B. Saunders.

Roberts, S.A., Cohen, M.D., & Fortar, J.O. (1973). Antenatal factors associated with neonatal hypocalcemic convulsions. *Lancet, 2,* 809–811.

Venkatamaran, P.S., Tsang, R.C., Greer, F.R., Noguchi, A., Larskazewski, P, & Steichen, J.J. (1985). Late infantile tetany and secondary hyperparathyroidism in infants fed humanized cow milk formula. *American Journal of Diseases of Childhood, 139,* 664–668.

137. Answer: (**A**) Hypercalcemic disorders (serum calcium >11 mg/dl, or 2.75 mmol/L) such as subcutaneous fat necrosis, Williams syndrome, and idiopathic hypercalcemia, are exceedingly rare in the newborn. Usually, hypercalcemia is of iatrogenic origin and results from excessive administration of calcium or vitamin D.

REFERENCES

DeMarini, S., Tsang, R.C., & Rath, L.L. (1993). Fluids, electrolytes, vitamins, and trace minerals: Basis of ingestion, digestion, elimination, and metabolism (pp. 393–413). In C. Kenner, A. Brueggemeyer, & L.P. Gunderson (eds.), *Comprehensive neonatal nursing: A physiologic perspective*. Philadelphia: W.B. Saunders.

Hahn, T.J. (1980). Drug induced disorders of vitamin D and mineral metabolism. *Clinics in Endocrinology and Metabolism, 9,* 107–129.

Kimberg, D.V. (1969). Effects of vitamin D. and steroid hormones on intestinal calcium transport. *New England Journal of Medicine, 280,* 1396–1405.

138. Answer: (**B**) Magnesium is distributed primarily in the skeleton and the intracellular spaces. It is involved in energy production, cell membrane function, mitochondrial function, and protein synthesis.

REFERENCES

DeMarini, S., Tsang, R.C., & Rath, L.L. (1993). Fluids, electrolytes, vitamins, and trace minerals: Basis of ingestion, digestion, elimination, and metabolism (pp. 393–413). In C. Kenner, A. Brueggemeyer, & L.P. Gunderson (eds.), *Comprehensive neonatal nursing: A physiologic perspective*. Philadelphia: W.B. Saunders.

Shaul, P.W., Mimouni, F., Tsang, R.C., & Specker, G.L. (1987). The role of magnesium in neonatal calcium homeostasis: Effects of magnesium infusion on calcitropic hormones and calcium. *Pediatric Research, 22,* 319–323.

139. Answer: (**A**) The metabolic functions of these vitamins include synthesis of neurotransmitters, heme, and prostaglandins and the interconversion of amino acids.

REFERENCES

DeMarini, S., Tsang, R.C., & Rath, L.L. (1993). Fluids, electrolytes, vitamins, and trace minerals: Basis of ingestion, digestion, elimination, and metabolism (pp. 393–413). In C. Kenner, A. Brueggemeyer, & L.P. Gunderson (eds.), *Comprehensive neonatal nursing: A physiologic perspective*. Philadelphia: W.B. Saunders.

Schanler, R.J. (1988). Water-soluble vitamins: C, B_1, B_2, B_6, niacin, biotin and pantothenic acid (pp. 236–252). In R.C. Tsang & B.L. Nichols (eds.), *Nutrition during infancy*. St. Louis: C.V. Mosby.

140. Answer: (**A**) Absorption of vitamin B_{12} occurs in the distal third of the ileum and requires the presence of intrinsic factor, a glycoprotein secreted by the stomach. Because both folic acid and vitamin B_{12} deficiency can cause megaloblastic anemia and because folic acid can interfere with vitamin B_{12} metabolism, the differential diagnosis becomes important.

REFERENCES

Dallman, P.R. (1988). Nutritional anemia of infancy: Iron, folic acid and vitamin B_{12} (pp. 175–189). In R.C. Tsang & B.L. Nichols (eds.), *Nutrition during infancy*. St. Louis: C.V. Mosby.

DeMarini, S., Tsang, R.C., & Rath, L.L. (1993). Fluids, electrolytes, vitamins, and trace minerals: Basis of ingestion, digestion, elimination, and metabolism (pp. 393–413). In C. Kenner, A. Brueggemeyer, & L.P. Gunderson (eds.), *Comprehensive neonatal nursing: A physiologic perspective*. Philadelphia: W.B. Saunders.

Kalser, M.H. (1985). Absorption of cobalamin (vitamin B_{12}), folate and other water-soluble vitamins (pp. 1553–1566). In J.E. Berk (ed.), *Gastroenterology*. (4th ed.). Philadelphia: W.B. Saunders.

141. Answer: (**B**) Retinol (vitamin A) is incorporated into chylomicrons and transported to the liver, where it is stored.

REFERENCES

DeMarini, S., Tsang, R.C., & Rath, L.L. (1993). Fluids, electrolytes, vitamins, and trace minerals: Basis of ingestion, digestion, elimination, and metabolism (pp. 393–413). In C. Kenner, A. Brueggemeyer, & L.P. Gunderson (eds.), *Comprehensive neonatal nursing: A physiologic perspective*. Philadelphia: W.B. Saunders.

Zachman, R.D. (1988). In RA.C. Tsang & B.L. Nichols (eds.), *Nutrition during infancy*. (pp. 253–263). St. Louis: C.V. Mosby.

142. Answer: (**A**) The purpose of the cardiac sphincter is to close after swallowing and prevent reflux of stomach contents into the esophagus.

REFERENCES

Lefrak-Okikawa, L. & Meier, P.P. (1993). Nutrition: Physiologic basis of metabolism and management of enteral and parenteral nutrition (pp. 414–433). In C. Kenner, A. Brueggemeyer, & L.P. Gunderson (eds.), *Comprehensive neonatal nursing: A physiologic perspective*. Philadelphia: W.B. Saunders.

Plaxico, D.T. & Loughlin, G.M. (1981). Nasopharyngeal reflux and neonatal apnea. *American Journal of Diseases of Children, 15,* 793–794.

143. Answer: (**B**) Vitamin K is required for the synthesis of coagulation Factors II, VII, IX, and X and for the conversion of inactive precursors into active clotting factors.

REFERENCES

DeMarini, S., Tsang, R.C., & Rath, L.L. (1993). Fluids, electrolytes, vitamins, and trace minerals: Basis of ingestion, digestion, elimination, and metabolism (pp. 393–413). In C. Kenner, A. Brueggemeyer, & L.P. Gunderson (eds.), *Comprehensive neonatal nursing: A physiologic perspective*. Philadelphia: W.B. Saunders.

Greer, F.R. & Suttie, J.W. (1988). Vitamin K and the newborn (pp. 289–297). In R.C. Tsang & B.L. Nichols (eds.), *Nutrition during infancy*. St. Louis: C.V. Mosby.

144. Answer: (**B**) The last phase of protein absorption, intestinal absorption, is a two-step process, during which the small polypeptides continue to break down into amino acids, and these substances are subsequently absorbed. This second mechanism is the direct absorption of macromolecules. It is most likely the mechanism that leads to some allergies later in life.

REFERENCES

Kerner, J.A. (1983). *Manual of pediatric parenteral nutrition* (pp. 63–68, 117–217). New York: Raven Press.

Lefrak-Okikawa, L. & Meier, P.P. (1993). Nutrition: Physiologic basis of metabolism and management of enteral and parenteral nutrition (pp. 414–433). In C. Kenner, A. Brueggemeyer, & L.P. Gunderson (eds.), *Comprehensive neonatal nursing: A physiologic perspective*. Philadelphia: W.B. Saunders.

Walker, W.A. (1985). Absorption of protein and protein fragments in the developing intestine: Role in immunologic allergic reaction. *Pediatrics* (suppl.), *75,* 167–171.

145. Answer: (**B**) Damage to the thoracic duct, which can occur in chest surgery, can then lead to the collection of chyle in the chest and require that dietary fat be modified or totally avoided until the leak resolves.

REFERENCES

Lebenthal, E. (ed.). (1989). *Textbook of gastroenterology and nutrition in infancy*. New York: Raven Press.

Lefrak-Okikawa, L. & Meier, P.P. (1993). Nutrition: Physiologic basis of metabolism and management of enteral and parenteral nutrition (pp. 414–433). In C. Kenner, A. Brueggemeyer, & L.P. Gunderson (eds.), *Comprehensive neonatal nursing: A physiologic perspective*. Philadelphia: W.B. Saunders.

Tsang, R.E. & Nichols, B.L. (eds.). (1988). *Nutrition during infancy*. Philadelphia: Hanley & Belfus.

146. Answer: (**B**) The main factors involved in the regulation of sodium reabsorption are the oncotic and hydrostatic pressure in the peritubular capillaries and the action of the hormone aldosterone, which increases the absorption of sodium in exchange with potassium or hydrogen.

REFERENCES

Bell, E.F., Warburton, D., Stonestreet, B.S., & Oh, W. (1980). Effect of fluid administration on the development of symptomatic patent ductus arteriosus and congestive heart failure in premature infants. *New England Journal of Medicine, 302,* 598–604.

DeMarini, S., Tsang, R.C., & Rath, L.L. (1993). Fluids, electrolytes, vitamins, and trace minerals: Basis of ingestion, digestion, elimination, and metabolism (pp. 393–413). In C. Kenner, A. Brueggemeyer, & L.P. Gunderson (eds.), *Comprehensive neonatal nursing: A physiologic perspective*. Philadelphia: W.B. Saunders.

Spitzer, A. (1982). The role of the kidney in sodium homeostasis during maturation. *Kidney International, 21,* 539–545.

Turnberg, L.A. (1971a). Abnormalities in intestinal electrolyte transport in congenital chloridorrhea. *Gut, 12,* 544–551.

Turnberg, L.A. (1971b). Potassium transport in the human small bowel. *Gut, 12,* 811–818.

Turnberg, L.A., Bieberdort, F.A., Mordowsky, S.G., & Gordtran, J.S. (1970). Interrelations of choloride, bicarbonate, sodium and hydrogen transport in human ileum. *Journal of Clinical Investigation, 49,* 557–567.

Weinberg, J., Weitzman, R., Zakauddin, S., & Leake, R. (1977). Inappropriate secretion of antidiuretic hormone in a premature infant. *Journal of Pediatrics, 90,* 111–114.

147. Answer: (**C**) The brush border villi of the neonate's intestines contain the enzymes that break down the disaccharides.

REFERENCES

Lebenthal, E. (ed.). (1989). *Textbook of gastroenterology and nutrition in infancy*. New York: Raven Press.

Lefrak-Okikawa, L. & Meier, P.P. (1993). Nutrition: Physiologic basis of metabolism and management of enteral and parenteral nutrition (pp. 414–433). In C. Kenner, A. Brueggemeyer, & L.P. Gunderson (eds.), *Comprehensive neonatal nursing: A physiologic perspective*. Philadelphia: W.B. Saunders.

Tsang, R.E. & Nichols, B.L. (eds.). (1988). *Nutrition during infancy*. Philadelphia: Hanley & Belfus.

148. Answer: (**B**) Wydase is used for the initial treatment of IV infiltration. Its action is to break down the cell membrane and dissipate the chemical irritant.

REFERENCES

Lefrak-Okikawa, L. & Meier, P.P. (1993). Nutrition: Physiologic basis of metabolism and management of enteral and parenteral nutrition (pp. 414–433). In C. Kenner, A. Brueggemeyer, & L.P. Gunderson (eds.), *Comprehensive neonatal nursing: A physiologic perspective*. Philadelphia: W.B. Saunders.

Zenk, K.E., Dungy, C.I., & Greene, G.R. (1981). Nafcillin extravasation injury. *American Journal of Diseases of Children, 135,* 1113–1114.

149. Answer: (**B**) Various obstetrical milestones also are used to estimate progressive gestational age. These include first auscultation of fetal heart tones by fetoscope (approximately 20 weeks), measurement of fundal height (directly related to weight of fetus and duration of pregnancy), and the mother's report of quickening (about 18 weeks in primigravidas and slightly earlier in multigravidas). Ultrasound can be used to monitor fetal growth and to identify certain abnormalities of development. Gestational age can be ascertained by ultrasound within a range of ±one week in early pregnancy (6–18 weeks), decreasing in certainty to ±three weeks from 29 weeks to term. Biparietal diameter can identify the growth retarded fetus. Laboratory tests, particularly on amniotic fluid obtained via amniocentesis, are increasingly accurate in estimating fetal development, but availability, cost, and risk factors generally limit their use to high-risk pregnancies. For example, the resting supine posture of a newborn less than about 28–30 weeks gestation will be hypotonic extension of all extremities. By 34 weeks, the legs are flexed ("frog-like"), while arms remain extended.

REFERENCES

Battaglia, F.C., & Lubchenco, L.O. (1967). A practical classification of newborn infants by weight and gestational age. *Journal of Pediatrics, 71*(2), 159–163.

Endo, A.S. & Nishioka, E. (1993). Neonatal assessment

(pp. 265–293). In C. Kenner, A. Brueggemeyer, & L.P. Gunderson (eds.), *Comprehensive neonatal nursing: A physiologic perspective*. Philadelphia: W.B. Saunders.

Petrucha, R. (1989). Fetal maturity/gestational age evaluation. *Journal of Perinatology, 9*(1), 100–101.

150. Answer: (**A**) Collaborative care environments require dedication on the part of professional providers to the process of identifying their patient care *values*. Ethical conflicts that exist are identified and discussed. Constancy is needed for the development of trust, a basic element of collaboration. For example, for a collaborative health care team to function effectively, there must be general agreement on the basic concepts of professional practice.

REFERENCES

Aradine, C.R. & Hansen, M.F. (1970). Interdisciplinary teamwork in family health care. *Nursing Clinics of North America, 5*(2), 211–222.

Gilles, C. (1991). Nonsurgical management of the infant with gastroesophageal reflux and respiratory problems. *Journal of the American Academy of Nursing Practice, 3*(1), 11–16.

Harrigan, R. & Perez, D. (1993). Collaborative practice in the NICU (pp. 9–13). In C. Kenner, A. Brueggemeyer, & L.P. Gunderson (eds.), *Comprehensive neonatal nursing: A physiologic perspective*. Philadelphia: W.B. Saunders.

151. Answer: (**A**) Rickets is caused by insufficient intake of calcium and phosphorus.

REFERENCES

DeMarini, S., Tsang, R.C., & Rath, L.L. (1993). Fluids, electrolytes, vitamins, and trace minerals: Basis of ingestion, digestion, elimination, and metabolism (pp. 393–413). In C. Kenner, A. Brueggemeyer, & L.P. Gunderson (eds.), *Comprehensive neonatal nursing: A physiologic perspective*. Philadelphia: W.B. Saunders.

Steichen, J.J., Gratton, T.L., & Tsang, R.C. (1980). Osteopenia of prematurity: The cause and possible treatment. *Journal of Pediatrics, 96*, 528–534.

152. Answer: (**A**) Preterm infants require approximately 120 cal/kg/day for tissue repair and growth.

REFERENCES

Lebenthal, E. (ed.). (1989). *Textbook of gastroenterology and nutrition in infancy*. New York: Raven Press.

Lefrak-Okikawa, L. & Meier, P.P. (1993). Nutrition: Physiologic basis of metabolism and management of enteral and parenteral nutrition (pp. 414–433). In C. Kenner, A. Brueggemeyer, & L.P. Gunderson (eds.), *Comprehensive neonatal nursing: A physiologic perspective*. Philadelphia: W.B. Saunders.

153. Answer: (**A**). Vitamin D is essential for normal metabolism of calcium and phosphorus.

REFERENCES

DeMarini, S., Tsang, R.C., & Rath, L.L. (1993). Fluids, electrolytes, vitamins, and trace minerals: Basis of ingestion, digestion, elimination, and metabolism (pp. 393–413). In C. Kenner, A. Brueggemeyer, & L.P. Gunderson (eds.), *Comprehensive neonatal nursing: A physiologic perspective*. Philadelphia: W.B. Saunders.

Tsang, R.C. (1983). The quandary of vitamin D in the newborn infant. *Lancet, 1*, 1370–1372.

154. Answer: (**C**) The formation of the gastrointestinal tract is largely dependent on the folding that the embryo undergoes at the end of the first month of development.

REFERENCES

Loper, D.L. (1983). Gastrointestinal development: Embryology, congenital anomalies, and impact on feedings. *Neonatal Network, 2*(1), 27–36.

McCollum, L.L. & Thigpen, J.L. (1993). Assessment and management of gastrointestinal dysfunction (pp. 434–479). In C. Kenner, A. Brueggemeyer, & L.P. Gunderson (eds.), *Comprehensive neonatal nursing: A physiologic perspective*. Philadelphia: W.B. Saunders.

Moore, K.L. (1989). *Before we are born: Basic embryology and birth defects* (3rd ed.). Philadelphia: W.B. Saunders.

Sadler, T.W. (1985). *Langman's medical embryology* (5th ed.). Baltimore: Williams & Wilkins.

155. Answer: (**A**) The mouth develops from a surface depression in the ectoderm called the stomodeum, or primitive mouth, and involves the most cranial part of the foregut, which is sometimes called the pharyngeal gut.

REFERENCES

Loper, D.L. (1983). Gastrointestinal development: Embryology, congenital anomalies, and impact on feedings. *Neonatal Network, 2*(1), 27–36.

McCollum, L.L. & Thigpen, J.L. (1993). Assessment and management of gastrointestinal dysfunction (pp. 434–479). In C. Kenner, A. Brueggemeyer, & L.P. Gunderson (eds.), *Comprehensive neonatal nursing: A physiologic perspective*. Philadelphia: W.B. Saunders.

Moore, K.L. (1989). *Before we are born: Basic embryology and birth defects* (3rd ed.). Philadelphia: W.B. Saunders.

Sadler, T.W. (1985). *Langman's medical embryology* (5th ed.). Baltimore: Williams & Wilkins.

156. Answer: (**A**) By the sixth week, the rate of growth of the intestinal tube outpaces the elongation of the body, causing the tube to bend ventrally. With the simultaneously rapid growth

of the liver, the space within the abdominal cavity becomes quickly limited. Consequently, at about seven weeks' gestation, loops of intestine begin to protrude into the umbilical cord.

REFERENCES

Loper, D.L. (1983). Gastrointestinal development: Embryology, congenital anomalies, and impact on feedings. *Neonatal Network, 2*(1), 27–36.

McCollum, L.L. & Thigpen, J.L. (1993). Assessment and management of gastrointestinal dysfunction (pp. 434–479). In C. Kenner, A. Brueggemeyer, & L.P. Gunderson (eds.), *Comprehensive neonatal nursing: A physiologic perspective*. Philadelphia: W.B. Saunders.

Moore, K.L. (1989). *Before we are born: Basic embryology and birth defects* (3rd ed.). Philadelphia: W.B. Saunders.

Sadler, T.W. (1985). *Langman's medical embryology* (5th ed.). Baltimore: Williams & Wilkins.

157. Answer: **(B)** By 12 weeks, the muscular layers of the intestine have appeared, and the primitive nerve cells, or neuroblasts, have completed their head-to-toe migration so the entire length of the gastrointestinal tract is innervated.

REFERENCES

Loper, D.L. (1983). Gastrointestinal development: Embryology, congenital anomalies, and impact on feedings. *Neonatal Network, 2*(1), 27–36.

McCollum, L.L. & Thigpen, J.L. (1993). Assessment and management of gastrointestinal dysfunction (pp. 434–479). In C. Kenner, A. Brueggemeyer, & L.P. Gunderson (eds.), *Comprehensive neonatal nursing: A physiologic perspective*. Philadelphia: W.B. Saunders.

Moore, K.L. (1989). *Before we are born: Basic embryology and birth defects* (3rd ed.). Philadelphia: W.B. Saunders.

Sadler, T.W. (1985). *Langman's medical embryology* (5th ed.). Baltimore: Williams & Wilkins.

158. Answer: **(C)** Neonatal asphyxia reflects an inability to establish adequate ventilation at birth with subsequent hypoxemia, respiratory and metabolic acidosis, cardiovascular deterioration with hypotension, bradycardia, and central nervous system (CNS) depression. Perinatal asphyxia implies a combination of hypoxemia, hypercapnia (increased P_{CO_2}) and circulatory insufficiency that can be induced by a variety of perinatal events. The fetal systemic responses to lack of oxygen include (1) in the presence of decreased oxygen the fetus cannot increase cardiac output as the adult can because the fetus's cardiac output is already two to three times per unit of body weight that of the adult. This is done by preferentially shunting and maintaining blood to the heart, brain and adrenals at the expense of organs such as GI tract, kidney, skin, and skeletal muscle. There is a drop in heart rate and decrease in oxygen consumption initially; (2) the fetal brain and heart receive about 7 percent of the cardiac output, but during fetal hypoxemia up to 26 percent of cardiac output. The placenta also receives a greater proportion of the cardiac output, up to 16 percent in the presence of hypoxemia in conjunction with acidosis; (3) with worsening fetal hypoxemia and acidosis, metabolism is converted to anaerobic glycolysis; and (4) metabolic acidosis secondary to poor tissue perfusion produces impaired myocardial function, decreases cardiac output, and causes hypotension. There is intense vasoconstriction that occurs during the shunting process and eventually results in fetal respiratory center depression.

REFERENCES

London, M.L. (1993). Resuscitation and stabilization of the neonate (pp. 231–246). In C. Kenner, A. Brueggemeyer, & L.P. Gunderson (eds.), *Comprehensive neonatal nursing: A physiologic perspective*. Philadelphia: W.B. Saunders.

Woods, J. (1983). Birth asphyxia: Pathophysiologic events and fetal adaptive changes. *Clinics in Perinatology, 10*(2), 473.

159. Answer: **(B)** Normally the rate of gastric emptying is controlled by the chemical composition and amount of chyme, but when the stomach is distended or subjected to hypertonic solutions or high loads of fat or acid, the gastric motility may actually decrease so more time can be devoted to digestion and absorption in the small intestine.

REFERENCES

Loper, D.L. (1983). Gastrointestinal development: Embryology, congenital anomalies, and impact on feedings. *Neonatal Network, 2*(1), 27–36.

McCollum, L.L. & Thigpen, J.L. (1993). Assessment and management of gastrointestinal dysfunction (pp. 434–479). In C. Kenner, A. Brueggemeyer, & L.P. Gunderson (eds.), *Comprehensive neonatal nursing: A physiologic perspective*. Philadelphia: W.B. Saunders.

Moore, K.L. (1989). *Before we are born: Basic embryol-*

ogy and birth defects (3rd ed.). Philadelphia: W.B. Saunders.

Sadler, T.W. (1985). *Langman's medical embryology* (5th ed.). Baltimore: Williams & Wilkins.

160. Answer: (**C**) Data for severe respiratory distress syndrome infants with birth weights less than 1500 grams reveal a mean time of passage of the first stool at 91 hours for those receiving early feedings versus an average of 168 hours for those with delayed feedings.

REFERENCES

Loper, D.L. (1983). Gastrointestinal development: Embryology, congenital anomalies, and impact on feedings. *Neonatal Network, 2*(1), 27–36.

McCollum, L.L. & Thigpen, J.L. (1993). Assessment and management of gastrointestinal dysfunction (pp. 434–479). In C. Kenner, A. Brueggemeyer, & L.P. Gunderson (eds.), *Comprehensive neonatal nursing: A physiologic perspective*. Philadelphia: W.B. Saunders.

Moore, K.L. (1989). *Before we are born: Basic embryology and birth defects* (3rd ed.). Philadelphia: W.B. Saunders.

Sadler, T.W. (1985). *Langman's medical embryology* (5th ed.). Baltimore: Williams & Wilkins.

161. Answer: (**A**) Gluconeogenesis is the mechanism by which lactate and amino acids are converted to glucose.

REFERENCES

Ampola, M.G. (1982). *Metabolic disease in pediatric practice*. Boston: Little, Brown.

Burman, D., Holton, J.B., & Pennock, C.A. (eds.). (1978). *Inherited disorders of carbohydrate metabolism*. Baltimore: University Park Press.

Cornblath, M., Wybregt, S.H., & Bacens, G.S. (1963). Studies of carbohydrate metabolism in the newborn infant. *Pediatrics, 32,* 1007.

Theorell, C.J. & Degenhardt, M. (1993). Assessment and management of metabolic dysfunction (pp. 480–526). In C. Kenner, A. Brueggemeyer, & L.P. Gunderson (eds.), *Comprehensive neonatal nursing: A physiologic perspective*. Philadelphia: W.B. Saunders.

162. Answer: (**B**) Although vomiting can be initiated by distention or irritative stimuli at any point along the length of the gut, the stomach and duodenum appear to be the most sensitive to these stimuli.

REFERENCES

Chang, J.H.T. (1980). Neonatal surgical emergencies: Part V—Intestinal obstruction. *Perinatology/Neonatology, 4*(2), 34–40.

Ghory, M.J. & Sheldon, C.A. (1985). Newborn surgical emergencies of the gastrointestinal tract. *Surgical Clinics of North America, 65*(5), 1083–1098.

McCollum, L.L. & Thigpen, J.L. (1993). Assessment and management of gastrointestinal dysfunction (pp. 434–479). In C. Kenner, A. Brueggemeyer, & L.P. Gunderson (eds.), *Comprehensive neonatal nursing: A physiologic perspective*. Philadelphia: W.B. Saunders.

163. Answer: (**B**) Percussion, although useful in the examination of the adult, is unreliable and difficult to perform in the infant because the internal abdominal organs are small and close together.

REFERENCES

McCollum, L.L. & Thigpen, J.L. (1993). Assessment and management of gastrointestinal dysfunction (pp. 434–479). In C. Kenner, A. Brueggemeyer, & L.P. Gunderson (eds.), *Comprehensive neonatal nursing: A physiologic perspective*. Philadelphia: W.B. Saunders.

Scanlon, J.W., Nelson, T., Grylack, L.J., & Smith, Y.F. (1979). *A system of newborn physical examination*. Baltimore: University Park Press.

164. Answer: (**B**) The Guthrie bacterial inhibition assay is considered the single most significant contribution to screening populations for metabolic diseases.

REFERENCES

Benson, P.F. (1983). Screening and management of potentially treatable genetic metabolic disorders. Boston: MTP Press.

Bickel, H., Guthrie, R., & Hammersen, G. (1980). *Neonatal screening for inborn errors of metabolism*. New York: Springer-Verlag.

Crawford, M. d'A., Gibbs, D.A., & Watts, R.W. E. (eds.). (1982). *Advances in the treatment of inborn errors of metabolism*. New York: Wiley.

Scriver, C.R., Beaudet, A.L., Sly, W.S., & Valle, D. (eds.). (1989). *The metabolic basis of inherited disease* (6th ed.). (Volume I and II). New York: McGraw-Hill.

Theorell, C.J. & Degenhardt, M. (1993). Assessment and management of metabolic dysfunction (pp. 480–526). In C. Kenner, A. Brueggemeyer, & L.P. Gunderson (eds.), *Comprehensive neonatal nursing: A physiologic perspective*. Philadelphia: W.B. Saunders.

Wapnir, R.A. (1985). Congenital metabolic disease diagnosis and treatment. New York: Marcel Dekker.

165. Answer: (**B**) As the primary regulator of blood glucose, the liver takes up glucose during times of abundance after meals and converts it mostly to glycogen.

REFERENCES

Ampola, M.G. (1982). *Metabolic disease in pediatric practice*. Boston: Little, Brown.

Burman, D., Holton, J.B., & Pennock, C.A. (eds.). (1978). *Inherited disorders of carbohydrate metabolism*. Baltimore: University Park Press.

Cornblath, M., Wybregt, S.H., & Bacens, G.S. (1963). Studies of carbohydrate metabolism in the newborn infant. *Pediatrics, 32,* 1007.

Theorell, C.J. & Degenhardt, M. (1993). Assessment and management of metabolic dysfunction (pp. 480–526). In C. Kenner, A. Brueggemeyer, & L.P. Gunderson (eds.), *Comprehensive neonatal nursing: A physiologic perspective.* Philadelphia: W.B. Saunders.

166. Answer: (**C**) The infant is usually more than 42 weeks' gestation with a birth weight greater than 4000 grams and may have a large posterior fontanelle owing to delayed ossification. The infant may appear lethargic and hypotonic, have difficulty feeding, and delay passing meconium.

REFERENCES

Gamblien, V., Bivens, K., Burton, K.S., Kissler, C.H., Kleeman, T.A., Freije, M. & Prows, C. (1993). Assessment and management of endocrine dysfunction (pp. 527–552). In C. Kenner, A. Brueggemeyer, & L.P. Gunderson (eds.), *Comprehensive neonatal nursing: A physiologic perspective.* Philadelphia: W.B. Saunders.

Goetzman, B.W. & Wenneberg, R.P. (1991). *Neonatal intensive care handbook* (2nd ed.). St. Louis: Mosby-Year Book.

Walfish, P.G. & Tseng, K.H. (1989). Thyroid physiology and pathology (pp. 367–375). In R. Collu, J. Duchame, & H. Guyda (eds.), *Pediatric endocrinology* New York: Raven Press.

167. Answer: (**B**) Breath hydrogen measurement is the most accurate, sensitive, and specific indirect test of detecting lactose deficiency.

REFERENCES

Ampola, M.G. (1982). *Metabolic disease in pediatric practice.* Boston: Little, Brown.

Burman, D., Holton, J.B., & Pennock, C.A. (eds.). (1978). *Inherited disorders of carbohydrate metabolism.* Baltimore: University Park Press.

Scriver, C.R., Beaudet, A.L., Sly, W.S., & Valle, D. (eds.). (1989). *The metabolic basis of inherited disease* (6th ed.). (Volume I and II). New York: McGraw-Hill.

Theorell, C.J. & Degenhardt, M. (1993). Assessment and management of metabolic dysfunction (pp. 480–526). In C. Kenner, A. Brueggemeyer, & L.P. Gunderson (eds.), *Comprehensive neonatal nursing: A physiologic perspective.* Philadelphia: W.B. Saunders.

Wapnir, R.A. (1985). Congenital metabolic disease diagnosis and treatment. New York: Marcel Dekker.

168. Answer: (**B**) The absence of transferase activity of erythrocytes is the basis for diagnosing galactosemia.

REFERENCES

Ampola, M.G. (1982). *Metabolic disease in pediatric practice.* Boston: Little, Brown.

Burman, D., Holton, J.B., & Pennock, C.A. (eds.). (1978). *Inherited disorders of carbohydrate metabolism.* Baltimore: University Park Press.

Levy, H. & Mammerson, G. (1978). Newborn screening for galactosemia and other galactose metabolic defects. *Journal of Pediatrics, 92*(6), 871–877.

Scriver, C.R., Beaudet, A.L., Sly, W.S., & Valle, D. (eds.). (1989). *The metabolic basis of inherited disease* (6th ed.). (Volume I and II). New York: McGraw-Hill.

Theorell, C.J. & Degenhardt, M. (1993). Assessment and management of metabolic dysfunction (pp. 480–526). In C. Kenner, A. Brueggemeyer, & L.P. Gunderson. (eds.), *Comprehensive neonatal nursing: A physiologic perspective.* Philadelphia: W.B. Saunders.

169. Answer: (**C**) The physical symptoms of glycogen storage disease are hepatomegaly and a large protruding abdomen that sharply contrast the thin extremities.

REFERENCES

Ampola, M.G. (1982). *Metabolic disease in pediatric practice.* Boston: Little, Brown.

Burman, D., Holton, J.B., & Pennock, C.A. (eds.). (1978). *Inherited disorders of carbohydrate metabolism.* Baltimore: University Park Press.

Scriver, C.R., Beaudet, A.L., Sly, W.S., & Valle, D. (eds.). (1989). *The metabolic basis of inherited disease* (6th ed.). (Volume I and II). New York: McGraw-Hill.

Theorell, C.J. & Degenhardt, M. (1993). Assessment and management of metabolic dysfunction (pp. 480–526). In C. Kenner, A. Brueggemeyer, & L.P. Gunderson (eds.), *Comprehensive neonatal nursing: A physiologic perspective.* Philadelphia: W.B. Saunders.

170. Answer: (**C**) Growth hormone is not thought to have an important role in fetal growth. Neonates with isolated growth hormone deficiency can have height and birth weight within normal range. It can result in hypoglycemia if growth hormone is deficient.

REFERENCES

Gamblien, V., Bivens, K., Burton, K.S., Kissler, C.H., Kleeman, T.A., Freije, M. & Prows, C. (1993). Assessment and management of endocrine dysfunction (pp. 527–552). In C. Kenner, A. Brueggemeyer, & L.P. Gunderson (eds.), *Comprehensive neonatal nursing: A physiologic perspective.* Philadelphia: W.B. Saunders.

Herber, S.M. & Kay, R. (1987). Aetiology of growth hormone deficiency. *Archives of Disease in Childhood, 62,* 735–736.

171. Answer: (**A**) Severe acidosis occurs only in (Type I) glucose-6-phosphatase deficiency.

REFERENCES

Ampola, M.G. (1982). *Metabolic disease in pediatric practice.* Boston: Little, Brown.

Burman, D., Holton, J.B., & Pennock, C.A. (eds.). (1978). *Inherited disorders of carbohydrate metabolism.* Baltimore: University Park Press.

Scriver, C.R., Beaudet, A.L., Sly, W.S., & Valle, D. (eds.). (1989). *The metabolic basis of inherited disease* (6th ed.). (Volume I and II). New York: McGraw-Hill.

Theorell, C.J. & Degenhardt, M. (1993). Assessment and management of metabolic dysfunction (pp. 480–

526). In C. Kenner, A. Brueggemeyer, & L.P. Gunderson (eds.), *Comprehensive neonatal nursing: A physiologic perspective.* Philadelphia: W.B. Saunders.

172. Answer: (**B**) In the newborn population, the most frequent cause of inappropriate ADH secretion is asphyxia, with signs including low serum osmolality; low serum potassium, chloride, and calcium; high urinary sodium in the face of severe hyponatremia; decreased free water clearance; and elevated urine specific gravity.

REFERENCES

Gamblien, V., Bivens, K., Burton, K.S., Kissler, C.H., Kleeman, T.A., Freije, M. & Prows, C. (1993). Assessment and management of endocrine dysfunction (pp. 527–552). In C. Kenner, A. Brueggemeyer, & L.P. Gunderson (eds.), *Comprehensive neonatal nursing: A physiologic perspective.* Philadelphia: W.B. Saunders.

Kinzie, B.J. (1987). Management of the syndrome of inappropriate secretion of antidiuretic hormone. *Clinical Pharmacy, 6,* 625–633.

Klaus, M.H. & Fanaroff, A.A. (1986). *Care of the high-risk neonate* (3rd ed.). Philadelphia: W.B. Saunders

173. Answer: (**B**) The most common signs of hypoglycemia are jitteriness, cyanosis, tachypnea, seizures, and apnea. Serum glucose levels need to be monitored frequently, and it may be necessary to provide the infant with early feedings or intravenous fluids to maintain a proper glucose level.

REFERENCES

Gamblien, V., Bivens, K., Burton, K.S., Kissler, C.H., Kleeman, T.A., Freije, M. & Prows, C. (1993). Assessment and management of endocrine dysfunction (pp. 527–552). In C. Kenner, A. Brueggemeyer, & L.P. Gunderson (eds.), *Comprehensive neonatal nursing: A physiologic perspective.* Philadelphia: W.B. Saunders.

Goetzman, B.W. & Wenneberg, R.P. (1991). *Neonatal intensive care handbook* (2nd ed.). St. Louis: Mosby-Year Book.

Perlman, R.H. (1983). The infant of the diabetic mother. *Primary Care, 10,* 751–760.

174. Answer: (**A**) The most common cause of ambiguous genitalia in the newborn is congenital adrenal hyperplasia.

REFERENCES

Gamblien, V., Bivens, K., Burton, K.S., Kissler, C.H., Kleeman, T.A., Freije, M. & Prows, C. (1993). Assessment and management of endocrine dysfunction (pp. 527–552). In C. Kenner, A. Brueggemeyer, & L.P. Gunderson (eds.), *Comprehensive neonatal nursing: A physiologic perspective.* Philadelphia: W.B. Saunders.

Griffin, J.E. & Wilson, J.D. (1986). Disorders of sexual differentiation. In P.C. Walsh, R.F. Gittes, A.D. Perlmutter, & T.A. Stamey (eds.), *Campbell's urology* (5th ed.). Philadelphia: W.B. Saunders.

Shapiro, E., Santiago, J.V., & Crane, J.P. (1989). Prenatal fetal adrenal suppression following in utero diagnosis of CAH. *Journal of Urology, 142*(Pt. 2), 663–666.

175. Answer: (**A**) Ionization requires an acid pH and occurs in the stomach.

REFERENCES

Costarino, A. & Baumgart, S. (1986). Modern fluid and electrolyte management of the critically ill premature infant. *Pediatric Clinics of North America, 33,* 153–158.

DeMarini, S., Tsang, R.C., & Rath, L.L. (1993). Fluids, electrolytes, vitamins, and trace minerals: Basis of ingestion, digestion, elimination, and metabolism (pp. 393–413). In C. Kenner, A. Brueggemeyer, & L.P. Gunderson (eds.), *Comprehensive neonatal nursing: A physiologic perspective.* Philadelphia: W.B. Saunders.

Pereira, G.R. & Zucker, A.H. (1986). Nutritional deficiencies in the neonate. *Clinics in Perinatology, 13,* 175–189.

176. Answer: (**B**) The chief symptom of ABO incompatibility is jaundice within the first 24 hours of life, with 90 percent of all affected infants being female.

REFERENCES

Maisels, M.J. (1990). Hyperbilirubinemia (pp. 258–262). In N.M. Nelson (ed.), *Current therapy in neonatal-perinatal medicine-2.* Philadelphia: B.C. Decker.

Shaw, N. (1993). Assessment and management of hematologic dysfunction (pp. 582–634). In C. Kenner, A. Brueggemeyer, & L.P. Gunderson (eds.), *Comprehensive neonatal nursing: A physiologic perspective.* Philadelphia: W.B. Saunders.

177. Answer: (**C**). Ribovirin administration is the drug of choice for respiratory syncytial virus.

REFERENCES

Lott, J.W., Nelson, K., Fahrner, R., & Kenner, C. (1993). Assessment and management of immunologic dysfunction (pp. 553–581). In C. Kenner, A. Brueggemeyer, & L. P. Gunderson (eds.), *Comprehensive neonatal nursing: A physiologic perspective.* Philadelphia: W.B. Saunders.

Prows, C.A. (1989). Ribavirin's risks in reproduction—How great are they? *MCN, 14*(6), 400–404.

Sweet, A.Y. (1991). Bacterial infections (pp. 84–167). In A.Y. Sweet & E.G. Brown (eds.), *Fetal and neonatal effects of maternal disease.* St. Louis: Mosby-Year Book.

Xanthou, M. (1987). Neonatal immunity (pp. 555–586). In L. Stern & P. Vert (eds.), *Neonatal medicine.* New York: Masson Publishing.

178. Answer: (**B**) A combination of ampicillin and gentamicin will provide adequate coverage for most gram-

positive and gram-negative organisms. Ampicillin and gentamicin provide antibacterial coverage against *Streptococci, Listeria monocytogenes,* and gram-negative enteric rods. These are the microorganisms most often associated with early onset sepsis.

REFERENCES

Lott, J.W. & Kilb, J.R. (1992). Selection of antimicrobials agents for treatment of neonatal sepsis: Which drug kills which bug. *Neonatal Pharmacology, 1*(1), 19–29, 1992.

Lott, J.W., Nelson, K., Fahrner, R., & Kenner, C. (1993). Assessment and management of immunologic dysfunction (pp. 553–581). In C. Kenner, A. Brueggemeyer, & L. P. Gunderson (eds.), *Comprehensive neonatal nursing: A physiologic perspective*. Philadelphia: W.B. Saunders.

Sweet, A.Y. (1991). Bacterial infections (pp. 84–167). In A.Y. Sweet & E.G. Brown (eds.), *Fetal and neonatal effects of maternal disease*. St. Louis: Mosby-Year Book.

179. Answer: (**A**) Vitamin E comprises several different compounds, named tocopherols, that are important biologic antioxidants; among these, α-tocopherol is believed to be most active. Vitamin E protects the polyunsaturated fatty acid of biologic membranes from peroxidation.

REFERENCES

DeMarini, S., Tsang, R.C., & Rath, L.L. (1993). Fluids, electrolytes, vitamins, and trace minerals: Basis of ingestion, digestion, elimination, and metabolism (pp. 393–413). In C. Kenner, A. Brueggemeyer, & L.P. Gunderson (eds.), *Comprehensive neonatal nursing: A physiologic perspective*. Philadelphia: W.B. Saunders.

Ehrenkranz, R.A., Ablow, R.C., & Warshaw, J.B. (1979). Prevention of bronchopulmonary dysplasia with vitamin E administration during the acute stages of respiratory distress syndrome. *Journal of Pediatrics, 95,* 873–878.

Finer, N.N., Schindler, R.F., Peters, K.L., & Grant, G.D. (1983). Vitamin E and retrolental fibroplasia. Improved visual outcome with early vitamin E. *Ophthalmology, 289,* 196–198.

Knight, M.E. & Roberts, R.J. (1986). Disposition of intravenously administered pharmacologic doses of vitamin E in newborn rabbits. *Journal of Pediatrics, 109,* 145–150.

180. Answer: (**A**) Nafcillin is very effective against gram-positive microorganisms, especially *Staphyloccocus aureus*. Gentamicin can be used in conjunction with nafcillin to provide broad-spectrum coverage.

REFERENCES

Lott, J.W. & Kilb, J.R. (1992). Selection of antimicrobials agents for treatment of neonatal sepsis: Which drug kills which bug. *Neonatal Pharmacology, 1*(1), 19–29, 1992.

Sweet, A.Y. (1991). Bacterial infections (pp. 84–167). In A.Y. Sweet & E.G. Brown (eds.), *Fetal and neonatal effects of maternal disease*. St. Louis: Mosby-Year Book.

181. Answer: (**A**) Factors affecting early RBC production are still unclear but erythropoietin has been identified as a major stimulant of erythropoiesis during the final months of gestation and throughout adult life.

REFERENCES

Oski, F. & Naiman, J. (1982c). Normal blood values in the newborn period. In F. Oski & J. Naiman (eds.), *Hematologic problems in the newborn. Vol IV. Major problems in clinical pediatrics* (3rd ed.). (pp. 1–31). Philadelphia: W.B. Saunders.

Shaw, N. (1993). Assessment and management of hematologic dysfunction (pp. 582–634). In C. Kenner, A. Brueggemeyer, & L.P. Gunderson (eds.), *Comprehensive neonatal nursing: A physiologic perspective*. Philadelphia: W.B. Saunders.

182. Answer: (**C**) Type B blood has B antigen on the cell surface and anti-A antibodies in the plasma. AB blood has A and B antigens on the cell surface and neither antibody in the plasma, whereas O type blood has neither antigen on the cell surface and both anti-A and B in the plasma. Though incompatibility can occur between A and B types, it is not seen as frequently as AO or BO because of the globulin composition of the antibodies. In the O type mother, the antibodies are usually IgG and can cross the placenta, whereas the antibodies of the type A or B mother frequently are IgM, which are too large to cross the placenta.

REFERENCES

Gomella, T.L. (1992). *Neonatalogy* (2nd ed.). Norwalk, CT: Appleton & Lange.

Polin, R.A. & Fox, W.W. (1992). *Fetal and neonatal physiology*. Philadelphia: W.B. Saunders.

Shaw, N. (1993). Assessment and management of hematologic dysfunction (pp. 582–634). In C. Kenner, A. Brueggemeyer, & L.P. Gunderson (eds.), *Comprehensive neonatal nursing: A physiologic perspective*. Philadelphia: W.B. Saunders.

183. Answer: (**B**) Other potential risks are maternal complications (i.e., premature rupture of membranes and abruption) and graft versus host phenomenon from transfusion of lymphocytes, which can be modified through the use of irradiated blood.

REFERENCES

Mollison, P. (1984). *Blood transfusion in clinical medicine* (7th ed.) (pp. 675). Oxford: Blackwell Scientific.

Gomella, T.L. (1992). *Neonatology* (2nd ed.). Norwalk, CT: Appleton & Lange.

Shaw, N. (1993). Assessment and management of hematologic dysfunction (pp. 582–634). In C. Kenner, A. Brueggemeyer, & L.P. Gunderson (eds.), *Comprehensive neonatal nursing: A physiologic perspective*. Philadelphia: W.B. Saunders.

184. Answer: (**C**) Glucuronyl transferase is the important hepatic enzyme required for the production of bilirubin glucuronide. About 95 percent of bilirubin glucuronide is excreted into bile and subsequently into the intestine.

REFERENCES

Oski, F. & Naiman, J. (1982b). Erythroblastosis fetalis (pp. 283–346). In F. Oski & J. Naiman (eds.), *Hematologic problems in the newborn. Vol IV. Major problems in clinical pediatrics*. (3rd ed.). Philadelphia: W.B. Saunders.

Shaw, N. (1993). Assessment and management of hematologic dysfunction (pp. 582–634). In C. Kenner, A. Brueggemeyer, & L.P. Gunderson (eds.), *Comprehensive neonatal nursing: A physiologic perspective*. Philadelphia: W.B. Saunders.

185. Answer: (**A**) Bilirubin removal is much less effective, with only 25 percent of the infant's total body bilirubin being removed during a double-volume exchange. This probably occurs because the major portion of bilirubin is in the extravascular compartment, an area not affected by the exchange of blood volume.

REFERENCES

Gomella, T.L. (1992). *Neonatology* (2nd ed.). Norwalk, CT: Appleton & Lange.

Polin, R.A. & Fox, W.W. (1992). *Fetal and neonatal physiology*. Philadelphia: W.B. Saunders.

Shaw, N. (1993). Assessment and management of hematologic dysfunction (pp. 582–634). In C. Kenner, A. Brueggemeyer, & L.P. Gunderson (eds.), *Comprehensive neonatal nursing: A physiologic perspective*. Philadelphia: W.B. Saunders.

186. Answer: (**C**) Vitamin K is not directly involved in the synthesis of these factors but is required for the conversion of precursor proteins, also produced by the liver, into active factors having coagulant capabilities.

REFERENCES

Gomella, T.L. (1992). *Neonatology* (2nd ed.). Norwalk, CT: Appleton & Lange.

Jackson, C. & Suttu, J. (1977). Recent developments in understanding the mechanism of vitamin K and vitamin K antagonist drug action and the consequences of vitamin K action in blood coagulation. *Progress In Hematology, 10*, 333.

Polin, R.A. & Fox, W.W. (1992). *Fetal and neonatal physiology*. Philadelphia: W.B. Saunders.

Shaw, N. (1993). Assessment and management of hematologic dysfunction (pp. 582–634). In C. Kenner, A. Brueggemeyer, & L.P. Gunderson (eds.), *Comprehensive neonatal nursing: A physiologic perspective*. Philadelphia: W.B. Saunders.

187. Answer: (**C**) Myeloschisis is a severe defect in which there is no cystic covering so the spinal cord is open and exposed.

REFERENCES

Blackburn, S.T. (1993). Assessment and management of neurologic dysfunction (pp. 635–689). In C. Kenner, A. Brueggemeyer, & L.P. Gunderson (eds.), *Comprehensive neonatal nursing: A physiologic perspective*. Philadelphia: W.B. Saunders.

Polin, R.A. & Fox, W.W. (1992). *Fetal and neonatal physiology*. Philadelphia: W.B. Saunders.

188. Answer: (**C**) Vitamin E is required in increasing amounts as the intake of polyunsaturated fatty acids increases.

REFERENCES

Gomella, T.L. (1992). *Neonatology* (2nd ed.). Norwalk, CT: Appleton & Lange.

Polin, R.A. & Fox, W.W. (1992). *Fetal and neonatal physiology*. Philadelphia: W.B. Saunders.

Shaw, N. (1993). Assessment and management of hematologic dysfunction (pp. 582–634). In C. Kenner, A. Brueggemeyer, & L.P. Gunderson (eds.), *Comprehensive neonatal nursing: A physiologic perspective*. Philadelphia: W.B. Saunders.

Tsang, R.C. & Nichols, B.L. (eds.). (1988). *Nutrition during infancy*. Philadelphia: Hanley & Belfus.

189. Answer: (**A**) Depolarization and repolarization of the nerve are produced by the movement of sodium and potassium across the cell membrane. The inward migration of Na^{2+} results in depolarization; repolarization is produced by the outward migration of K^{+}.

REFERENCES

Blackburn, S.T. (1993). Assessment and management of neurologic dysfunction (pp. 635–689). In C. Kenner, A. Brueggemeyer, & L.P. Gunderson (eds.), *Comprehensive neonatal nursing: A physiologic perspective*. Philadelphia: W.B. Saunders.

Polin, R.A. & Fox, W.W. (1992). *Fetal and neonatal physiology*. Philadelphia: W.B. Saunders.

190. Answer: (**C**) Seizures associated with sever birth asphyxia, grade III or IV intraventricular hemorrhage, herpes infection, some bacterial meningitides, and CNS malformations have the poorest prognosis.

REFERENCES

Blackburn, S.T. (1993). Assessment and management of neurologic dysfunction (pp. 635–689). In C. Kenner, A. Brueggemeyer, & L.P. Gunderson (eds.), *Comprehensive neonatal nursing: A physiologic perspective*. Philadelphia: W.B. Saunders.

Gomella, T.L. (1992). *Neonatalogy* (2nd ed.). Norwalk, CT: Appleton & Lange.

Polin, R.A. & Fox, W.W. (1992). *Fetal and neonatal physiology*. Philadelphia: W.B. Saunders.

191. Answer: **(C)** The clinical signs that correlate most closely with CT evidence of hemorrhage are (1) a falling hematocrit, or failure of the hematocrit to rise after a transfusion; (2) full anterior fontanel; (3) changes in activity level; and (4) decreased tone.

REFERENCES

Blackburn, S.T. (1993). Assessment and management of neurologic dysfunction (pp. 635–689). In C. Kenner, A. Brueggemeyer, & L.P. Gunderson (eds.), *Comprehensive neonatal nursing: A physiologic perspective*. Philadelphia: W.B. Saunders.

Volpe, J.J. (1987). *Neurology of the newborn* (2nd ed.). Philadelphia: W.B. Saunders.

192. Answer: **(C)** Infants with uncomplicated linear fractures require no special management. They should be observed closely.

REFERENCES

Blackburn, S.T. (1993). Assessment and management of neurologic dysfunction (pp. 635–689). In C. Kenner, A. Brueggemeyer, & L.P. Gunderson (eds.), *Comprehensive neonatal nursing: A physiologic perspective*. Philadelphia: W.B. Saunders.

Gomella, T.L. (1992). *Neonatalogy* (2nd ed.). Norwalk, CT: Appleton & Lange.

Merenstein, G. B. & Gardner, S.L. (1993). *Handbook of neonatal intensive care* (2nd ed.). St. Louis: Mosby.

193. Answer: **(C)** Vitamin C deficiency is associated with transient tyrosinemia and neonatal scurvy.

REFERENCES

DeMarini, S., Tsang, R.C., & Rath, L.L. (1993). Fluids, electrolytes, vitamins, and trace minerals: Basis of ingestion, digestion, elimination, and metabolism (pp. 393–413). In C. Kenner, A. Brueggemeyer, & L.P. Gunderson (eds.), *Comprehensive neonatal nursing: A physiologic perspective*. Philadelphia: W.B. Saunders.

Schanler, R.J. (1988). Water-soluble vitamins: C, B_1, B_2, B_6, niacin, biotin and pantothenic acid (pp. 236–252). In R.C. Tsang & B.L. Nichols (eds.), *Nutrition during infancy*. St. Louis: C.V. Mosby.

194. Answer: **(C)** Median and sciatic nerve injuries are generally postnatal iatrogenic events. Median nerve injury can be a complication of brachial or radial arterial punctures.

REFERENCES

Blackburn, S.T. (1993). Assessment and management of neurologic dysfunction (pp. 635–689). In C. Kenner, A. Brueggemeyer, & L.P. Gunderson (eds.), *Comprehensive neonatal nursing: A physiologic perspective*. Philadelphia: W.B. Saunders.

Gomella, T.L. (1992). *Neonatalogy* (2nd ed.). Norwalk, CT: Appleton & Lange.

Merenstein, G.B. & Gardner, S.L. (1993). *Handbook of neonatal intensive care* (2nd ed.). St. Louis: Mosby.

195. Answer: **(A)** The most common malformations are stenosis of the aqueduct of Sylvius, Dandy-Walker syndrome, and Arnold-Chiari malformation. Aqueductal (Sylvius) stenosis is the most common malformation associated with hydrocephalus, accounting for about two thirds of infants with congenital hydrocephalus.

REFERENCES

Blackburn, S.T. (1993). Assessment and management of neurologic dysfunction (pp. 635–689). In C. Kenner, A. Brueggemeyer, & L.P. Gunderson (eds.), *Comprehensive neonatal nursing: A physiologic perspective*. Philadelphia: W.B. Saunders.

Gomella, T.L. (1992). *Neonatalogy* (2nd ed.). Norwalk, CT: Appleton & Lange.

Merenstein, G.B. & Gardner, S.L. (1993). *Handbook of neonatal intensive care* (2nd ed.). St. Louis: Mosby.

196. Answer: **(B)** Achondroplasia, while once used to describe any form of dwarfism, is now recognized as one distinct type of dwarfism with characteristic features. Achondroplasia, the most common type of dwarfism, has an autosomal dominant pattern of inheritance. The majority of cases occur by spontaneous mutation. Achondroplasia occurs in three of every 1 million live births.

REFERENCES

Butler, J. (1993). Assessment and management of musculoskeletal dysfunction (pp. 690–705). In C. Kenner, A. Brueggemeyer, & L.P. Gunderson (eds.), *Comprehensive neonatal nursing: A physiologic perspective*. Philadelphia: W.B. Saunders.

Fanaroff, A.A. & Martin, R.J. (1992). *Neonatal-perinatal medicine* (5th ed.). St. Louis: Mosby.

Gardner, R.J.M. (1977). A new estimate of the achondroplasia mutation rate. *Clinical Genetics, 11*, 31.

197. Answer: **(C)** The last layer, that which actually lines the lumen of the gut, is known as the mucosa and con-

tains most of the exocrine gland cells and epithelial cells.

REFERENCES

Loper, D.L. (1983). Gastrointestinal development: Embryology, congenital anomalies, and impact on feedings. *Neonatal Network, 2*(1), 27–36.

McCollum, L.L. & Thigpen, J.L. (1993). Assessment and management of gastrointestinal dysfunction (pp. 434–479). In C. Kenner, A. Brueggemeyer, & L.P. Gunderson (eds.), *Comprehensive neonatal nursing: A physiologic perspective*. Philadelphia: W.B. Saunders.

Moore, K.L. (1989). *Before we are born: Basic embryology and birth defects* (3rd ed.). Philadelphia: W.B. Saunders.

Sadler, T.W. (1985). *Langman's medical embryology* (5th ed.). Baltimore: Williams & Wilkins.

198. Answer: (**C**) Achondroplasia, while once used to describe any form of dwarfism, is now recognized as one distinct type of dwarfism with characteristic features. Achondroplasia, the most common type of dwarfism, has an autosomal dominant pattern of inheritance. Most cases occur by spontaneous mutation. Achondroplasia occurs in three of every 1 million live births (Gardner, 1977).

Distal arthrogryposis is inherited by an autosomal dominant pattern. Parents with an infant with distal arthrogryposis can have a risk calculation done by a genetics counselor to give them an idea of their potential for having another child with this same condition.

Differences in incidence rates of CDH can be attributed to genetic, ethnic, and environmental influences. Other influential factors include the age of the infant at the time of examination, the expertise of the examiner, and the definition used by the examiner for the diagnosis of CDH.

REFERENCES

Butler, J. (1993). Assessment and management of musculoskeletal dysfunction (pp. 690–705). In C. Kenner, A. Brueggemeyer, & L.P. Gunderson (eds.), *Comprehensive neonatal nursing: A physiologic perspective*. Philadelphia: W.B. Saunders.

Gardner, R.J.M. (1977). A new estimate of the achondroplasia mutation rate. *Clinical Genetics, 11*, 31.

Clark, D.R. & Eteson, D.J. (1991). Congenital anomalies (pp. 159–191). In H.W. Taeusch, R.A. Ballard, & M.E. Avery (eds.), *Schaffer and Avery's diseases of the newborn*. (6th ed.). Philadelphia: W.B. Saunders.

199. Answer: (**B**) In the neonatal period, the neonatal nurse specialist is greatly assisted in diagnosing CDH through the Ortolani and Barlow maneuvers. The Ortolani procedure determines dislocation in the hip of a newborn, whereas the Barlow procedure is used to determine whether the hip is dislocatable (Barlow, 1962; Ortolani, 1976). In practice, both procedures are done in sequence. For examination, the infant is placed on a firm surface in the supine position. The infant should be relaxed and quiet. Examine only one hip at a time.

REFERENCES

Barlow, T.G. (1962). Early diagnosis and treatment of congenital dislocation of the hip. *Journal of Bone and Joint Surgery, 44B*, 292–301.

Butler, J. (1993). Assessment and management of musculoskeletal dysfunction (pp. 690–705). In C. Kenner, A. Brueggemeyer, & L.P. Gunderson (eds.), *Comprehensive neonatal nursing: A physiologic perspective*. Philadelphia: W.B. Saunders.

Ortolani, M. (1976). The classic: Congenital hip dysplasia in the light of early and very early diagnosis. *Clinical Orthopedics and Related Research, 119*, 6–10.

200. Answer: (**A**) The Barlow procedure is used to determine whether the hip is dislocatable (Barlow, 1962; Ortolani, 1976).

REFERENCES

Barlow, T.G. (1962). Early diagnosis and treatment of congenital dislocation of the hip. *Journal of Bone and Joint Surgery, 44B*, 292–301.

Butler, J. (1993). Assessment and management of musculoskeletal dysfunction (pp. 690–705). In C. Kenner, A. Brueggemeyer, & L.P. Gunderson (eds.), *Comprehensive neonatal nursing: A physiologic perspective*. Philadelphia: W.B. Saunders.

Ortolani, M. (1976). The classic: Congenital hip dysplasia in the light of early and very early diagnosis. *Clinical Orthopedics and Related Research, 119*, 6–10.

201. Answer: (**B**) The goal of collaborative management is to achieve and maintain reduction of the unstable hip. This goal may be achieved with hip splinting. The sooner treatment is implemented, the greater are the chances for successful outcome.

REFERENCES

Butler, J. (1993). Assessment and management of musculoskeletal dysfunction (pp. 690–705). In C. Kenner, A. Brueggemeyer, & L.P. Gunderson (eds.), *Comprehensive neonatal nursing: A physiologic perspective*. Philadelphia: W.B. Saunders.

Gomella, T.L. (1992). *Neonatalogy* (2nd ed.). Norwalk, CT: Appleton & Lange.

202. Answer: (**A**) The classic clubfoot, talipes equinovarus, refers to a dysmorphic appearing foot with hindfoot equinus, forefoot adduction, and midfoot supination. The term clubfoot also may be used to describe milder talipes conditions including talipes calcaneous, and talipes varus.

REFERENCES

Butler, J. (1993). Assessment and management of musculoskeletal dysfunction (pp. 690–705). In C. Kenner, A. Brueggemeyer, & L.P. Gunderson (eds.), *Comprehensive neonatal nursing: A physiologic perspective.* Philadelphia: W.B. Saunders.

Gomella, T.L. (1992). *Neonatalogy* (2nd ed.). Norwalk, CT: Appleton & Lange.

203. Answer: (**C**) The precise mechanism for the development of clubfoot has not been established. Some researchers allude to the theory of intrauterine malposition, whereas others, noting a higher incidence of clubfoot in families with a positive history of the disorder, ascribe to a genetic causation (Fine, Gwinn, & Young, 1968; MacLeod & Patriguin, 1974; & Tachdijian, 1985). Gaining popularity is the theory that clubfoot is a multifactorial disorder indicating a genetic predisposition coupled with environmental forces such as oligohydramnios, primiparity, macrosomia, and multiple fetuses (Palmer, Conneally, & Yu, 1974; Wynne-Davies, 1972).

REFERENCES

Butler, J. (1993). Assessment and management of musculoskeletal dysfunction (pp. 690–705). In C. Kenner, A. Brueggemeyer, & L.P. Gunderson (eds.), *Comprehensive neonatal nursing: A physiologic perspective.* Philadelphia: W.B. Saunders.

Fine, R.N., Gwinn, J.L., & Young, E.F. (1968). Smith-Lemli-Opitz syndrome: Radiologic and postmortem findings. *American Journal of Diseases of Childhood, 115,* 482–488.

MacLeod, P. & Patriguin, H. (1974). The whistling face syndrome: Cranio-carpo-tarsal dysplasia. Report of a case and survey of the literature. *Clinical Pediatrics, 13,* 184–189.

Tachdijian, M. (1985). Congenital deformities: Congenital talipes equinovarus (pp. 139–170). In M. Tachdijian (ed.), *The child's foot.* Philadelphia: W.B. Saunders.

Palmer, R.M., Conneally, P.M., & Yu, P.L. (1974). Studies of the inheritance of idiopathic talipes equinovarus. *Orthopedic Clinics of North America, 5,* 99–108.

Wynne-Davies, R. (1964). Family studies and cause of congenital clubfoot. *Journal of Bone and Joint Surgery, 46B,* 445–465.

204. Answer: (**C**) The type and timing of treatment depends on the classification. Surgery is directed toward promoting normal function and appearance. Fingers of unequal length should be separated within 6–12 months of age to prevent curvature of the longer finger deviated toward the shorter finger. If more than two adjacent digits are involved, surgery should be performed in stages to prevent vascular compromise of the middle digits.

REFERENCES

Butler, J. (1993). Assessment and management of musculoskeletal dysfunction (pp. 690–705). In C. Kenner, A. Brueggemeyer, & L.P. Gunderson (eds.), *Comprehensive neonatal nursing: A physiologic perspective.* Philadelphia: W.B. Saunders.

Gomella, T.L. (1992). *Neonatalogy* (2nd ed.). Norwalk, CT: Appleton & Lange.

205. Answer: (**C**) Amniotic band syndrome with an incidence ranging from 1 in 5000 to 1 in 15,000 live births is characterized by uncommon, asymmetric fetal deformities (Ossipoff & Hall, 1977). Deformities attributed to the amniotic band syndrome include congenital limb amputation, syndactyly, constriction bands, clubfeet, craniofacial defects such as cleft lip and palate, and visceral defects such as gastroschisis and omphalocele.

The exogenous, and seemingly more popular, theory contends that early amniotic rupture allows the fetus to move into close approximation to the chorion by entering the chorionic activity. The ruptured amnion then forms fibrous strings or bands. These bands can adhere to the skin causing alterations of normal morphogenesis, that is, cleft lip/palate, omphalocele, or disrupt the vascular integrity resulting in gastroschisis.

REFERENCES

Butler, J. (1993). Assessment and management of musculoskeletal dysfunction (pp. 690–705). In C. Kenner, A. Brueggemeyer, & L.P. Gunderson (eds.), *Comprehensive neonatal nursing: A physiologic perspective.* Philadelphia: W.B. Saunders.

Ossipoff, V. & Hall, B.D. (1977). Etiologic factors in the amniotic band syndrome: A study of 24 patients. *Birth Defects, 13,* 117–132.

206. Answer: (**B**) The kidney performs several critical functions for the neonate: (1) secretion; (2) reabsorption, and (3) excretion.

REFERENCES

Kenner, C. & Brueggemeyer, A. (1993). Assessment and management of genitourinary dysfunction (pp. 706–741). In C. Kenner, A. Brueggemeyer, & L.P. Gunderson (eds.), *Comprehensive neonatal nursing: A physiologic perspective*. Philadelphia: W.B. Saunders.

Vander, A.J. (1985). Renal physiology (3rd ed.). New York: McGraw-Hill.

207. Answer: (**A**) Tubular secretion is the process by which substances are moved from the epithelial lining of the tubule's capillaries into the interstitial fluid and finally into the lumen.

REFERENCES

Kenner, C. & Brueggemeyer, A. (1993). Assessment and management of genitourinary dysfunction (pp. 706–741). In C. Kenner, A. Brueggemeyer, & L.P. Gunderson (eds.), *Comprehensive neonatal nursing: A physiologic perspective*. Philadelphia: W.B. Saunders.

Vander, A.J. (1985). Renal physiology (3rd ed.). New York: McGraw-Hill.

208. Answer: (**B**) Kidney function with production of fetal urine is established by the eighth week of gestation.

REFERENCES

Kenner, C. & Brueggemeyer, A. (1993). Assessment and management of genitourinary dysfunction (pp. 706–741). In C. Kenner, A. Brueggemeyer, & L.P. Gunderson (eds.), *Comprehensive neonatal nursing: A physiologic perspective*. Philadelphia: W.B. Saunders.

Gomella, T.L. (1992). *Neonatology* (2nd ed.). Norwalk, CT: Appleton & Lange.

Polin, R.A. & Fox, W.W. (1992). *Fetal and neonatal physiology*. Philadelphia: W.B. Saunders.

Vander, A.J. (1985). Renal physiology (3rd ed.). New York: McGraw-Hill.

209. Answer: (**A**) It is the glomerulus, Bowman's capsule, and tubules that constitute a nephron, a part of the excretory system and site of urine formation.

REFERENCES

José, P.A., Stewart, C.L., Tina, L.U., & Calcano, P.L. (1987). Renal disease (pp. 795–849). In G.B. Avery (ed.), *Neonatology: Pathophysiology and management of the newborn* (3rd ed.). Philadelphia: W.B. Saunders.

Kenner, C. & Brueggemeyer, A. (1993). Assessment and management of genitourinary dysfunction (pp. 706–741). In C. Kenner, A. Brueggemeyer, & L.P. Gunderson (eds.), *Comprehensive neonatal nursing: A physiologic perspective*. Philadelphia: W.B. Saunders.

Moore, K. (1988). *The developing human: Clinically oriented embryology* (4th ed.). Philadelphia: W.B. Saunders.

210. Answer: (**C**) Hydraulic pressure with the capillary depends on renal blood flow.

REFERENCES

Kenner, C. & Brueggemeyer, A. (1993). Assessment and management of genitourinary dysfunction (pp. 706–741). In C. Kenner, A. Brueggemeyer, & L.P. Gunderson (eds.), *Comprehensive neonatal nursing: A physiologic perspective*. Philadelphia: W.B. Saunders.

Vander, A.J. (1985). Renal physiology (3rd ed.). New York: McGraw-Hill.

211. Answer: (**C**) The ultimate goal of the renin-angiotensin cycle is to maintain systemic blood flow adequate enough to supply the body's vital organs.

REFERENCES

Kenner, C. & Brueggemeyer, A. (1993). Assessment and management of genitourinary dysfunction (pp. 706–741). In C. Kenner, A. Brueggemeyer, & L.P. Gunderson (eds.), *Comprehensive neonatal nursing: A physiologic perspective*. Philadelphia: W.B. Saunders.

Vander, A.J. (1985). Renal physiology (3rd ed.). New York: McGraw-Hill.

212. Answer: (**A**) Calcium absorption occurs through a carrier-mediated mechanism and passive diffusion. The carrier-mediated mechanism depends on a vitamin D_3 metabolite.

REFERENCES

Lebenthal, E. (ed.). (1989). *Textbook of gastroenterology and nutrition in infancy*. New York: Raven Press.

Lefrak-Okikawa, L. & Meier, P.P. (1993). Nutrition: Physiologic basis of metabolism and management of enteral and parenteral nutrition (pp. 414–433). In C. Kenner, A. Brueggemeyer, & L.P. Gunderson (eds.), *Comprehensive neonatal nursing: A physiologic perspective*. Philadelphia: W.B. Saunders.

Tsang, R.E. & Nichols, B.L. (eds.). (1988). *Nutrition during infancy*. Philadelphia: Hanley & Belfus.

213. Answer: (**C**) The safest and one of the most useful tests to determine renal anomalies is the use of ultrasonography.

REFERENCES

Gomella, T.L. (1992). *Neonatology* (2nd ed.). Norwalk, CT: Appleton & Lange.

Kenner, C. & Brueggemeyer, A. (1993). Assessment and management of genitourinary dysfunction (pp. 706–741). In C. Kenner, A. Brueggemeyer, & L.P. Gunderson (eds.), *Comprehensive neonatal nursing: A physiologic perspective*. Philadelphia: W.B. Saunders.

Vander, A.J. (1985). Renal physiology (3rd ed.). New York: McGraw-Hill.

214. Answer: (**B**) IgG is the immunoglobulin that is transferred most readily across the placenta. The IgG effectively protects the infant against Group A *Streptococcus* and *Treponema pallidum*.

REFERENCES

Faden, H. & Rosales, S. (1984). Infections in the compromised neonate (pp. 185–202). In P.L. Ocra (ed.), *Neonatal infections: Nutritional and immunologic interactions*. Orlando, FL: Grune & Stratton.

Kenner, C. & Brueggemeyer, A. (1993). Assessment and management of genitourinary dysfunction (pp. 706–741). In C. Kenner, A. Brueggemeyer, & L.P. Gunderson (eds.), *Comprehensive neonatal nursing: A physiologic perspective*. Philadelphia: W.B. Saunders.

215. Answer: (**A**) Hydronephrosis is the accumulation of urine within the renal pelvis and calices to the point of overdistention. Hydronephrosis often follows obstruction of urine flow at the junction of the ureteropelvis, ureterovesical valve, or urethrovesical valve.

REFERENCES

Kenner, C. & Brueggemeyer, A. (1993). Assessment and management of genitourinary dysfunction (pp. 706–741). In C. Kenner, A. Brueggemeyer, & L.P. Gunderson (eds.), *Comprehensive neonatal nursing: A physiologic perspective*. Philadelphia: W.B. Saunders.

Vander, A.J. (1985). Renal physiology (3rd ed.). New York: McGraw-Hill.

216. Answer: (**B**) The single most significant concern is infection.

REFERENCES

Baley, J. & Silverman, R. (1988). Systemic candidiasis: Cutaneous manifestations in low birth weight infants. *Pediatrics, 82*(2), 211–215.

Baley, J., Kliegman, R., Boxerbaum, B., & Fanaroff, A. (1986). Fungal colonization in the very low birth weight infant. *Pediatrics, 78,* 225–232.

D'Angio, C., McGowan, K., Baumgart, S., Geme, J., & Harris, M.C. (1989). Surface colonization with coagulase-negative staphylococci in premature neonates. *Journal of Pediatrics, 114,* 1029–1034.

Kuller, J.M. & Lund, C.H. (1993). Assessment and management of integumentary dysfunction (pp. 742–781). In C. Kenner, A. Brueggemeyer, & L.P. Gunderson (eds.), *Comprehensive neonatal nursing: A physiologic perspective*. Philadelphia: W.B. Saunders.

Patrick, C. (1990). Coagulase-negative staphylococci: Pathogens with increasing clinical significance. *Journal of Pediatrics, 116,* 497–507.

Patrick, C., Kaplan, S., Baker, C., Parisi, J., & Mason, E. (1989). Persistent bacteremia due to coagulase-negative staphylococci in premature neonates. *Pediatrics, 84,* 977–985.

217. Answer: (**B**) Normally, the tympanic membrane appears translucent in character. White shadows of the ossicles can usually be seen through the membrane. Otitis media does occur in the first days of life and can be diagnosed by otoscopic exam. Otitis media often presents as a poorly mobile, bulging, yellow, opacified tympanic membrane.

REFERENCES

Haubrich, K. (1993). Assessment and management of auditory dysfunction (pp. 782–808). In C. Kenner, A. Brueggemeyer, & L.P. Gunderson (eds.), *Comprehensive neonatal nursing: A physiologic perspective*. Philadelphia: W.B. Saunders.

Schwartz, R. & Rodriguez, W.J. (1981). Acute otitis media in children eight years old and older: A reappraisal of the role of *Hemophilus influenzae*. *American Journal of Otolaryngology, 2*(1), 19–21.

218. Answer: (**A**) During weeks 26–29 of gestation, subcutaneous fat begins to be deposited and starts to smooth out the many wrinkles in the skin.

REFERENCES

Ackerman, A. (1985). Structure and function of the skin. In S. Moschella & H. Hurley (eds.), *Dermatology* (2nd ed.). (Vol. II). Philadelphia: W.B. Saunders.

Kuller, J.M. & Lund, C.H. (1993). Assessment and management of integumentary dysfunction (pp. 742–781). In C. Kenner, A. Brueggemeyer, & L.P. Gunderson (eds.), *Comprehensive neonatal nursing: A physiologic perspective*. Philadelphia: W. B. Saunders.

219. Answer: (**A**) Photosensitivity in the full-term infant can be due to melanin production that is low. The infant will sunburn easily.

REFERENCES

Kuller, J.M. & Lund, C.H. (1993). Assessment and management of integumentary dysfunction (pp. 742–781). In C. Kenner, A. Brueggemeyer, & L.P. Gunderson (eds.), *Comprehensive neonatal nursing: A physiologic perspective*. Philadelphia: W. B. Saunders.

Shalita, A. (1981). *Principles of infant skin care* (pp. 6–18). Skillman, NJ: Johnson & Johnson Baby Products.

220. Answer: (**A**) Sensorineural hearing loss can present as a congenital inner ear abnormality, resulting in congenital deafness. Other conditions that can result in sensorineural hearing loss include trauma to the inner ear from injury, effects of certain drugs, prolonged exposure to loud noise, infec-

tions, infectious conditions such as measles, and effects of aging.

REFERENCES

Beachy, P. & Deacon, J. (eds.). (1993). *Core curriculum for neonatal intensive care.* Philadelphia: W.B. Saunders.

Haubrich, K. (1993). Assessment and management of auditory dysfunction (pp. 782–808). In C. Kenner, A. Brueggemeyer, & L.P. Gunderson (eds.), *Comprehensive neonatal nursing: A physiologic perspective.* Philadelphia: W.B. Saunders.

Hoekelman, R.A., Friedman, S.B., Nelson, N.M., & Seidel, H.M. (1992). *Primary pediatric care* (2nd ed.). St. Louis: C.V. Mosby.

221. Answer: (**A**) Cutis marmorata or mottling is a normal physiologic vascular response to cool air.

REFERENCES

Avery, G. (1987). *Neonatology* (3rd ed.). Philadelphia: J.B. Lippincott.

Kuller, J.M. & Lund, C.H. (1993). Assessment and management of integumentary dysfunction (pp. 742–781). In C. Kenner, A. Brueggemeyer, & L.P. Gunderson (eds.), *Comprehensive neonatal nursing: A physiologic perspective.* Philadelphia: W. B. Saunders.

222. Answer: (**A**) Caput succedaneum is a diffuse, generalized edema of the scalp caused by local pressure and trauma during labor. The borders are not well defined, and the swelling crosses suture lines.

REFERENCES

Kuller, J. (1990). In M. Auvenshine & M. Enriquez (eds.), *Comprehensive maternity nursing: Perinatal and women's health* (2nd ed). Boston: Jones and Bartlett.

Kuller, J.M. & Lund, C.H. (1993). Assessment and management of integumentary dysfunction (pp. 742–781). In C. Kenner, A. Brueggemeyer, & L.P. Gunderson (eds.), *Comprehensive neonatal nursing: A physiologic perspective.* Philadelphia: W. B. Saunders.

223. Answer: (**C**) Dysphagia can occur from facial and pharyngeal scarring, which is secondary to erosions on the buccal mucosa, tongue, palate, esophagus, and pharynx.

REFERENCES

Hymes, D. (1983). Epidermolysis bullosa in the neonate. *Neonatal Network, 1*(4), 36–39.

Kuller, J.M. & Lund, C.H. (1993). Assessment and management of integumentary dysfunction (pp. 742–781). In C. Kenner, A. Brueggemeyer, & L.P. Gunderson (eds.), *Comprehensive neonatal nursing: A physiologic perspective.* Philadelphia: W. B. Saunders.

224. Answer: (**B**) Vibroacoustic stimulation by use of an artificial larynx attached to the mother's abdomen has been reported to test well-being in the fetus.

REFERENCES

Haubrich, K. (1993). Assessment and management of auditory dysfunction (pp. 782–808). In C. Kenner, A. Brueggemeyer, & L.P. Gunderson (eds.), *Comprehensive neonatal nursing: A physiologic perspective.* Philadelphia: W. B. Saunders.

Jensen, O.H. (1984). Fetal heart rate response to a controlled sound stimulus as a measure of fetal well-being. *Acta Obstetrica et Gynecologica Scandinavica, 63*(2), 97–101.

225. Answer: (**B**) Blueberry muffin syndrome is a result of erythropoiesis in the dermis of infants with cytomegalovirus or rubella.

REFERENCES

Fanaroff, A.A. & Martin, R.J. (1992). *Neonatal-perinatal medicine* (5th ed.). St. Louis: C.V. Mosby.

Gomella, T.L. (1992). *Neonatology* (2nd ed.). Norwalk, CT: Appleton & Lange.

Kuller, J.M. & Lund, C.H. (1993). Assessment and management of integumentary dysfunction (pp. 742–781). In C. Kenner, A. Brueggemeyer, & L.P. Gunderson (eds.), *Comprehensive neonatal nursing: A physiologic perspective.* Philadelphia: W. B. Saunders.

Merenstein, G. B. & Gardner, S. L. (1993). *Handbook of neonatal intensive care* (pp. 338–339). (2nd ed.). St. Louis: Mosby.

Solmon, L. & Esterly, N. (1987). The skin (pp. 1172–1199). In A.A. Fanaroff & R.J. Martin (eds.), *Neonatal-perinatal medicine: Diseases of the fetus and infant* (4th ed.). St. Louis: C.V. Mosby.

226. Answer: (**B**) Avoid the use of plasticized polymers such as Skin Gel, Skin Prep, and Bard Protective Film because the effects of absorption are unknown.

REFERENCES

Kuller, J. & Tobin, C. (1990). Skin care management of the low-birthweight infant. In L. Gunderson & C. Kenner (eds.), *Care of the 24–25 week gestational age infant.* Petaluma, CA: Neonatal Network.

Kuller, J.M. & Lund, C.H. (1993). Assessment and management of integumentary dysfunction (pp. 742–781). In C. Kenner, A. Brueggemeyer, & L.P. Gunderson (eds.), *Comprehensive neonatal nursing: A physiologic perspective.* Philadelphia: W. B. Saunders.

227. Answer: (**C**) Environmental sounds have their greatest impact in shaping auditory ability from the time that the inner ear and the eighth cranial nerve become functional to the time of central nervous system (CNS) maturation—approximately five months' gestation to between 18 and 28 months of age.

REFERENCES

Haubrich, K. (1993). Assessment and management of auditory dysfunction (pp. 782–808). In C. Kenner, A. Brueggemeyer, & L.P. Gunderson (eds.), *Comprehensive neonatal nursing: A physiologic perspective.* Philadelphia: W. B. Saunders.

Hoekelman, R.A., Friedman, S.B., Nelson, N.M., & Seidel, H.M. (1992). *Primary pediatric care* (2nd ed.). St. Louis: C.V. Mosby.

Webster, D.B. & Webster, M. (1979). Effects of neonatal conductive hearing loss on brain stem auditory nuclei. *Annals of Otology, Rhinology and Laryngology, 88*(5, Pt.1), 684–688.

228. Answer: (**A**) A further report by Balkany et al (1978) reported that 30 percent of a random 125 infants from the NICU were found to have middle ear effusion. They also found that endotracheal intubation of longer than seven days contributed to the incidence of middle ear effusion. This finding has implications for the long-term auditory development of the neonate and supports the need for visualization of the middle ear as part of the septic work-up of all neonates.

REFERENCES

Balkany, T.J., Bereman, S.A., Simmons, M.A., & Jafek, B.W. (1978). Middle ear effusion in neonates. *Laryngoscope 88,* 398–405.

Haubrich, K. (1993). Assessment and management of auditory dysfunction (pp. 782–808). In C. Kenner, A. Brueggemeyer, & L.P. Gunderson (eds.), *Comprehensive neonatal nursing: A physiologic perspective.* Philadelphia: W. B. Saunders.

229. Answer: (**B**) The incidence of sensorineural hearing loss in children with severe perinatal asphyxia has been reported to be approximately four percent.

REFERENCES

Fanaroff, A.A. & Martin, R.J. (1992). *Neonatal-perinatal medicine* (5th ed.). St. Louis: C.V. Mosby.

Haubrich, K. (1993). Assessment and management of auditory dysfunction (pp. 782–808). In C. Kenner, A. Brueggemeyer, & L.P. Gunderson (eds.), *Comprehensive neonatal nursing: A physiologic perspective.* Philadelphia: W. B. Saunders.

Stein, L., Ozdamar, O., Kraus, N. & Paton, J., (1983). Follow-up of infants screened by auditory brainstem response in the neonatal intensive care unit. *Journal of Pediatrics, 63,* 447–453.

230. Answer: (**A**) In early childhood the onset of infantile congenital syphilis is usually between the 8th and 20th year. Hearing loss is sudden, bilateral, symmetrical, profound and with no accompanying symptoms.

REFERENCES

Haubrich, K. (1993). Assessment and management of auditory dysfunction (pp. 782–808). In C. Kenner, A. Brueggemeyer, & L.P. Gunderson (eds.), *Comprehensive neonatal nursing: A physiologic perspective.* Philadelphia: W.B. Saunders.

Schuknecht, H.J. (1974). *Pathology of the ear.* Cambridge: Harvard University Press.

231. Answer: (**B**) Epicanthal folds, true vertical folds extending from the nasal fold into the upper eyelid, are commonly noted in infants with Down syndrome. Twisted hair (pili torti) has been associated with sensorineural hearing loss. Defects of the neck that may be associated with hearing defects are brachial cleft fistulae and mildly webbed or shortened neck.

REFERENCES

Feingold, M. (1982). Clinical evaluation of a patient with a genetic birth defect syndrome. *Alabama Journal of Medical Science 19*(2), 151–156.

Haubrich, K. (1993). Assessment and management of auditory dysfunction (pp. 782–808). In C. Kenner, A. Brueggemeyer, & L.P. Gunderson (eds.), *Comprehensive neonatal nursing: A physiologic perspective.* Philadelphia: W.B. Saunders.

232. Answer: (**A**) Infants can be fitted with hearing aids before three months of age. Attention to these early factors, identification, amplification, and education does not necessarily ensure but certainly facilitates speech and language acquisition even in the most profoundly hearing impaired child.

REFERENCES

Haubrich, K. (1993). Assessment and management of auditory dysfunction (pp. 782–808). In C. Kenner, A. Brueggemeyer, & L.P. Gunderson (eds.), *Comprehensive neonatal nursing: A physiologic perspective.* Philadelphia: W.B. Saunders.

Markiden, A. (1986). Age at fitting of hearing aids and speech intelligibility. *British Journal of Audiology, 20,* 165–168.

233. Answer: (**B**) Capillary hemangioma of the lid, a blood vessel tumor, usually appears before the age of six months. They tend to enlarge, stabilize, and then regress by five years of age (Duane & Jaeger, 1988). The tumor tends to be elevated and reddish-purple in color. Capillary hemangiomas are often termed strawberry nevi because of their appearance. They may interfere with vision in some cases.

REFERENCES

Duane, T.D. & Jaeger, E.A. (1988). *Clinical ophthalmology*. (Vols. 1, 2, 4, 5). Philadelphia: J.B. Lippincott.
Heveston, E.M. & Ellis, F.D. (1980). *Pediatric ophthalmology practice*. St. Louis: C.V. Mosby.
Werner, R.B. & Werner, R. (1993). Assessment and management of ophthalmic dysfunction (pp. 809–820). In C. Kenner, A. Brueggemeyer, & L.P. Gunderson (eds.), *Comprehensive neonatal nursing: A physiologic perspective*. Philadelphia: W.B. Saunders.

234. Answer: (**A**) An allele is any possible alternative loci on same gene or alternative gene form.

REFERENCES

Cohen, F.L. (1984). *Clinical genetics in nursing practice*. Philadelphia: J.B. Lippincott.
Connor, J. & Ferguson-Smith, M. (1987). *Essential medical genetics*. Oxford: Blackwell Scientific.
Cummings, M. (1988). *Human heredity: Principles and issues*. New York: West Publishing.
Thompson, S. & Thompson, M. (1986). *Genetics in medicine* (4th ed). Philadelphia: W.B. Saunders.

235. Answer: (**B**) Cataracts due to galactosemia are important to recognize and treat early. The cataract has the appearance of an oil droplet. This disease can be suspected by the appearance of reducing substances when the urine is tested by Clinitest. Early detection and proper treatment can halt the progression of galactosemia cataracts and cause regression of mild cataracts due to this metabolic defect.

REFERENCES

Duane, T.D. & Jaeger, E.A. (1988). *Clinical ophthalmology* (Vols. 1, 2, 4, 5). Philadelphia: J.B. Lippincott.
Heveston, E.M. & Ellis, F.D. (1980). *Pediatric ophthalmology practice*. St. Louis: C.V. Mosby.
Werner, R.B. & Werner, R. (1993). Assessment and management of ophthalmic dysfunction (pp. 809–820). In C. Kenner, A. Brueggemeyer, & L.P. Gunderson (eds.), *Comprehensive neonatal nursing: A physiologic perspective*. Philadelphia: W.B. Saunders.

236. Answer: (**C**) The ideal biophysical sensor would require no direct patient contact or any type of external stimulus to produce a detectable response. Such a sensor is the infrared thermometer, which can transduce skin temperature directly from the emission characteristics of electromagnetic energies from the skin.

REFERENCES

Donnelly, M.M. (1993). Monitoring neonatal biophysical parameters (pp. 823–845). In C. Kenner, A. Brueggemeyer, & L.P. Gunderson (eds.), *Comprehensive neonatal nursing: A physiologic perspective*. Philadelphia: W.B. Saunders.
Gomella, T.L., Cunningham, M.D., & Eyal, F.G. (1992). *Neonatology: Management, procedures, on-call problems, diseases, drugs*. Norwalk, CT: Appleton & Lange.

237. Answer: (**B**) High-intensity optical radiation from phototherapy or examination lights can affect the transducers or conditioning and processing devices.

REFERENCES

Donnelly, M.M. (1993). Monitoring neonatal biophysical parameters (pp. 823–845). In C. Kenner, A. Brueggemeyer, & L.P. Gunderson (eds.), *Comprehensive neonatal nursing: A physiologic perspective*. Philadelphia: W.B. Saunders.
Gomella, T.L., Cunningham, M.D., & Eyal, F.G. (1992). *Neonatology: Management, procedures, on-call problems, diseases, drugs*. Norwalk, CT: Appleton & Lange.
King, J.D. & Jung, A.L. (1990). Phototherapy. In N. Nelson (ed.), *Current therapy in neonatal-perinatal medicine, No. 2* (pp. 461–464). Philadelphia: B.C. Decker.

238. Answer: (**A**) The relative energies of the reflected light can be correlated to the concentration of total bilirubin at the measurement site. Measurement accuracy ultimately depends on the optical properties of the skin. Darker and more mature skin has more melanin, which interferes with accurate transcutaneous measurement.

REFERENCES

Donnelly, M.M. (1993). Monitoring neonatal biophysical parameters (pp. 823–845). In C. Kenner, A. Brueggemeyer, & L.P. Gunderson (eds.), *Comprehensive neonatal nursing: A physiologic perspective*. Philadelphia: W.B. Saunders.
Gomella, T.L., Cunningham, M.D., & Eyal, F.G. (1992). *Neonatology: Management, procedures, on-call problems, diseases, drugs*. Norwalk, CT: Appleton & Lange.
King, J.D. & Jung, A.L. (1990). Phototherapy. In N. Nelson (ed.), *Current therapy in neonatal-perinatal medicine, No. 2* (pp. 461–464). Philadelphia: B.C. Decker.

239. Answer: (**A**) Certain infections such as cytomegalovirus, toxoplasmosis, and syphilis have a distinct radiographic and ultrasonic presentation if the exposure occurred in utero rather than in the neonatal period.

REFERENCES

Fanaroff, A.A. & Martin, R.J. (eds.). (1992). *Neonatal-perinatal medicine* (5th ed.). St. Louis: C.V. Mosby.
Gyll, C. & Blake, N. (1986). *Pediatric diagnostic imaging*. London: William Heinemann Medical Books.
Haller, J.O. & Slovis, T.L. (1984). *Introduction to radiol-*

ogy in clinical pediatrics. Chicago: Year Book Medical Publishers.
Kirks, D.R. (1984). *Practical pediatric imaging*. Boston: Little, Brown.
Swischuk, L.E. (1984). *Imaging of the newborn, infant, and young child* (3rd ed.). Baltimore: Williams & Wilkins.
Theorell, C.J. (1993). Diagnostic imaging (pp. 846–871). In C. Kenner, A. Brueggemeyer, & L.P. Gunderson (eds.), *Comprehensive neonatal nursing: A physiologic perspective*. Philadelphia: W.B. Saunders.

240. Answer: (**B**) An overexposed film results in a progressive loss of pulmonary vascular markings until the lungs have a black "burned out" appearance.

REFERENCES

Swischuk, L.E. (1984). *Imaging of the newborn, infant, and young child* (3rd ed.). Baltimore: Williams & Wilkins.
Theorell, C.J. (1993). Diagnostic imaging (pp. 846–871). In C. Kenner, A. Brueggemeyer, & L.P. Gunderson (eds.), *Comprehensive neonatal nursing: A physiologic perspective*. Philadelphia: W.B. Saunders.
Wesenberg, R.L. (1983). *The newborn chest*. Hagerstown, MD: Harper & Row.

241. Answer: (**C**) As an imaging modality, magnetic resonance imaging has several advantages over computed tomography: (1) magnetic resonance, like ultrasonography does not use ionizing radiation to produce the image, but rather uses magnetic fields and radiowaves; (2) the magnetic resonance image depends on three separate molecular parameters that are sensitive to changes in structure and bioactivity rather than on x-ray photon interaction with tissue electrons, as in CT; (3) the region of the body imaged in magnetic resonance imaging is not limited by the gantry geometry as in CT, but can be controlled electronically, allowing imaging in transverse planes as well as in true sagittal, coronal, and oblique planes; and (4) magnetic resonance images are free of high-intensity artifacts produced in CT scans by sharp, dense bone or metallic surgical clips.

REFERENCES

Dubowitz, L.M.S. & Bydder, G.M. (1985). Nuclear magnetic resonance imaging in the diagnosis and follow-up of neonatal cerebral injury. *Clinics in Perinatology, 12*, 243–260.
Friedman, B.R., Jones, J.P., Chaves-Munoz, J., Salmon, A.P., & Merritt, C.R.B. (1989). *Principles of MRI*. New York: McGraw-Hill.
Moss, A.A., Ring, E.G., & Higgins, C.B. (eds.) (1984). NMR, CT and interventional radiology. San Francisco: University of California Printing Department.
Theorell, C.J. (1993). Diagnostic imaging (pp. 846–871). In C. Kenner, A. Brueggemeyer, & L.P. Gunderson (eds.), *Comprehensive neonatal nursing: A physiologic perspective*. Philadelphia: W.B. Saunders.

242. Answer: (**B**) Echocardiography is a commonly used noninvasive diagnostic procedure. Using high-frequency sound waves, vibrations are sent to the heart. Structures within the heart then reflect energy that is transmitted into a visual image. Single-dimension echocardiography allows for evaluation of anatomical structures including valves, chambers, and vessels. Two-dimensional echocardiography provides more in-depth information about relationships between the heart and great vessels. Doppler echocardiography is used in various forms to evaluate characteristics of blood flow through the heart, valves, and great vessels.

REFERENCES

Gomella, T.L., Cunningham, M.D., & Eyal, F.G. (1992). *Neonatology: Management, procedures, on-call problems, diseases, drugs*. Norwalk, CT: Appleton & Lange.
Harjo, J. & Jones, M.A. (1993). Diagnostic tests and laboratory values (pp. 872–884). In C. Kenner, A. Brueggemeyer, & L.P. Gunderson (eds.), *Comprehensive neonatal nursing: A physiologic perspective*. Philadelphia: W.B. Saunders.
Streeter, N.S. (1986). *High risk neonatal care*. Gaithersburg, MD: Aspen Publishers.

243. Answer: (**B**) Follow-up x-rays may be desirable to evaluate the emptying ability of the stomach and intestinal motility as the contrast material moves through the small bowel. Again, care of the infant will include assessment of temperature, cardiac and respiratory status throughout the procedure. The nurse should be alert for reflux or vomiting, which can be accompanied by aspiration. Evacuation of contrast from the bowel remains a concern after UBL series and should be monitored by the nurse. It is also possible for fluid to be pulled out of the vascular compartment and into the bowel. The side effects then are fluid loss and hypotension. It is imperative that the health care team assess the infant for signs of these complications.

REFERENCES

Gomella, T.L., Cunningham, M.D., & Eyal, F.G. (1992). *Neonatology: Management, procedures, on-call prob-*

lems, diseases, drugs. Norwalk, CT: Appleton & Lange.

Harjo, J. & Jones, M.A. (1993). Diagnostic tests and laboratory values (pp. 872–884). In C. Kenner, A. Brueggemeyer, & L.P. Gunderson (eds.), *Comprehensive neonatal nursing: A physiologic perspective.* Philadelphia: W.B. Saunders.

244. Answer: (**B**) Fetal surgery should be done only when the natural progression of the disease will possibly result in fetal demise or neonatal death if surgery is not undertaken at this time.

REFERENCES

Bergman, K., Kenner, C., Levine, A.H., & Inturrisi, M. (1993). Fetal therapy (pp. 887–902). In C. Kenner, A. Brueggemeyer, & L.P. Gunderson (eds.), *Comprehensive neonatal nursing: A physiologic perspective.* Philadelphia: W.B. Saunders.

Elias, S. & Annas, G.J. (1987). *Reproductive genetics and the law.* Chicago: Year Book Medical Publishers.

Manning, F.A. (1986). International fetal surgery registry: 1985 update. *Clinical Obstetrics and Gynecology, 29,* 551–557.

245. Answer: (**B**) Some of the physiologic differences between healthy pregnant women and healthy adults are (1) a decrease in peripheral vascular resistance (cardiac output increase with no increase in blood pressure, indicating a decrease in peripheral vascular resistance); (2) a decrease in functional residual capacity (FRC) and increase in alveolar ventilation, therefore the rapidity of induction with inhalation anesthetics is increased; (3) an increase of oxygen consumption (a decreased FRC combined with an increased oxygen consumption makes pregnant women more likely to become hypoxic); and (4) hypotension due to aortocaval compression (by lying supine, a pregnant woman in the second and third trimester may develop hypotension as the result of aortocaval compression by the gravid uterus).

REFERENCES

Bergman, K., Kenner, C., Levine, A.H., & Inturrisi, M. (1993). Fetal therapy (pp. 887–902). In C. Kenner, A. Brueggemeyer, & L.P. Gunderson (eds.), *Comprehensive neonatal nursing: A physiologic perspective.* Philadelphia: W.B. Saunders.

Harrison, M.R., Golbus, M.S., & Filly, R.A. (1989). *The unborn patient: Prenatal diagnosis and treatment.* Orlando, FL: Grune & Stratton.

246. Answer: (**C**) Hydrocephalus is the accumulation of fluid within the ventricles of the brain, resulting in an enlargement of the cranial cavity. The condition is due to either an actual defect in the structure of the ventricles themselves (e.g. Arnold-Chiari malformation, communicating hydrocephalus) that affects the movement or absorption of cerebral spinal fluid (CSF), or an obstruction along the circulatory pathway of the CSF, especially at the aqueduct of Sylvius or the fourth ventricle, as in Dandy-Walker malformation, noncommunicating hydrocephalus. Both malformations can accompany a meningomyelocele or neural tube defect. Aqueductal stenosis is the usual cause of hydrocephalus. Bladder outlet obstruction can also be relieved by fetal surgery.

REFERENCES

Bergman, K., Kenner, C., Levine, A.H., & Inturrisi, M. (1993). Fetal therapy (pp. 887–902). In C. Kenner, A. Brueggemeyer, & L.P. Gunderson (eds.), *Comprehensive neonatal nursing: A physiologic perspective.* Philadelphia: W.B. Saunders.

Harrison, M.R., Golbus, M.S., & Filly, R.A. (1989). *The unborn patient: Prenatal diagnosis and treatment.* Orlando, FL: Grune & Stratton.

Manning, F.A., Harrison, M.R., & Rodeck, C. (1986). Catheter shunts for fetal hydronephrosis and hydrocephalus. *New England Journal of Medicine, 315,* 336–340.

247. Answer: (**C**) Alterations in acid-base balance can be caused by various factors in the surgical neonate. Major areas that can result in acidosis include inadequate respiratory support and fluid or electrolyte imbalances. The effects of sepsis and tissue necrosis also are significant causes of acidosis. Acidosis in the surgical neonate can be respiratory, metabolic, or mixed.

REFERENCES

Harjo, J. & Jones, M.A. (1993). The surgical neonate (pp. 903–912). In C. Kenner, A. Brueggemeyer, & L.P. Gunderson (eds.), *Comprehensive neonatal nursing: A physiologic perspective.* Philadelphia: W.B. Saunders.

Kenner, C., Brueggemeyer, A., & Harjo, J. (1988). *Neonatal surgery: A nursing perspective.* Orlando, FL: Grune & Stratton.

248. Answer: (**A**) Dobutamine achieves organ perfusion by increasing cardiac output. Dopamine, used in low to moderate doses, causes vasodilatation with resultant improvement in cardiac, renal, GI, and cerebral blood flow.

REFERENCES

Harjo, J. & Jones, M.A. (1993). The surgical neonate (pp. 903–912). In C. Kenner, A. Brueggemeyer, & L.P. Gunderson (eds.), *Comprehensive neonatal nursing: A physiologic perspective.* Philadelphia: W.B. Saunders.
Kenner, C., Brueggemeyer, A., & Harjo, J. (1988). *Neonatal surgery: A nursing perspective.* Orlando, FL: Grune & Stratton.

249. Answer: (**A**) It was not until the discovery that up to 80 percent of fibers that transmit pain information remain unmyelinated in the adult that the potential for infants with immature (largely unmyelinated) nervous systems to perceive pain was recognized and fully appreciated.

REFERENCES

Franck, L.S. (1993). Identification, management, and prevention of pain in the neonate (pp. 913–925). In C. Kenner, A. Brueggemeyer, & L.P. Gunderson (eds.), *Comprehensive neonatal nursing: A physiologic perspective.* Philadelphia: W.B. Saunders.
Price, D.D. & Dubner, R. (1977). Neurons that subserve the sensory-discriminative aspects of pain. *Pain, 3,* 307–338.

250. Answer: (**B**) Magnesium transfer from mother to fetus theoretically might be impaired in the presence of placental malfunction, and placental insufficiency appears to predispose the infant to neonatal hypomagnesemia (serum magnesium <1.5 mg/dl, or <0.61 mmol/L).

REFERENCES

DeMarini, S., Tsang, R.C., & Rath, L.L. (1993). Fluids, electrolytes, vitamins, and trace minerals: Basis of ingestion, digestion, elimination, and metabolism (pp. 393–413). In C. Kenner, A. Brueggemeyer, & L.P. Gunderson (eds.), *Comprehensive neonatal nursing: A physiologic perspective.* Philadelphia: W.B. Saunders.
Paunier, L., Ingeborg, C.R., Kooh, S.Y., Cohen, P.E., & Fraser, D. (1968). Primary hypomagnesemia with secondary hypocalcemia in an infant. *Pediatrics, 41,* 385–402.

251. Answer: (**B**) Because it is difficult to interpret the behavioral language of infants, distinguishing irritable, restless behavior due to pain from agitation due to other causes is one of the most challenging tasks of infant pain management.

REFERENCES

Fanaroff, A.A. & Martin, R.J. (eds.). (1992). *Neonatal-perinatal medicine* (5th ed.). St. Louis: C.V. Mosby.
Franck, L.S. (1993). Identification, management, and prevention of pain in the neonate (pp. 913–925). In C. Kenner, A. Brueggemeyer, & L.P. Gunderson (eds.), *Comprehensive neonatal nursing: A physiologic perspective.* Philadelphia: W.B. Saunders.

252. Answer: (**A**) The current definition of pain, adopted in 1979 by the International Association for the Study of Pain, holds that "pain is an unpleasant sensory and emotional experience associated with actual or potential tissue damage, or described in terms of such damage" (Merskey, 1979, p. 250.).

REFERENCES

Franck, L.S. (1993). Identification, management, and prevention of pain in the neonate (pp. 913–925). In C. Kenner, A. Brueggemeyer, & L.P. Gunderson (eds.), *Comprehensive neonatal nursing: A physiologic perspective.* Philadelphia: W.B. Saunders.
Merskey, H. (1979). Pain terms: A list with definitions and notes on usage. Recommended by the IASP Subcommittee on Taxonomy, *Pain, 6,* 249–252.

253. Answer: (**C**) The discovery of the importance of neural plasticity in the development of the CNS was the second factor contributing to the emergence of an imperative for the study and treatment of infant pain. It was not until the 1980s that the relationship between functional interaction with the environment and development of brain structures was fully realized. Interaction between the developing infant and the environment, particularly during periods of rapid brain growth, has been shown to have profound effects on the speed and amount of neuronal regression and on the structural connectivity at the neuronal level.

REFERENCES

Franck, L.S. (1993). Identification, management, and prevention of pain in the neonate (pp. 913–925). In C. Kenner, A. Brueggemeyer, & L.P. Gunderson (eds.), *Comprehensive neonatal nursing: A physiologic perspective.* Philadelphia: W.B. Saunders.
Gollin, E.S. (ed.). (1981). *Developmental plasticity: Behavioral and biological aspects of variations in development.* New York: Academic Press.

254. Answer: (**B**) Infants have the neurologic capability to feel pain before birth, even premature birth. The evidence for this statement comes from research in many fields within the biologic sciences.

REFERENCES

Anand, K.J.S. & Carr, D.B. (1989). The neuroanatomy, neurophysiology, and neurochemistry of pain, stress, and analgesia in newborns and children. *Pediatric Clinics of North America, 36,* 795–822.

Franck, L.S. (1991). *Pain control in critical care nursing*. Gaithersburg, MD: Aspen Publishers.
Franck, L.S. (1993). Identification, management, and prevention of pain in the neonate (pp. 913–925). In C. Kenner, A. Brueggemeyer, & L.P. Gunderson (eds.), *Comprehensive neonatal nursing: A physiologic perspective*. Philadelphia: W.B. Saunders.

255. Answer: (**B**) The fetus produces endorphins in response to asphyxia, acidosis, and maternal drug addiction.

REFERENCES

Anand, K.J.S. & Carr, D.B. (1989). The neuroanatomy, neurophysiology, and neurochemistry of pain, stress, and analgesia in newborns and children. *Pediatric Clinics of North America, 36,* 795–822.
Franck, L.S. (1991). *Pain control in critical care nursing*. Gaithersburg, MD: Aspen Publishers.
Franck, L.S. (1993). Identification, management, and prevention of pain in the neonate (pp. 913–925). In C. Kenner, A. Brueggemeyer, & L.P. Gunderson (eds.), *Comprehensive neonatal nursing: A physiologic perspective*. Philadelphia: W.B. Saunders.

256. Answer: (**B**) The newborn's sympathetic response to pain is immature, thus is less predictable than that of the adult.

REFERENCES

Brazy, J.A. (1988). Effects of crying on cerebral blood flow and cytochromosome aa3. *Journal of Pediatrics, 112,* 457–461.
Franck, L.S. (1993). Identification, management, and prevention of pain in the neonate (pp. 913–925). In C. Kenner, A. Brueggemeyer, & L.P. Gunderson (eds.), *Comprehensive neonatal nursing: A physiologic perspective*. Philadelphia: W.B. Saunders.

257. Answer: (**B**) The hormonal-metabolic changes seen in term infants are greater in magnitude but shorter in duration than in adults undergoing similar surgery.

REFERENCES

Anand, K.J.S. (1990). Neonatal stress responses to anesthesia and surgery. *Clinics in Perinatology, 17,* 207–214.
Franck, L.S. (1993). Identification, management, and prevention of pain in the neonate (pp. 913–925). In C. Kenner, A. Brueggemeyer, & L.P. Gunderson (eds.), *Comprehensive neonatal nursing: A physiologic perspective*. Philadelphia: W.B. Saunders.

258. Answer: (**B**) The rate of absorption of drug from an intramuscular site is directly related to the blood flow to that site. Therefore, IM drug administration to a cold or vasoconstricted neonate is not appropriate or likely to be effective.

REFERENCES

Rowland, M. (1978). Drug administration and regimens (pp. 25–70). In K.L. Melmon & H.F. Morelli (eds.), *Clinical pharmacology basic principles in therapeutics* (2nd ed.). New York: Macmillan.
Stull, J.C., Erenberg, A., & Leff, R.D. (1988). Flow rate variability from electronic infusion devices. *Critical Care Medicine, 16,* 888–891.
Ward, R.M. (1993). Neonatal pharmacology (pp. 926–939). In C. Kenner, A. Brueggemeyer, & L.P. Gunderson (eds.), *Comprehensive neonatal care: A physiologic perspective*. Philadelphia: W.B. Saunders.

259. Answer: (**B**) The effects of post-term pregnancy on the fetus and neonate include (1) failure of growth; (2) dehydration; (3) dry, cracked, wrinkled, parchment-like skin due to reduction of subcutaneous fat; (4) long, thin arms and legs; (5) advanced hardness of skull; (6) absence of vernix and lanugo; (7) skin maceration, especially in folds; (8) brownish-green discoloration of the skin secondary to meconium staining; and (9) increased appearance of alertness (Gilbert & Harmon, 1986).

REFERENCES

Creasy, R. & Resnick, M. (1989). *Maternal fetal medicine: Principles and practice*. Philadelphia: W.B. Saunders.
Gilbert, E. & Harmon, J. (1986). *High risk pregnancy and delivery*. St. Louis: C.V. Mosby.
Harmon, J.S. (1993). High-risk pregnancy (pp. 157–170). In C. Kenner, A. Brueggemeyer, & L.P. Gunderson (eds.), *Comprehensive neonatal nursing: A physiologic perspective*. Philadelphia: W.B. Saunders.
Moore, K. (1989). *The developing human* (4th ed.). Philadelphia: W.B. Saunders.

260. Answer: (**B**) *First pass effect* (elimination) is the removal of a large portion of a drug dose during the first circulation through an organ. This usually applies to drugs administered and absorbed enterally, which then circulate through the portal vein to the liver where they are extensively metabolized or removed from the circulation.

REFERENCES

Roberts, R.J. (1984). *Drug therapy in infants* (pp. 3–29). Philadelphia: W.B. Saunders.
Rowland, M. (1978). Drug administration and regimens. In K.L. Melmon & H.F. Morelli (eds.), *Clinical pharmacology basic principles in therapeutics* (2nd ed.) (pp. 25–70). New York: Macmillan.
Ward, R.M. (1993). Neonatal pharmacology (pp. 926–939). In C. Kenner, A. Brueggemeyer, & L.P. Gunderson (eds.), *Comprehensive neonatal care: A physiologic perspective*. Philadelphia: W.B. Saunders.

261. Answer: (**B**) Peak and trough drug concentrations are used frequently in therapeutic drug monitoring. The trough concentration is the lowest concentration just before administration of the next dose. Practically, this concentration can be obtained within 30 to 60 minutes of drug administration. The peak concentration refers to the concentration immediately after the end of the distribution (alpha) phase.

REFERENCES

Ward, R.M. (1993). Neonatal pharmacology (pp. 926–939). In C. Kenner, A. Brueggemeyer, & L.P. Gunderson (eds.), *Comprehensive neonatal care: A physiologic perspective*. Philadelphia: W.B. Saunders.
Yeh, T.F. (1991). *Neonatal therapeutics*. St. Louis: C.V. Mosby.

262. Answer: (**A**) The goals of monitoring drug concentrations are to avoid concentrations that are toxic and to achieve concentrations that are effective at the site of drug action.

REFERENCES

Kauffman, R.E. (1981). The clinical interpretation and application of drug concentration data. *Pediatric Clinics of North America, 28,* 35–45.
Sheiner, L.B. & Tozer, T.N. (1978). Clinical pharmacokinetics: The use of plasma concentrations of drugs (pp. 71–109). In K.L. Melmon & H.F. Morelli (eds.), *Clinical pharmacology basic principles in therapeutics* (2nd ed.) (pp. 71–109). New York: Macmillan Publishing Company, Inc.
Ward, R.M. (1993). Neonatal pharmacology (pp. 926–939). In C. Kenner, A. Brueggemeyer, & L.P. Gunderson (eds.), *Comprehensive neonatal care: A physiologic perspective*. Philadelphia: W.B. Saunders.

263. Answer: (**C**) Table 1.

REFERENCES

American Academy of Pediatrics Committee on Drugs. (1989). The transfer of drugs and other chemicals into human milk. *Pediatrics, 84,* 924–936.
Ward, R.M. (1993). Neonatal pharmacology (pp. 926–939). In C. Kenner, A. Brueggemeyer, & L.P. Gunderson (eds.), *Comprehensive neonatal care: A physiologic perspective*. Philadelphia: W.B. Saunders.

264. Answer: (**B**) The current theory is that HIV is an RNA virus that has a gp120 surface molecule that attaches to the CD4+ receptor sites on the cell's surface. The term retrovirus refers to the ability of the virus to enter the target cell via the receptor site, and then during cell division the virus's RNA material is copied into the DNA.

Table 1. Drugs Contraindicated During Nursing

Drugs-Contraindicated	Drugs of Abuse-Contraindicated
Bromocriptine	Amphetamine
Cocaine	Cocaine
Cyclophosphamide	Heroin
Cyclosporine	Marijuana
Doxorubicin	Nicotine (smoking)
Ergotamine	Phencyclidine
Lithium	
Methotrexate	
Phencyclidine (PCP)	
Phenindione	

Source: American Academy of Pediatrics Committee on Drugs (1989). The transfer of drugs and other chemicals into human milk. *Pediatrics, 84,* 924–936.

REFERENCES

Centers for Disease Control (1991). Centers for Disease Control HIV/AIDS. *Surveillance Report,* March.
Fahrner, R. (1992). Pediatric HIV infection and AIDS (pp. 408–425). In P.L. Jackson & J.A. Vessery (eds.), *Primary care of the child with a chronic condition*. St. Louis: C.V. Mosby.
Gunderson, L.P. & Gumm, B. (1993). Neonatal acquired immunodeficiency syndrome: Human immunodeficiency virus infection and acquired immunodeficiency syndrome in the infant (pp. 940–967). In C. Kenner, A. Brueggemeyer, & L.P. Gunderson (eds.), *Comprehensive neonatal care: A physiologic perspective*. Philadelphia: W.B. Saunders.

265. Answer: (**A**) Once the neonate has been stabilized in the delivery room, then transfer to either the regular nursery or intensive care nursery. In the nursery, routine neonatal care can be implemented depending on the infant's gestational age, Apgar score, and current physical status. Isolation is not necessary for the HIV exposed neonate. If, however, the infant has enteritis, draining wounds, congenital syphilis, cytomegalovirus, herpes, rubella, or other viral infections, the neonate should be placed in isolation for these disease entities and not the HIV itself.

REFERENCES

Gunderson, L.P. & Gumm, B. (1993). Neonatal acquired immunodeficiency syndrome: Human immunodeficiency virus infection and acquired immunodeficiency syndrome in the infant (pp. 940–967). In C. Kenner, A. Brueggemeyer, & L.P. Gunderson (eds.), *Comprehensive neonatal care: A physiologic perspective*. Philadelphia: W.B. Saunders.
Mendez, H. & Jule, J.E. (1990). Care of the infant born exposed to human immunodeficiency virus. *Obstetrics*

and Gynecology Clinics of North America, 17(3), 637–649.

266. Answer: (**A**) The period of latency is different for the infant than the adult. The latency period for the infant is much shorter than the six months to 10 years for the adult. Rubinstein and Bernstein (1986) reported that six months was the average age between exposure to HIV and the development of HIV symptoms in the infant.

REFERENCES

De Wolf, F., Goudsmit, J., & Paul, D.A. (1987). Risk of ARC and AIDS in homosexual men with persistent HIV antigenaemia. *British Medical Journal, 295,* 569–572.
Fahrner, R. (1992). Pediatric HIV infection and AIDS (pp. 408–425). In P.L. Jackson & J.A. Vessery (eds.), *Primary care of the child with a chronic condition.* St. Louis: Mosby.
Gunderson, L.P. & Gumm, B. (1993). Neonatal acquired immunodeficiency syndrome: Human immunodeficiency virus infection and acquired immunodeficiency syndrome in the infant (pp. 940–967). In C. Kenner, A. Brueggemeyer, & L.P. Gunderson (eds.), *Comprehensive neonatal care: A physiologic perspective.* Philadelphia: W.B. Saunders.
Mendez, H. & Jule, J.E. (1990). Care of the infant born exposed to human immunodeficiency virus. *Obstetrics and Gynecology Clinics of North America,* 17(3), 637–649.
Pizzo, P.A. (1990). Pediatric AIDS: Problems within problems. *Journal of Infectious Disease, 161,* 316–325.
Rubinstein, A. & Bernstein, L. (1986). The epidemiology of pediatric acquired immunodeficiency syndrome. *Clinical Immunology and Immunopathology, 40,* 115–121.

267. Answer: (**C**) Early signs and symptoms in the infant are recurrent bacterial infections with sepsis, candida (thrush), and failure to thrive.

REFERENCES

Gunderson, L.P. & Gumm, B. (1993). Neonatal acquired immunodeficiency syndrome: Human immunodeficiency virus infection and acquired immunodeficiency syndrome in the infant (pp. 940–967). In C. Kenner, A. Brueggemeyer, & L.P. Gunderson (eds.), *Comprehensive neonatal care: A physiologic perspective.* Philadelphia: W.B. Saunders.
Mendez, H. & Jule, J.E. (1990). Care of the infant born exposed to human immunodeficiency virus. *Obstetrics and Gynecology Clinics of North America,* 17(3), 637–649.

268. Answer: (**B**) Prophylactic administration of hepatitis B vaccine should be undertaken. Older infants and children should receive all scheduled immunizations and polio vaccine before transplantation evaluation when possible. Influenza immunizations are administered to older children but not to neonates.

REFERENCES

A-Kader, H.H., Ryckman, F.C., & Balistreri, W.F. (1991). Liver transplantation in the pediatric population: Indications and monitoring. *Clinical Transplant, 5,* 161.
Kalayoglu, M., Stratta, R.J., Sollinger, H.W., Hoffmann, R.M., D'Alessandro, A.M., Pirsch, J.D. & Belzer, F.O. (1989). Liver transplantation in infants and children. *Journal of Pediatric Surgery, 24,* 70–76.
Ryckman, F.C. & Pedersen, S.H. (1993). Hepatic and renal transplantation in infants and children (pp. 968–980). In C. Kenner, A. Brueggemeyer, & L.P. Gunderson (eds.), *Comprehensive neonatal care: A physiologic perspective.* Philadelphia: W.B. Saunders.
Shaw, B.W., Starzl, T.E., Iwatsuki, S., & Gordon, R.D. (1989). An overview of orthotopic transplantation of the liver (pp. 347–363). In E. Wickland (ed.), *Principles of organ transplantation.* Philadelphia: W.B. Saunders.

269. Answer: (**B**) For the infant, the ELISA and Western blot may not be useful in detecting the presence of HIV owing to the fact that maternal antibodies for HIV (IgG) cross the placenta and may be found in the infant's serum for up to 15 months after birth. The maternal antibodies can give a false-positive test rather than an actual indicator of how the infant's immune system is responding to the HIV infection.

REFERENCES

American Academy of Pediatrics (AAP) (1988). *Report of the Committee on Infectious Disease.* (21st ed., pp. 91–115). Elk Grove, IL: Author.
American Academy of Pediatrics and American College of Obstetricians and Gynecologists. (1988). Guidelines for perinatal care (2nd ed.). Elk Grove, IL: American Academy of Pediatrics.
Gunderson, L.P. & Gumm, B. (1993). Neonatal acquired immunodeficiency syndrome: Human immunodeficiency virus infection and acquired immunodeficiency syndrome in the infant (pp. 940–967). In C. Kenner, A. Brueggemeyer, & L.P. Gunderson (eds.), *Comprehensive neonatal care: A physiologic perspective.* Philadelphia: W.B. Saunders.
Husson, R.N., Corneau, A.M., & Hoff, R. (1990). Diagnosis of human immunodeficiency virus infection in infant's and children. *Pediatrics, 86*(1), 1–10.

270. Answer: (**A**) Transplantation of the liver in infants and children has been recognized for many years to be the only possible solution to many inherited metabolic diseases and primary abnormalities of liver function. At present, liver transplantation is offered to all children with progressive liver failure, regardless of age or weight.

REFERENCES

A-Kader, H.H., Ryckman, F.C., & Balistreri, W.F. (1991). Liver transplantation in the pediatric population: Indications and monitoring. *Clinical Transplant, 5,* 161.

Annual Report on the U.S. Scientific Registry for Organ Transplantation Network (1988–89). Richmond, VA: United Network for Organ Sharing.

Ryckman, F.C. & Pedersen, S.H. (1993). Hepatic and renal transplantation in infants and children (pp. 968–980). In C. Kenner, A. Brueggemeyer, & L.P. Gunderson (eds.), *Comprehensive neonatal care: A physiologic perspective.* Philadelphia: W.B. Saunders.

Starzl, T.E., Iwatsuki, S., & Shaw, B.W. (1986). Liver transplantation (pp. 373–382). In K.J. Welch, J.G. Randolph, M.M. Ravitch, J.A. O'Neill, & M.I. Rowe (eds.), *Pediatric surgery* (4th ed.), Chicago: Year Book Medical Publishers.

271. Answer: (**A**) "Boarder babies" is a term used to describe infants who live in the hospital without medical necessity; they simply do not have a safe place to go.

REFERENCES

Boarder Babies: (1991, January-February). Winning the battle. *Discharge Planning Update,* p. 15.

Gunderson, L.P. & Gumm, B. (1993). Neonatal acquired immunodeficiency syndrome: Human immunodeficiency virus infection and acquired immunodeficiency syndrome in the infant (pp. 940–967). In C. Kenner, A. Brueggemeyer, & L.P. Gunderson (eds.), *Comprehensive neonatal care: A physiologic perspective.* Philadelphia: W.B. Saunders.

Mendez, H. & Jule, J.E. (1990). Care of the infant born exposed to human immunodeficiency virus. *Obstetrics and Gynecology Clinics of North America,* 17(3), 637–649.

272. Answer: (**A**) Most patients with progressive cirrhosis develop the common complications of portal hypertension: esophageal varices, gastrointestinal hemorrhage, and hypersplenism.

REFERENCES

A-Kader, H.H., Ryckman, F.C., & Balistreri, W.F. (1991). Liver transplantation in the pediatric population: Indications and monitoring. *Clinical Transplant, 5,* 161.

Ryckman, F.C. & Pedersen, S.H. (1993). Hepatic and renal transplantation in infants and children (pp. 968–980). In C. Kenner, A. Brueggemeyer, & L.P. Gundreson (eds.), *Comprehensive neonatal care: A physiologic perspective.* Philadelphia: W.B. Saunders.

273. Answer: (**B**) Acute cellular rejection occurs in up to 95 percent of patients treated by conventional immunosuppressive protocols using prednisone, cyclosporine, and azathioprine (Ryckman et al, 1991). When sequential induction immunotherapy using orthoclone OKT-3, prednisone, and azathioprine is combined with the delayed introduction of cyclosporine, the incidence of rejection is decreased to 46 percent (Ryckman et al, 1991; Starzl & Demetris, 1990).

REFERENCES

A-Kader, H.H., Ryckman, F.C., & Balistreri, W.F. (1991). Liver transplantation in the pediatric population: Indications and monitoring. *Clinical Transplant, 5,* 161.

Ryckman, F.C. & Pedersen, S.H. (1993). Hepatic and renal transplantation in infants and children (pp. 968–980). In C. Kenner, A. Brueggemeyer, & L.P. Gunderson (eds.), *Comprehensive neonatal care: A physiologic perspective.* Philadelphia: W.B. Saunders.

Ryckman, F.C., Schroeder, T.J., Pedersen, S.H., Fisher, R.A., Farrell, M.K., Heubi, J.E., Ziegler, M.M., & Balistreri, W.F. (1991). The use of monoclonal immunosuppressive therapy in pediatric renal and liver transplantation. *Clinical Transplantation, 5,* 189.

Starzl, T.E. & Demetris, A.J. (1990). Liver transplantation. A 31-year perspective. Part III. In S.A. Wells, Jr. (ed.), *Current problems in surgery.* Chicago: Year Book Medical Publishers.

Todo, S., Fung, J.J., Starzl, T.E., Tzakis, A., Demetris, A.J., Kormos, R., Jain, A., Alessiani, M., Takaya, S., & Shapiro, R. (1990). Liver, kidney, and thoracic organ transplantation under FK 506. *Annals of Surgery, 212,* 295–307.

274. Answer: (**A**) To reduce the complications from rapidly introduced therapy, nurses must take an active role. Evaluation should be preceded by literature review or telephone survey to determine what is published about the practice and to gain as much information as possible. Nurses need to ask pertinent questions related to nursing practice and seek nursing information from units where the practice was initially researched or if the practice has existed for a period. If no information about the nursing implications of the therapy exists, a prospective approach must occur. They must be encouraged to report all complications and must be given a mechanism to facilitate reporting.

REFERENCES

Bassen, J.I. (1986). From problem reporting to technological solutions. *Medical Instrumentation, 20,* 17–26.

Golonka, L. (1986). Trends in health care and use of technology by nurses. *Medical Instrumentation, 20,* 8–10.

Lefrak-Okikawa, L. (1993). Iatrogenic complications of the neonatal intensive care unit (pp. 981–996). In C. Kenner, A. Brueggemeyer, & L.P. Gunderson (eds.), *Comprehensive neonatal care: A physiologic perspective.* Philadelphia: W.B. Saunders.

Raju, T.N., Thornton, J.P., Kecskes, S., Perry, M., &

Geldman, S. (1989). Medication errors in neonatal and paediatric intensive-care units. *Lancet, 2,* 374–376.
Jain, L. & Vidyasagar, D. (1989). Iatrogenic disorders in modern neonatology. *Clinics in Perinatology, 16,* 255–273.

275. Answer: (**C**) There has yet to be a readily identifiable withdrawal pattern among infants born to women abusing cocaine. The infants are often irritable and difficult to handle. Infants who are cocaine exposed have a significant depression of interactive behavior. They also exhibit poor organizational responses to external stimuli. This makes these infants difficult to console and frustrating for the caregiver. The researchers conclude that the effects of cocaine are self-limiting as opposed to being a permanent manifestation of cocaine exposure. Heroin-exposed infants weigh significantly less than nonexposed infants.

REFERENCES

Chasnoff, I. (1988). Newborn infants with drug withdrawal symptoms. *Pediatrics in Review, 9*(9), 273–277.
Cherukuri, S., Minkoff, H., Feldman, J., Parekh, A., & Glass, L. (1988). Cohort study of alkaloidal cocaine ("crack") in pregnancy. *Obstetrics and Gynecology, 72*(2), 17–151.
Doberazak, T., Shanzer, S., Senie, R., & Kandell, S. (1988). Neonatal neurologic and electroencephalographic effects of intrauterine cocaine exposure. *Journal of Pediatrics, 113,* 354–358.
Flandermeyer, A.A. (1993). The drug-exposed neonate (pp. 997–1033). In C. Kenner, A. Brueggemeyer, & L.P. Gunderson (eds.), *Comprehensive neonatal care: A physiologic perspective.* Philadelphia: W.B. Saunders.
Schneider, J. & Chasnoff, I. (1987). Cocaine abuse during pregnancy: Its effects on infant motor development—A clinical perspective. *Topics in Acute Care, Trauma, & Rehabilitation, 2*(1), 59–69.
Zelson, C., Lee, S., & Casalino, M. (1973). Neonatal narcotic addiction. *New England Journal of Medicine, 289*(23), 1216–1220.
Zelson, C., Rubio, E., & Wasserman, E. (1971). Neonatal narcotic addiction: 10 year observation. *Pediatrics, 48*(2), 178–189.

276. Answer: (**A**) If nurses have sole responsibility for the introduction of certain kinds of equipment, two steps will smooth the process of evaluation. The first step involves asking a series of standard questions to all sales representatives before deciding on a device to evaluate. The second step involves creating a "critical function" list for any device before evaluation.

REFERENCES

Bassen, J.I. (1986). From problem reporting to technological solutions. *Medical Instrumentation, 20,* 17–26.
Golonka, L. (1986). Trends in health care and use of technology by nurses. *Medical Instrumentation, 20,* 8–10.
Lefrak-Okikawa, L. (1993). Iatrogenic complications of the neonatal intensive care unit (pp. 981–996). In C. Kenner, A. Brueggemeyer, & L.P. Gunderson (eds.), *Comprehensive neonatal care: A physiologic perspective.* Philadelphia: W.B. Saunders.

277. Answer: (**B**) Pregnant women and their fetuses are slower to metabolize cocaine as a consequence of a lower level of plasma cholinesterase activity. According to Chasnoff, Burns and Burns (1987), if a woman has ingested cocaine two to three days before delivery, the adult urine will contain metabolites for 24 hours and the neonate's urine will continue to test positive for four to seven days. However, the more immature the fetal liver, the longer cocaine's metabolites may linger in the fetal system.

REFERENCES

Chasnoff, I., Burns, K., & Burns, W. (1987). Cocaine use in pregnancy: Perinatal morbidity and mortality. *Neurotoxicology and Teratology, 9*(4), 291–293.
Flandermeyer, A.A. (1993). The drug-exposed neonate (pp. 997–1033). In C. Kenner, A. Brueggemeyer, & L.P. Gunderson (eds.), *Comprehensive neonatal care: A physiologic perspective.* Philadelphia: W.B. Saunders.
Pritchard, J. (1955). Plasma cholinesterase activity in normal pregnancy and in eclamptogenic toxemia. *South American Journal of Obstetrics and Gynecology, 70,* 1083.
Udell, B. (1989). Crack cocaine (pp. 5–8). In Ross Laboratories (ed.), *Special currents: Cocaine babies.* Columbus, OH: Ross Laboratories.

278. Answer: (**C**) Opiates, heroin, and methadone are generally accepted as not being teratogenic. Therefore, the pregnant woman is maintained on methadone until delivery. There is a cross dependence between heroin and methadone so fetal withdrawal is prevented. The benefits of methadone over heroin is that methadone can be prescribed by exact dose, given orally, and it does not exert the mood-altering effects of heroin. Most infants born to women addicted to heroin undergo withdrawal. Alcohol is considered teratogenic, producing characteristic facies.

REFERENCES

Boobis, S. & Sullivan, F. (1986). Effects of life-style on reproduction (pp. 373–425). In S. Fabro & A. Sciall (eds.), *Drug and chemical action in pregnancy: Pharmacologic and toxicologic principles*. New York: Marcel Dekker.

Flandermeyer, A.A. (1993). The drug-exposed neonate (pp. 997–1033). In C. Kenner, A. Brueggemeyer, & L.P. Gunderson (eds.), *Comprehensive neonatal care: A physiologic perspective*. Philadelphia: W.B. Saunders.

Naeye, R., Blanc, W., LeBlanc, W., & Khatamee, M. (1973). Fetal complications of maternal heroin addiction: Abnormal growth, infections, and episodes of stress. *The Journal of Pediatrics, 83*(96), 1055–1061.

Reddy, A., Harper, R., & Stern, G. (1971). Observations on heroin and methadone withdrawal in the newborn. *Pediatrics, 48*(3), 353–358.

Zelson, C., Rubio, E., & Wasserman, E. (1971). Neonatal narcotic addiction: 10 year observation. *Pediatrics, 48*(2), 178–189.

279. Answer: (**A**) Fetal alcohol syndrome (FAS) is on the severe end of the continuum, and Fetal Alcohol Effects (FAE) refers to mild symptomatology. Ernhart et al (1987) found a "critical period for alcohol teratogenicity was confirmed to be around the time of conception" (p. 33). A critical period refers to a time during fetal development when developing tissue is highly vulnerable to a teratogen. Typically, it occurs when cells are rapidly dividing and differentiating. Other investigators (Hanson, Streissguth, & Smith, 1978; Warren & Bast, 1988) observed a consistent pattern between alcohol consumption shortly after conception and an increased incidence of fetal alcohol syndrome (FAS). FAS is diagnosed by reported maternal alcohol consumption during pregnancy and characteristic neonatal features. These findings revolve around three areas: (1) prenatal and postnatal growth deficiency, (2) dysmorphic characteristics, and (3) CNS dysfunction.

REFERENCES

Ernhart, C., Sokol, R., Martier, S., Moron, P., Nadler, D., Ager, J., & Wolf, A. (1987). Alcohol teratogenicity in the human: A detailed assessment of specificity, critical period, and threshold. *American Journal of Obstetrics and Gynecology, 156*(1), 33–39.

Flandermeyer, A.A. (1993). The drug-exposed neonate (pp. 997–1033). In C. Kenner, A. Brueggemeyer, & L.P. Gunderson (eds.), *Comprehensive neonatal care: A physiologic perspective*. Philadelphia: W.B. Saunders.

Hanson, J., Jones, K., & Smith, D. (1976). Fetal alcohol syndrome: Experience with 41 patients. *JAMA, 235*(14), 1458–1460.

Hanson, J., Streissguth, A., & Smith, D. (1978). The effects of moderate alcohol consumption during pregnancy on fetal growth and morphogenesis. *Journal of Pediatrics, 92*(3), 457–460.

Jones, K. & Smith, D. (1973). Recognition of the fetal alcohol syndrome in early infancy. *Lancet, 1,* 999–1001.

Jones, K., Smith, D., Ulleland, C., & Streissguth, A. (1973). Pattern of malformation in offspring of chronic alcoholic mothers. *Lancet, 1,* 1267–1271.

Lipson, T. (1988). Fetal alcohol syndrome. *Australian Family Physician, 17*(5), 385–386.

Streissguth, A., Clarren, S., & Jones, K. (1985). A natural history of the fetal alcohol syndrome: A 10-year follow-up of 11 patients. *Alcohol Health and Research World,* Fall, 13–19.

Streissguth, A. & LaDue, R. (1985). Psychological and behavioral effects in children prenatally exposed to alcohol. *Alcohol Health and Research World,* Fall, 6–12.

Warren, K. & Bast, R. (1988). Alcohol-related birth defects: An update. *Public Health Reports, 103*(6), 638–642.

280. Answer: (**C**) The clinician should avoid dwelling on what damage may have already been sustained and instead focus on the potential good that could occur from detoxification or in the case of heroin transference to methadone. Infants who have been exposed should be fed smaller quantities more frequently. Three-hour feeds are often tolerated well; however, this can be individually assessed. Accurate intake and output should be recorded. An indwelling, small diameter (e.g., 5 Fr) nasogastric (NG) feeding tube is often helpful. The feeding situation requires special consideration with respect to infant state and readiness. As previously discussed, the infant needs to set the pace for the interaction with the caregiver. If the infant is fragile with respect to state control, the caregiver may need to slowly initiate contact. Holding the infant in a flexed position, with their hands past midline also is helpful. Other soothing techniques include handholding, vertical rocking, and use of a pacifier. Daily weight and head circumference should be done to track growth.

REFERENCES

Flandermeyer, A.A. (1993). The drug-exposed neonate (pp. 997–1033). In C. Kenner, A. Brueggemeyer, & L.P. Gunderson (eds.), *Comprehensive neonatal care: A physiologic perspective*. Philadelphia: W.B. Saunders.

Griffith, D. (1988). The effects of perinatal cocaine exposure on infant neurobehavior and early mother-infant interactions (pp. 105–113). In I. Chasnoff (ed.), *Drugs, alcohol, pregnancy, and parenting*. Higham, MA: Kluwer Academic Publishers.

Schneider, J. & Chasnoff, I. (1987) Cocaine abuse during pregnancy: Its effects on infant motor development—A clinical perspective. *Topics in Acute Care, Trauma, & Rehabilitation, 2*(1), 59–69.

281. Answer: (**C**) Data bases need not hold only patient data but can provide for effective storage and easy retrieval of reference information used by clinicians. Policies, procedures, drug information, and other reference information can be accessed by the clinician when and where the information is needed by using computer terminals located in the patient care area. Some units have developed computer programs to verify drug and (total parenteral nutrition) TPN orders or calculate resuscitation drugs precisely for each individual infant's weight; others have automated the physician orders. Drug calculation and TPN preparation are examples of tedious, problem-prone systems that represent high risk to the patient if errors occur.

REFERENCES

Duncan, R.G. & Pomerance, J.J. (1982). Computer assistance in delivery of patient care in a neonatal intensive care unit (pp. 337–351). In T.R. Harris & J.P. Bahr (eds.), *The uses of computers in perinatal medicine*. New York: Praeger.

Franck, L.S. (1993). Use of computers in neonatal nursing (pp. 1034–1045). In C. Kenner, A. Brueggemeyer, & L.P. Gunderson (eds.), *Comprehensive neonatal care: A physiologic perspective*. Philadelphia: W.B. Saunders.

Harper, R.G., Carrera, E., Weiss, S., & Luongo, M. (1985). A complete computerized program for nutritional management in the neonatal intensive care nursery. *Journal of Perinatology, 2*(2), 161–162.

Prophet, C.M. (1989). Patient care planning: An interdisciplinary approach (pp. 827–833). In L. Kingsland (ed.), *Proceedings, Thirteenth annual symposium on computer applications in medical care*. Washington, DC: IEEE Computer Society Press.

Simpson, R.L. (1991). The joint commission did what you wouldn't. *Nursing Management, 22*(10), 26–27.

Thomas, L.W. (1987). Computerized order calculation and label generation for neonatal parenteral nutrient solutions. *Journal of Medical Systems, 12*(2), 115–120.

282. Answer: (**B**) Soothing interventions for the immature or ill infant include containment and swaddling, providing time out for recovery, reducing stimulation, holding the infant's hands or feet, prone positioning, and providing sucking opportunities.

REFERENCES

Als, H. (1986). A synactive model of neonatal behavioral organization: Framework for the assessment of neurobehavioral development in the premature infant and for the support of infants and parents in the neonatal intensive care environment. *Physical and Occupational Therapy in Pediatrics, 6,* 3–53.

Blackburn, S.T. & VandenBerg, K.A. (1993). Assessment and management of neonatal neurobehavioral development (pp. 1094–1133). In C. Kenner, A. Brueggemeyer, & L.P. Gunderson (eds.), *Comprehensive neonatal care: A physiologic perspective*. Philadelphia: W.B. Saunders.

Lawhon, G. (1986). Management of stress in premature infants (pp. 319–328). In D.J. Angelini, C.M. Knapp, & R.M. Gibes (eds.), *Perinatal/neonatal nursing: A clinical handbook*. Boston: Blackwell Scientific.

VandenBerg, K. (1990a). The management of oral nippling in the sick neonate: The disorganized feeder. *Neonatal Network, 9*(1), 9–16.

VandenBerg, K. (1990b). Behaviorally supportive care for the extremely premature infant. In L.P. Gunderson & C. Kenner (eds.), *Care of the 24–25 gestational age infant (small baby protocol)*. Petaluma, CA: Neonatal Network.

283. Answer: (**A**) A PC system to assist physicians in classifying dysmorphic syndromes in children is one use of computers in medicine. The physician enters the pertinent clinical data into the computer, and the program presents the most likely syndromes that match the clinical data as well as the probability of occurrence. Another system provides an algorithm for determining ventilator setting based on arterial blood gas data. This system also builds a patient data base to allow for retrospective trend analysis. The computer provides decision support for planning and documenting nursing care based on patient medical and/or nursing diagnoses. A key feature of the system is its use of semantic network of associations rather than decision rules to select from the knowledge base. The developers believe this methodology more accurately represents the practice of nursing in which numerous parallel goals are proposed and disparate activities are coordinated.

REFERENCES

Boyarsky, A. (1987). Computerized ventilation management system for neonates. *Journal of Perinatology, 7*(1), 21–29.

Evans, S. (September, 1990). PACE/CPC: Nursing care planning and decision support for the 1990's. *Healthcare Informatics,* 26–27.

Franck, L.S. (1993). Use of computers in neonatal nursing (pp. 1034–1045). In C. Kenner, A. Brueggemeyer,

& L.P. Gunderson (eds.), *Comprehensive neonatal care: A physiologic perspective.* Philadelphia: W.B. Saunders.

Wiener, F. & Anneren, G. (1989). PC-based system for classifying dysmorphic syndromes in children. *Computer Methods and Programs in Biomedicine, 28,* 111–117.

284. Answer: (**C**) Examples of computer assisted instruction (CAI) programs for perinatal medicine include evaluation of the cyanotic premature infant and bereavement. This approach is beginning to be applied to patient and family education and reduces the need for reading and typing skills. Sweeney and Gulind (1988) describe a system for providing breast and bottle feeding instruction using video disc technology.

JCAHO recently mandated nursing involvement in computer system selection. Nursing representatives do not need to be experts in computer science but should have a clear understanding of the task for which the computer will be used and be able to articulate the right questions and understand the solutions proposed.

REFERENCES

Ball, M.J. & Hannah, K.J. (1988). What is informatics and what does it mean for nursing (pp. 260–266). In M.J. Ball, K.J. Hannah, U. Gerdin-Jelger, & H. Peterson (eds.), *Nursing informatics: Where care and technology meet.* New York: Springer-Verlag.

Franck, L.S. (1993). Use of computers in neonatal nursing (pp. 1034–1045). In C. Kenner, A. Brueggemeyer, & L.P. Gunderson (eds.), *Comprehensive neonatal care: A physiologic perspective.* Philadelphia: W.B. Saunders.

Lambrecht, M.E. (1989). Death: Perspectives for clinical practice videodisc series. In L. Kingsland (ed.), *Proceedings, Thirteenth annual symposium on computer applications in medical care* (pp. 1052–1054). Washington, DC: IEEE Computer Society Press.

Sweeney, M.A. & Gulino, C. (1988). From variables to videodiscs: Interactive video in the clinical setting. *Computers in nursing, 6*(4), 157–163.

Tinsley, L.R., Ashton, G.C., Boychuk, R.B., & Easa, D.J. (1989). Cyanotic premature babies: A video disc-based program. In L. Kingsland (ed.), *Proceedings, Thirteenth annual symposium on computer applications in medical care* (pp. 796–801). Washington, DC: IEEE Computer Society Press.

285. Answer: (**A**) Within the home environment, the parent–infant interaction was found to be the best predictive factor for later positive development in preterm infants.

REFERENCES

Barnard, K.E., Hammond, M., Booth, C.L., Bee, H.L., Mitchell, S.K., & Spieker, S.J. (1989). Measurement and meaning of parent-child interaction. In F. Morrison, C. Lord, & D. Keating (eds.), *Applied developmental psychology* (Vol. III). New York: Academic Press.

Barrera, M.E., Rosenbaum, P.L., & Cunningham, C.E. (1986). Early home intervention with low birth weight infants and their parents. *Child Development, 57,* 20–33.

Bendersky, M. & Lewis, M. (1986). The impact of birth order on mother-infant interactions in preterm and sick infants. *Developmental and Behavioral Pediatrics, 7*(4), 242–246.

Crnic, K.A. & Greenberg, M.T. (1987). Transactional relationships between perceived family style, risk status and mother-child interaction in two-year-olds. *Journal of Pediatric Psychology, 12*(3), 343–362.

Field, T. M. (1987). Interaction and attachment in normal and atypical infants. *Journal of Consulting and Clinical Psychology, 55*(6), 853–859.

Greenberg, M.T. & Crnic, K.A. (1988). Longitudinal predictors of developmental status and social interaction in premature and full-term infants at age two. *Child Development, 59,* 554–570.

Johnson-Crowley, N. (1993). Systematic assessment and home follow-up: A basis for monitoring the neonate's integration into the family unit (pp. 1055–1076). In C. Kenner, A. Brueggemeyer, & L.P. Gunderson (eds.), *Comprehensive neonatal care: A physiologic perspective.* Philadelphia: W.B. Saunders.

Ramey, C.T., Farram, D.C., & Campbell, F.A. (1979). Predicting IQ from mother–infant interactions. *Child Development, 50,* 804–814.

Schraeder, B.D., Rappaport, J. & Courtwright, L. (1987). Preschool development of very low birthweight infants. *Image: Journal of Nursing Scholarship, 19*(4), 174–177.

286. Answer: (**B**) The nursing child assessment sleep-activity (NCASA) record is a 24-hour record that requires the parent (or caregiver) to keep an hour-by-hour record of the infant's sleep and activity for one week. This record is set in graph form, with each square representing 60 minutes. Caregivers record sleep, awake times when the child is content and when the child is fussy or crying, feeding, play times, and any other activity for which the parent or nurse identifies a need.

REFERENCES

Barnard, K.E. (1987). *Nursing child assessment learner manual.* Seattle, WA: NCAST Publications.

Johnson-Crowley, N. (1993). Systematic assessment and home follow-up: A basis for monitoring the neonate's integration into the family unit (pp. 1055–1076). In C. Kenner, A. Brueggemeyer, & L.P. Gunderson (eds.), *Comprehensive neonatal care: A physiologic perspective.* Philadelphia: W.B. Saunders.

287. Answer: (**B**) Another phenomenon reported to be associated with preterm infants is child abuse. The reasons for the increased risk of abuse seem to be

the combination of infant behavioral characteristics (irritability, lack of clear cues, and low social responsiveness) and certain parental experiences and characteristics (lack of social support, history of violence as a child or with a spouse, insensitivity to their child, annoyance or anger when the infant cries). However, rather than reacting with a lack of responsiveness to the infant (parental burnout), an increase in infant stimulation (super parent syndrome), or overprotectiveness (vulnerable child syndrome), the parent instead abuses the child.

REFERENCES

Beckwith, L. (1990). Adaptive and maladaptive parenting-implications for intervention. In S.J. Meisels & J.P. Shonkoff (eds.), *Handbook of early childhood intervention*. Cambridge: Cambridge University Press.

Clark, M.C. (1989). In what ways, if any, are child abusers different from other parents? *Health Visit, 62*(9), 268–270.

Elmer, E. & Gregg, G. (1967). Developmental characteristics of abused children. *Pediatrics, 40,* 596–602.

Johnson-Crowley, N. (1993). Systematic assessment and home follow-up: A basis for monitoring the neonate's integration into the family unit (pp. 1055–1076). In C. Kenner, A. Brueggemeyer, & L.P. Gunderson (eds.), *Comprehensive neonatal care: A physiologic perspective*. Philadelphia: W.B. Saunders.

Klein, M. & Stern, L. (1979). Low birthweight and the battered child syndrome. *American Journal of Diseases of Children, 122,* 15–18.

Ricciuti, H.N. (1983). Interaction of multiple factors contributing to high-risk parenting. In V.J. Sasserrath (ed.), *Minimizing high-risk parenting-Pediatric Round Table: 7*. Skillman, N.J.: Johnson & Johnson Baby Products.

Schmitt, B. & Kempe, H. (1975). Neglect and abuse of children (pp. 108–111). In V. Vaughan & R. McKay (eds.), *Nelson textbook of pediatrics*. Philadelphia: W.B. Saunders.

288. Answer: (**A**) Contingent interaction between the infant and caregiver depends on three characteristics: (1) readability or clarity of behaviors and cues; (2) predictability of the other in anticipating behavior from immediately preceding behaviors; and (3) responsiveness or reactions of the other with appropriate behaviors within a short latency period.

REFERENCES

Blackburn, S.T. & VandenBerg, K. A. (1993). Assessment and management of neonatal neurobehavioral development (pp. 1094–1133). In C. Kenner, A. Brueggemeyer, & L.P. Gunderson (eds.), *Comprehensive neonatal care: A physiologic perspective*. Philadelphia: W.B. Saunders.

Sammons, W.A.H. & Lewis, J.M. (1985). *Premature babies: A different beginning*. St. Louis: C.V. Mosby.

289. Answer: (**B**) The protocols designed as part of the NSTEP-P program are intended to complement a health agency's current strategy of care. Nurses are encouraged to use their agency's routines and to incorporate any existing preterm follow-up programs in the community. Although comprehensive in scope, the NSTEP-P program is not designed to take the place of physician visits. In fact, an important part of this program is to monitor families to make sure they continue to see their physicians for well-child check-ups or for specific health concerns.

REFERENCES

Johnson-Crowley, N. & Sumner, G.A. (1987a). Concept manual: Nursing systems toward effective parenting-preterm. Seattle, WA: NCAST Publications.

Johnson-Crowley, N. & Sumner, G.A. (1987b). Protocol manual: Nursing systems toward effective parenting-preterm. Seattle, WA: NCAST Publications.

Johnson-Crowley, N. (1993). Systematic assessment and home follow-up: A basis for monitoring the neonate's integration into the family unit (pp. 1055–1076). In C. Kenner, A. Brueggemeyer, & L.P. Gunderson (eds.), *Comprehensive neonatal care: A physiologic perspective*. Philadelphia: W.B. Saunders.

290. Answer: (**B**) The organization of sleeping and waking, as indicated by individual state criteria or the overall patterning of states, can be used to predict the developmental outcome of infants.

REFERENCES

Adam, K. & Oswald, I. (1984). Sleep helps healing. *British Medical Journal, 289,* 1400–1401.

Holditch-Davis, D. (1993). Neonatal sleep-wake states (pp. 1075–1093). In C. Kenner, A. Brueggemeyer, & L.P. Gunderson (eds.), *Comprehensive neonatal care: A physiologic perspective*. Philadelphia: W.B. Saunders.

291. Answer: (**B**) When children in the home require health care support personnel, family dynamics have been noted to change dramatically. An unusual phenomenon has been reported by Byers and Fabian (1988) of the University of Colorado Children's Hospital Home Care Program. Skilled caregivers have observed that some parents and families become so dependent on home care personnel that they are unable or unwilling to participate in the child's care. This has been termed

the "parent drop-out syndrome" (Byers & Fabian, 1988).

REFERENCES

Byers, J.E. & Fabian, A.M. (1988). The parent drop-out syndrome. *Caring, 7*(6), 36–38.

Hall, L.H. (1993). Home care (pp. 1148–1158). In C. Kenner, A. Brueggemeyer, & L.P. Gunderson (eds.), *Comprehensive neonatal care: A physiologic perspective*. Philadelphia: W.B. Saunders.

Lima, L. & Seliger, J. (1990). Early intervention keeps medically fragile babies at home. *Children Today, 19*(1), 28–32.

Tooley, W. (1988). In R.A. Ballard (ed.), *Pediatric care of the ICN graduate* (pp. xii). Philadelphia: W.B. Saunders.

292. Answer: (**A**) Included in this program is an observation tool (Level 1 NIDCAP-naturalistic behavioral observation), which is extremely useful for the NICU nurse. This assessment involves an observation of the infant before, during, and after a routine caregiving episode.

REFERENCES

Als, H. (1982). Toward a synactive theory of development: Promise for the assessment and support of infant individuality. *Infant Mental Health Journal, 3,* 229–243.

Als, H., Lester, B.M., Tronick, E.Z., & Brazelton, T.B. (1982). Assessment of preterm infant behavior (APIB). In H.E. Fitzgerald & M. Yogman (eds.), *Theory and research in behavioral pediatrics*. New York: Plenum Press.

Blackburn, S.T. & VandenBerg, K.A. (1993). Assessment and management of neonatal neurobehavioral development (pp. 1094–1133). In C. Kenner, A. Brueggemeyer, & L.P. Gunderson (eds.), *Comprehensive neonatal care: A physiologic perspective*. Philadelphia: W.B. Saunders.

293. Answer: (**B**) Infant stress signals include autonomic system cues such as respiratory pauses, tachypnea, gasping, color changes, tremors, startles, twitches, yawning, gagging, spitting up, hiccoughing, straining, sneezing, coughing, sighing. Infant stability signals include state system cues such as clear, robust sleep states; rhythmic, robust crying, active self-quieting/consoling; focused, shiny-eyed alertness with intent or animated facial express; "Ooh" face; cooing; and attentional smiling.

REFERENCES

Als, H. (1982). Toward a synactive theory of development: Promise for the assessment and support of infant individuality. *Infant Mental Health Journal, 3,* 229–243.

Als, H., Lester, B.M., Tronick, E.Z., & Brazelton, T.B. (1982). Assessment of preterm infant behavior (APIB). In H.E. Fitzgerald & M. Yogman (eds.), *Theory and research in behavioral pediatrics*. New York: Plenum Press.

Blackburn, S.T. & VandenBerg, K.A. (1993). Assessment and management of neonatal neurobehavioral development (pp. 1094–1133). In C. Kenner, A. Brueggemeyer, & L.P. Gunderson (eds.), *Comprehensive neonatal care: A physiologic perspective*. Philadelphia: W.B. Saunders.

294. Answer: (**B**) The second trimester is the time of beginning bind-in or attachment. Claiming begins during the third trimester.

REFERENCES

Kemp, V.H. & Page, C.K. (1987). Maternal prenatal attachment in normal and high-risk pregnancies. *JOGNN, 16*(3), 179–184.

Kenner, C. & Bagwell, G.A. (1993). Assessment and management of the transition to home (pp. 1134–1147). In C. Kenner, A. Brueggemeyer, & L.P. Gunderson (eds.), *Comprehensive neonatal care: A physiologic perspective*. Philadelphia: W.B. Saunders.

Mehren, E. (1991). *Born too soon: The story of Emily*. New York: Doubleday Book.

Rubin, R. (1973). Cognitive style in pregnancy (pp. 22–33). In M.H. Browning & E.P. Lewis. (eds.), *Maternal and newborn care: Nursing interventions*. New York: The American Journal of Nursing Company.

295. Answer: (**B**) Parents of sick or preterm infants often express the loss of their expected child once the reality of the neonatal problem shatters their hopes and fantasies. But as time goes on, parents continue to grieve but in the form of anticipating that the infant would eventually die if she or he was sick enough to require special or NICU care. Although the infant may or may not die, they anticipate this potential. This anticipatory grief is a normal coping process. There also seems to be a component of grief for the loss of their expected parenting role. They mourn the loss of their normal, familiar role.

REFERENCES

Kemp, V.H. & Page, C.K. (1987). Maternal prenatal attachment in normal and high-risk pregnancies. *JOGNN, 16*(3), 179–184.

Kenner, C.A. (1988). *Parent transition from the newborn intensive care unit (NICU) to home*. Unpublished Doctoral Dissertation. Indianapolis, IN: Indiana University.

Kenner, C. & Bagwell, G.A. (1993). Assessment and management of the transition to home (pp. 1134–1147). In C. Kenner, A. Brueggemeyer, & L.P. Gunderson (eds.), *Comprehensive neonatal care: A physiologic perspective*. Philadelphia: W.B. Saunders.

Mehren, E. (1991). *Born too soon: The story of Emily*. New York: Doubleday Book.

Sammons, W.A.H. & Lewis, J.M. (1985). *Premature babies: A different beginning*. St. Louis: C.V. Mosby.

296. Answer: (**A**) Hospice care is a philosophy of caring when cure is no longer a reasonable expectation. This care is not just terminal care but rather an effort to maximize the present quality of life without giving up all interest in a cure. Hospice provides comfort measures and focuses on alleviation of symptoms. Whether the infant is terminally or chronically ill, the ultimate goal is to provide an environment that comforts the child and supports the family.

REFERENCES

Hall, L.H. (1993). Home care (pp. 1148–1158). In C. Kenner, A. Brueggemeyer, & L.P. Gunderson (eds.), *Comprehensive neonatal care: A physiologic perspective*. Philadelphia: W.B. Saunders.
Martin, B.B. (1985). Home care for terminally ill children and their families (pp. 65–86). In C.A. Corr & D.M. Corr (eds.), *Hospice approaches to pediatric care*. New York: Springer-Verlag.
Rhymes, J. (1990). Hospice care in America. *Journal of American Medical Association, 264,* 369–372.

297. Answer: (**C**) Institutions dedicated to the care of the terminally ill have become an important alternative care approach and an accepted part of the health care field in the United States. Hospice facilities caring for children are currently increasing in number, but access to hospice care still has several barriers. Most facilities require a physician's certification that the child will die within six months. Another serious barrier is the lack of financial reimbursement for care or the inadequacy of the reimbursement to cover the cost of hospice care (Rhymes, 1990).

REFERENCES

Hall, L.H. (1993). Home care (pp. 1148–1158). In C. Kenner, A. Brueggemeyer, & L.P. Gunderson (eds.), *Comprehensive neonatal care: A physiologic perspective*. Philadelphia: W.B. Saunders.
Martin, B.B. (1985). Home care for terminally ill children and their families (pp. 65–86). In C.A. Corr & D.M. Corr (eds.), *Hospice approaches to pediatric care* New York: Springer-Verlag.
Rhymes, J. (1990). Hospice care in America. *Journal of American Medical Association, 264,* 369–372.

298. Answer: (**A**) Legislation to control the development of advanced practice in neonatal nursing should not be sought. This is a responsibility of the professional organization, and it has been accepted by the National Association of Neonatal Nurses.

REFERENCES

Harrigan, R.C. & Perez, D. (1993). Neonatal nursing and its role in comprehensive care (pp. 3–8). In C. Kenner, A. Brueggemeyer, & L.P. Gunderson (eds.), *Comprehensive neonatal nursing: A physiologic perspective*. Philadelphia: W.B. Saunders.
Johnson, P.J., Jung, A.L., & Boros, S.J. (1979). Neonatal nurse practitioners: Part 1. A new expanded nursing role. *Perinatology/Neonatology,* January-February, 34–36.

299. Answer: (**B**) Autosomal recessive patterns of inheritance are associated with many normal characteristics and variations in body structure and function such as Rh negative blood type and blue eyes. In addition, this pattern of inheritance has been demonstrated in a variety of genetically transmitted conditions, which include albinism, sickle cell anemia, and cystic fibrosis.

REFERENCES

Cohen, F.L. (1984). *Clinical genetics in nursing practice*. Philadelphia: J.B. Lippincott.
Connor, J. & Ferguson-Smith, M. (1987). *Essential medical genetics*. Oxford: Blackwell Scientific.
Cummings, M. (1988). *Human heredity: Principles and issues*. New York: West Publishing.
Thompson, S. & Thompson, M. (1986). *Genetics in medicine* (4th ed.). Philadelphia: W.B. Saunders
Workman, M.L., Kenner, C., & Hilse, M. (1993). Human genetics (pp. 101–131). In C. Kenner, A. Brueggemyer, & L.P. Gunderson (eds.), *Comprehensive neonatal nursing: A physiologic perspective*. Philadelphia: W.B. Saunders.

300. Answer: (**B**) The timing of the closure of the aortic and pulmonary valves is determined by the volume of blood ejected from the aorta and pulmonary artery and the resistance against which the ventricles must pump. In the immediate newborn period, the right and left ventricles pump similar quantities of blood and the pulmonary pressure is close to aortic pressure, the valves (A & P) close almost simultaneously. As the pulmonary resistance falls, the pulmonary resistance decreases and becomes lower than the aortic pressure, causing a splitting of S2 as the valves on the left side of the heart (aortic) close before the valve leaflets on the right side of the heart (pulmonary). Thus, pulmonary vascular resistance is one factor associated

with the timing of the closure. The other two answers are accurate but not complete. Factors that prolong right ventricular ejection time or shorten left ventricular ejection time would affect the S2 by increasing the time between the closing of one valve until the closing of the other valve. Thus, these changes are also factors associated with the timing of the closure.

REFERENCES

Johnson, G.L. (1990). Clinical examination (pp. 223–235). In W.A. Long (ed.), *Fetal and neonatal cardiology*. Philadelphia: W.B. Saunders.

Lott, J.W. (1993). Assessment and management of cardiovascular dysfunction (pp. 355–391). In C. Kenner, A. Brueggemeyer, & L.P. Gunderson (eds.), *Comprehensive neonatal nursing: A physiologic perspective*. Philadelphia: W.B. Saunders.

Park, M.K. (1984). Physical examination (pp. 9–33). *Pediatric cardiology for practitioners*. Chicago: Year Book Medical Publishers.

ANSWERS TO REVIEW TEST 2

1. Answer: (**A**) The nurse begins to act as an informal mentor as an outgrowth.

REFERENCES

France, M.H., & McDowell, C. (1983). A systematic career development model: An overview. *Canadian Vocational Journal, 19*(1), 31–34.

Harrigan, R.C. & Perez, D. (1993). Neonatal nursing and its role in comprehensive care (pp. 3–8). In C. Kenner, A. Brueggemeyer, & L.P. Gunderson (eds.), *Comprehensive neonatal nursing: A physiologic perspective*. Philadelphia: W.B. Saunders.

Perez, R. (1981). *Protocols for perinatal nursing practice*. St. Louis: C.V. Mosby.

2. Answer: (**A**) Rickets or osteopenia of prematurity, a common disorder in VLBW infants, is not believed to be generally caused by dietary deficiency or abnormality of metabolism of vitamin D but by an insufficient intake of calcium and phosphorus.

REFERENCES

DeMarini, S., Tsang, R.C., & Rath, L.L. (1993). Fluids, electrolytes, vitamins, and trace minerals: Basis of ingestion, digestion, elimination, and metabolism (pp. 393–413). In C. Kenner, A. Brueggemeyer, & L.P. Gunderson (eds.), *Comprehensive neonatal nursing: A physiologic perspective*. Philadelphia: W.B. Saunders.

Steichen, J.J., Gratton, T.L, & Tsang, R.C. (1980). Osteopenia of prematurity: The cause and possible treatment. *Journal of Pediatrics, 96,* 528–534.

3. Answer: (**A**) Signs and symptoms of placental abruption include (1) uterine tenderness or rigidity and low back pain, (2) dark-red vaginal bleeding, (3) fetal symptoms of stress, and (4) maternal signs of shock and disseminating intravascular coagulation (DIC).

   Signs and symptoms of previa rarely occur before the early third trimester. The initial onset of symptoms is usually mild, and their recurrence is unpredictable. The signs and symptoms of previa include (1) painless bleeding, usually bright red and initially slight in amount, (2) high presenting fetal part, and (3) subsequent recurrences of bleeding in increasing significant amounts and associated signs of fetal stress (Gilbert & Harmon, 1986).

REFERENCES

Creasy, R. & Resnick, M. (1989). *Maternal fetal medicine: Principles and practice*. Philadelphia: W.B. Saunders.

Gilbert, E. & Harmon, J. (1986). *High risk pregnancy and delivery*. St. Louis: C.V. Mosby.

Harmon, J.S. (1993). High-risk pregnancy (pp. 157–170). In C. Kenner, A. Brueggemeyer, & L.P. Gunderson (eds.), *Comprehensive neonatal nursing: A physiologic perspective*. Philadelphia: W.B. Saunders.

Moore, K. (1989). *The developing human* (4th ed.). Philadelphia: W.B. Saunders.

4. Answer: (**B**) Outreach education addresses the functioning of the perinatal staff as a team. Members have defined roles on the team and within the system. Accountability for one's actions is an individual's responsibility (The National Foundation, March of Dimes, 1976). Regular assessment of the team's functioning provides the opportunity to learn of current problems, discuss potential solutions, and evaluate progress. The impact of the outreach programs is seen in the improvement of care and the decrease of morbidity and mortality in the region (Jones & Modica, 1989).

REFERENCES

Jones, D.B. & Modica, M.M. (1989). Assessment strategies for the outreach educator. *The Journal of Perinatal & Neonatal Nursing, 2*(3), 1–9.

National Perinatal Information Center, Inc. (1988). *The perinatal partnership: An approach to organizing care in the 1990s* (Project No. 12129). Providence, RI: Cooke, Schwartz, & Gagoron.

Ryan, G.M. (1975). Toward improving the outcome of pregnancy. Recommendations for the regional development of perinatal health services. *Journal of Obstetrics and Gynecology, 46*(4), 375–384.

Wolfe, L.S. (1993). Regionalization of care (pp. 171–181). In C. Kenner, A. Brueggemeyer, & L.P. Gunderson (eds.), *Comprehensive neonatal care: A physiologic perspective*. Philadelphia: W.B. Saunders.

5. Answer: (**B**) Certain fetal or maternal conditions can affect the quantity

of amniotic fluid. Fetal renal malfunctions can lead to less amniotic fluid, whereas gastrointestinal anomalies can cause greater amniotic fluid (polyhydramnios). Certain maternal conditions, especially nutritional deficiencies, are often associated with a smaller placenta and lower amniotic fluid volume (oligohydramnios). This, in turn, can lead to nutritional growth retardation of the fetus. The most common occurrence of decreased amniotic fluid is with postterm pregnancy, in which both fetal and maternal contribution to the volume is reduced.

REFERENCES

Creasy, R. & Resnick, M. (1989). *Maternal fetal medicine: Principles and practice*. Philadelphia: W.B. Saunders.
Gilbert, E. & Harmon, J. (1986). *High risk pregnancy and delivery*. St. Louis: C.V. Mosby.
Harmon, J.S. (1993). High-risk pregnancy (pp. 157–170). In C. Kenner, A. Brueggemeyer, & L.P. Gunderson (eds.), *Comprehensive neonatal nursing: A physiologic perspective*. Philadelphia: W.B. Saunders.
Moore, K. (1989). *The developing human* (4th ed.). Philadelphia: W.B. Saunders.

6. Answer: (**B**) Amniotic fluid has a number of functions. It (1) permits symmetrical growth and development; (2) prevents adherence of the amnion to the embryo; (3) cushions the fetus against jolts by distributing any impacts the mother may receive; (4) helps to control fetal body temperature by maintaining a relatively constant temperature; (5) enables the fetus to move freely, thus aiding musculoskeletal development; (6) protects the umbilical cord; and (7) provides antimicrobial protection (Moore, 1989). These functions can be impaired in the presence of oligohydramnios or polyhydramnios.

REFERENCES

Creasy, R. & Resnick, M. (1989). *Maternal fetal medicine: Principles and practice*. Philadelphia: W.B. Saunders.
Gilbert, E. & Harmon, J. (1986). *High risk pregnancy and delivery*. St. Louis: C.V. Mosby.
Harmon, J.S. (1993). High-risk pregnancy (pp. 157–170). In C. Kenner, A. Brueggemeyer, & L.P. Gunderson (eds.), *Comprehensive neonatal nursing: A physiologic perspective*. Philadelphia: W.B. Saunders.
Moore, K. (1989). *The developing human* (4th ed.). Philadelphia: W.B. Saunders.

7. Answer: (**C**) To meet the growing needs of the fetus for maternal storage of fat and protein, there should be an increase of 300 to 500 calories per day above normal caloric requirements. The formation and storage of fat and lean body tissue act as a reserve for the fetus during the last part of pregnancy and provide an energy source for labor, delivery, and lactation. Social habits such as alcohol intake, smoking, and drug abuse will interfere with adequate absorption of nutrients in the fetus and the mother (Gilbert & Harmon, 1986).

REFERENCES

Creasy, R. & Resnick, M. (1989). *Maternal fetal medicine: Principles and practice*. Philadelphia: W.B. Saunders.
Gilbert, E. & Harmon, J. (1986). *High risk pregnancy and delivery*. St. Louis: C.V. Mosby.
Harmon, J.S. (1993). High-risk pregnancy (pp. 157–170). In C. Kenner, A. Brueggemeyer, & L.P. Gunderson (eds.), *Comprehensive neonatal nursing: A physiologic perspective*. Philadelphia: W.B. Saunders.
Moore, K. (1989). *The developing human* (4th ed.). Philadelphia: W.B. Saunders.

8. Answer: (**A**) Mature sex cells (gametes have only 23 chromosomes, half of each pair). This number is known as the haploid number (1N) of chromosomes for humans.

REFERENCES

Cohen, F.L. (1984). *Clinical genetics in nursing practice*. Philadelphia: J.B. Lippincott.
Connor, J. & Ferguson-Smith, M. (1987). *Essential medical genetics*. Oxford: Blackwell Scientific.
Cummings, M. (1988). *Human heredity: Principles and issues*. New York: West Publishing.
Thompson, S. & Thompson, M. (1986). *Genetics in medicine*. (4th ed.). Philadelphia: W.B. Saunders.
Workman, M.L., Kenner, C., & Hilse, M. (1993). Human genetics (pp. 101–131). In C. Kenner, A. Brueggemeyer, & L.P. Gunderson (eds.), *Comprehensive neonatal nursing: A physiologic perspective*. Philadelphia: W.B. Saunders.

9. Answer: (**B**) The actual cause of placental abruption is unknown. Conditions associated with abruption are (Gilbert & Harmon, 1986) (1) PIH or chronic hypertension, present in four percent of patients; (2) maternal age over 35 years; (3) multiparity greater than five pregnancies; (4) previous abruption; 10 percent increased risk after one abruption and 25 percent increased risk after two abruptions; (5) trauma from a direct blow to the

abdomen or needle puncture during an amniocentesis; (6) short umbilical cord; (7) folic acid deficiency; and (8) cigarette smoking, cocaine use, and polysubstance abuse, causing vasoconstriction of spiral arterioles and leading to decidual necrosis.

REFERENCES

Creasy, R. & Resnick, M. (1989). *Maternal fetal medicine: Principles and practice.* Philadelphia: W.B. Saunders.

Gilbert, E. & Harmon, J. (1986). *High risk pregnancy and delivery.* St. Louis: C.V. Mosby.

Harmon, J.S. (1993). High-risk pregnancy (pp. 157–170). In C. Kenner, A. Brueggemeyer, & L.P. Gunderson (eds.), *Comprehensive neonatal nursing: A physiologic perspective.* Philadelphia: W.B. Saunders.

Moore, K. (1989). *The developing human* (4th ed.). Philadelphia: W.B. Saunders.

10. Answer: (**C**) Vitamin A deficiency can occur with any form of fat malabsorption (decreased absorption), in preterm infants (low hepatic stores and decreased intake), in infants on parenteral nutrition (adherence of retinal to plastic tubing), and in infants with BPD. Shenai, Chityl, and Stahlman (1985) reported lower concentrations of serum retinol in infants with BPD than in controls without BPD. In infants with BPD, vitamin A deficiency is not absolute but relative, possibly owing to increased vitamin A requirements.

REFERENCES

DeMarini, S., Tsang, R.C., & Rath, L.L. (1993). Fluids, electrolytes, vitamins, and trace minerals: Basis of ingestion, digestion, elimination, and metabolism (pp. 393–413). In C. Kenner, A. Brueggemeyer, & L.P. Gunderson (eds.), *Comprehensive neonatal nursing: A physiologic perspective.* Philadelphia: W.B. Saunders.

Shenai, J.P., Chityl, F., & Stahlman, M.T. (1985). Vitamin A status of neonates with bronchopulmonary dysplasia. *Pediatric Research, 19,* 185–188.

Zachman, R.D. (1988). In R.A.C. Tsang & B.L. Nichols (eds.), *Nutrition during infancy* (pp. 253–263). St. Louis: C.V. Mosby.

11. Answer: (**B**) Nurses in particular feel that replicating or repeating a study is cheating and has no value. This is not true. Studies need to be repeated to support the findings from the original study. Replication of studies is an easy way to begin to learn the research process and often is less frustrating for the beginning researcher that does not feel capable of designing an original study.

REFERENCES

Brink, P.J. & Wood, M.J. (eds.). (1989). *Advanced design in nursing research.* Newbury Park, California: Sage Publications.

Franck, L.S., Gunderson, L.P., & Kenner, C. (1993). Collaborative research in neonatal nursing (pp. 52–66). In C. Kenner, A. Brueggemeyer, & L.P. Gunderson (eds.), *Comprehensive neonatal nursing: A physiologic perspective.* Philadelphia: W.B. Saunders.

12. Answer: (**C**) Vitamin D in its active form, 1,25-dihydroxyvitamin D, is essential for the active process.

REFERENCES

Costarino, A. & Baumgart, S. (1986). Modern fluid and electrolyte management of the critically ill premature infant. *Pediatric Clinics of North America, 33,* 153–158.

DeMarini, S., Tsang, R.C., & Rath, L.L. (1993). Fluids, electrolytes, vitamins, and trace minerals: Basis of ingestion, digestion, elimination, and metabolism (pp. 393–413). In C. Kenner, A. Brueggemeyer, & L.P. Gunderson (eds.), *Comprehensive neonatal nursing: A physiologic perspective.* Philadelphia: W.B. Saunders.

Specker, B.L., Greer, F., & Tsang, R.C. (1988). Vitamin D (pp. 264–276). In R.C. Tsang & B.L. Nichols (eds.), *Nutrition during infancy.* St. Louis: C.V. Mosby.

Specker, B.L., Valanis, B., Hertzberg, V., Edwards, N., & Tsang, R.C. (1985). Sunshine exposure and serum 25-hydroxyvitamin D concentrations in exclusively breast-fed infants. *Journal of Pediatrics, 107,* 372–376.

13. Answer: (**C**) In law a negligence suit can be brought when the careless (as opposed to the intentional) acts of an individual bring about harm to a person to whom one has a duty of care. The legal elements necessary to prove negligence are duty, breach of duty, injury, and causation.

REFERENCES

American Nurses' Association. (1984). *Code for nurse with interpretive statements.* Kansas City, MO: Author.

Driscoll, K.M. (1993). Legal aspects of perinatal care (pp. 36–51). In C. Kenner, A. Brueggemeyer, & L.P. Gunderson (eds.), *Comprehensive neonatal nursing: A physiologic perspective.* Philadelphia: W.B. Saunders.

Pegalis, S.E. & Wachsman, H.F. (1990). *American law of medical malpractice.* (Cum. Suppl.). Rochester, NY: Lawyers Co-Operative Publishing.

14. Answer: (**A**) Pellagra (rough skin) is the consequence of niacin deficiency. Signs include dermatitis and inflammation of the mucous membranes, diarrhea, and dementia.

REFERENCES

DeMarini, S., Tsang, R.C., & Rath, L.L. (1993). Fluids, electrolytes, vitamins, and trace minerals: Basis of ingestion, digestion, elimination, and metabolism (pp. 393–413). In C. Kenner, A. Brueggemeyer, & L.P. Gunderson (eds.), *Comprehensive neonatal nursing: A physiologic perspective.* Philadelphia: W.B. Saunders.

Schanler, R.J. (1988). Water-soluble vitamins: C, B_1, B_2, B_6, niacin, biotin and pantothenic acid (pp. 236–252). In R.C. Tsang & B.L. Nichols (eds.), *Nutrition during infancy.* St. Louis: C.V. Mosby.

15. Answer: (**A**) Thirty percent of preterm infants (37 weeks' gestation), 35 percent of birth-asphyxiated infants, 50 percent of infants of insulin-dependent diabetic mothers, and 90 percent of VLBW infants (>1500 grams) develop hypocalcemia in the first days of life. Several factors appear to be involved: abrupt termination of maternal calcium supply, temporary functional hypoparathyroidism (infants of diabetic mothers), increased calcitonin concentrations (asphyxia, preterm infants), and 1,25-dihydroxyvitamin D resistance (VLBW infants).

REFERENCES

DeMarini, S., Tsang, R.C., & Rath, L.L. (1993). Fluids, electrolytes, vitamins, and trace minerals: Basis of ingestion, digestion, elimination, and metabolism (pp. 393–413). In C. Kenner, A. Brueggemeyer, & L.P. Gunderson (eds.), *Comprehensive neonatal nursing: A physiologic perspective.* Philadelphia: W.B. Saunders.

Tsang, R.C., Kleinman, L.I., Sutherland, J.M., & Light, I.J. (1972). Hypocalcemia in infants of diabetic mothers. *Journal of Pediatrics, 80,* 384–395.

Tsang, R.C. & Oh, W. (1970). Neonatal hypocalcemia in low birthweight infants. *Pediatrics, 45,* 773–781.

Venkatamaran, P.S., Tsang, R.C., Steichen, J.J., Grey, I., Neylan, M., & Fleischmann., A.R. (1986). Early neonatal hypocalcemia in extremely preterm infants. *American Journal of Diseases of Childhood, 140,* 1004–1008.

16. Answer: (**A**) Long chain fatty acids require bile acids for absorption. Because of the slow rate of bile acid synthesis and the increased rate of turnover, this process is extremely inefficient in preterm infants.

REFERENCES

Lebenthal, E. (ed.). (1989). *Textbook of gastroenterology and nutrition in infancy.* New York: Raven Press.

Lefrak-Okikawa, L. & Meier, P.P. (1993). Nutrition: Physiologic basis of metabolism and management of enteral and parenteral nutrition (pp. 414–433). In C. Kenner, A. Brueggemeyer, & L.P. Gunderson (eds.), *Comprehensive neonatal nursing: A physiologic perspective.* Philadelphia: W.B. Saunders.

Tsang, R.E. & Nichols, B.L. (eds.). (1988). *Nutrition during infancy.* Philadelphia: Hanley & Belfus.

17. Answer: (**B**) Alpha, or a type I error, refers to the rejection of the null hypothesis when in fact it is true. Beta, or type II error, refers to accepting a false null hypothesis when in fact it is true.

REFERENCES

Brink, P.J. & Wood, M.J. (eds.). (1989). *Advanced design in nursing research.* Newbury Park, CA: Sage Publications.

Franck, L.S., Gunderson, L.P., & Kenner, C. (1993). Collaborative research in neonatal nursing (pp. 52–66). In C. Kenner, A. Brueggemeyer, & L.P. Gunderson (eds.), *Comprehensive neonatal nursing: A physiologic perspective.* Philadelphia: W.B. Saunders.

18. Answer: (**A**) A case manager is a coordinator of formal and informal health services for an individual child and family. Leadership is decentralized, flexible, and task-oriented.

REFERENCES

Aradine, C.R. & Hansen, M.F. (1970). Interdisciplinary teamwork in family health care. *Nursing Clinics of North America, 5*(2), 211–222.

Gilles, C. (1991). Nonsurgical management of the infant with gastroesophageal reflux and respiratory problems. *Journal of the American Academy of Nursing Practice, 3*(1), 11–16.

Harrigan, R. & Perez, D. (1993). Collaborative practice in the NICU (pp. 9–13). In C. Kenner, A. Brueggemeyer, & L.P. Gunderson (eds.), *Comprehensive neonatal nursing: A physiologic perspective.* Philadelphia: W.B. Saunders.

Temkin-Greener, H. (1983). Interprofessional perspectives on teamwork in health care: A case study. *Milbank Memorial Fund Quarterly/Health and Society, 61*(4), 641–657.

19. Answer: (**C**) Calcium is the most abundant mineral in the human body. It is an essential component of the skeleton and plays an important role in muscle contraction, neural transmission, and blood coagulation. Phosphorus is essential for bone mineralization, erythrocyte function, cell metabolism, and the generation and storage of energy.

REFERENCES

Costarino, A. & Baumgart, S. (1986). Modern fluid and electrolyte management of the critically ill premature infant. *Pediatric Clinics of North America, 33,* 153–158.

DeMarini, S., Tsang, R.C., & Rath, L.L. (1993). Fluids, electrolytes, vitamins, and trace minerals: Basis of ingestion, digestion, elimination, and metabolism (pp. 393–413). In C. Kenner, A. Brueggemeyer, &

L.P. Gunderson (eds.), *Comprehensive neonatal nursing: A physiologic perspective*. Philadelphia: W.B. Saunders.

Tsang, R.C., Chen, I., Hayes, W., Atkinson, W., Atherton, H., & Edwards, N. (1974). Neonatal hypocalcemia in infants with birth asphyxia. *Journal of Pediatrics, 84,* 428–433.

Tsang, R.C. & Oh, W. (1970). Neonatal hypocalcemia in low birthweight infants. *Pediatrics, 45,* 773–781.

20. Answer: (**A**) IRBs were developed to ensure the rights and welfare of research subjects. The function of the IRB is to review, approve, disapprove, or request revision of research protocols for the purposes of protection of human subjects and to uphold the ethical principles of research.

REFERENCES

Brink, P.J. & Wood, M.J. (eds.). (1989). *Advanced design in nursing research*. Newbury Park, CA: Sage Publications.

Franck, L.S., Gunderson, L.P., & Kenner, C. (1993). Collaborative research in neonatal nursing (pp. 52–66). In C. Kenner, A. Brueggemeyer, & L.P. Gunderson (eds.), *Comprehensive neonatal nursing: A physiologic perspective*. Philadelphia: W.B. Saunders.

21. Answer: (**B**) Employers have a right to know whether a nurse who claims to be a specialist is indeed so qualified, and they have a responsibility to verify credentials of neonatal nurse specialists.

REFERENCES

Harper, R.G., Little, G.A., & Sia, C.G. (1982). The scope of nursing practice in level III neonatal intensive care units. *Pediatrics, 70,* 875–878.

Harrigan, R.C. & Perez, D. (1993). Neonatal nursing and its role in comprehensive care (pp. 3–8). In C. Kenner, A. Brueggemeyer, & L.P. Gunderson (eds.), *Comprehensive neonatal nursing: A physiologic perspective*. Philadelphia: W.B. Saunders.

22. Answer: (**C**) During the pancreatic or intraluminal phase, the polysaccharides are broken down into mono- and disaccharides. Amylase is the primary enzyme responsible for this process, and it is secreted by the pancreas into the small intestine. At term, amylase is only at 10 percent of adult levels.

REFERENCES

Lebenthal, E. (ed.). (1989). *Textbook of gastroenterology and nutrition in infancy*. New York: Raven Press.

Lefrak-Okikawa, L. & Meier, P.P. (1993). Nutrition: Physiologic basis of metabolism and management of enteral and parenteral nutrition (pp. 414–433). In C. Kenner, A. Brueggemeyer, & L.P. Gunderson (eds.), *Comprehensive neonatal nursing: A physiologic perspective*. Philadelphia: W.B. Saunders.

Tsang, R.E. & Nichols, B.L. (eds.). (1988). *Nutrition during infancy*. Philadelphia: Hanley & Belfus.

23. Answer: (**C**) Increased renal loss of chloride is the characteristic feature of Bartter's syndrome, which has as its underlying mechanism a defect in tubular reabsorption of chloride. Increased urinary chloride and prostaglandin concentrations are diagnostic, and therapy with indomethacin (a prostaglandin antagonist) is usually effective.

REFERENCES

Bartter, F.C. (1986). On the pathogenesis of Bartter's syndrome. *Mineral and Electrolyte Metabolism, 3,* 61–65.

Costarino, A. & Baumgart, S. (1986). Modern fluid and electrolyte management of the critically ill premature infant. *Pediatric Clinics of North America, 33,* 153–158.

DeMarini, S., Tsang, R.C., & Rath, L.L. (1993). Fluids, electrolytes, vitamins, and trace minerals: Basis of ingestion, digestion, elimination, and metabolism (pp. 393–413). In C. Kenner, A. Brueggemeyer, & L.P. Gunderson (eds.), *Comprehensive neonatal nursing: A physiologic perspective*. Philadelphia: W.B. Saunders.

Perkin, R.M. & Levin, D.L. (1980). Common fluid and electrolyte problems in the pediatric intensive care unit. *Pediatric Clinics of North America, 27,* 558–567.

Spitzer, A., Berstein, J., Edelman, C.M., & Boichis, H. (1987). The kidney and urinary tract (pp. 981–1015). In A.A. Fanaroff & R.J. Martin (eds.), *Neonatal-perinatal medicine*. St. Louis: C.V. Mosby.

24. Answer: (**C**) Together the Code for Nurses and the Social Policy Statement provide the mandate for nurses' participation in ethical deliberations.

REFERENCES

ANA. (1985). *Code for nurses with interpretive statements*. Kansas City, MO: American Nurses' Association.

ANA. (1985). *Social policy statement for nurses*. Kansas City, MO: American Nurses' Association.

Southwell, S. M, & Archer-Dusté, H. (1993). Ethical aspects of perinatal care (pp. 14–35). In C. Kenner, A. Brueggemeyer, & L.P. Gunderson (eds.), *Comprehensive neonatal nursing: A physiologic perspective*. Philadelphia: W.B. Saunders.

25. Answer: (**B**) Chronic administration of furosemide is often necessary in BPD and can cause chloride deficiency with secondary metabolic alkalosis. Alkalosis, in turn, causes hypoventilation and increased $PaCo_2$. This

clinical picture can simulate pulmonary edema, but in this case the treatment should not include additional diuretic therapy (as in pulmonary edema) but rather correction of the hypochloremia.

REFERENCES

Blanchard, P.W., Brown, T.M., & Coates, A.L. (1987). Pharmacotherapy in bronchopulmonary dysplasia. *Clinics in Perinatology, 14,* 881–910.

Costarino, A. & Baumgart, S. (1986). Modern fluid and electrolyte management of the critically ill premature infant. *Pediatric Clinics of North America, 33,* 153–158.

DeMarini, S., Tsang, R.C., & Rath, L.L. (1993). Fluids, electrolytes, vitamins, and trace minerals: Basis of ingestion, digestion, elimination, and metabolism (pp. 393–413). In C. Kenner, A. Brueggemeyer, & L.P. Gunderson (eds.), *Comprehensive neonatal nursing: A physiologic perspective.* Philadelphia: W.B. Saunders.

Perkin, R.M. & Levin, D.L. (1980). Common fluid and electrolyte problems in the pediatric intensive care unit. *Pediatric Clinics of North America, 27,* 558–567.

26. Answer: (**B**) *Cognitive* activities include early identification and evaluation of risk factors. The neonatal nurse uses specific screening tools to identify problems and then initiates appropriate action and referral. The nurse provides appropriate anticipatory guidance and teaching for the family related to the neonate's health and developmental status. *Generative* activities include developing new behaviors and modifying environments or roles to help parents and neonates adjust to their developmental and health needs. *Nurturant* nursing behaviors provide surveillance of physiological variables, comfort for infants, and teaching for the family about the infants' illnesses.

REFERENCES

Harrigan, R.C. & Perez, D. (1993). Neonatal nursing and its role in comprehensive care (pp. 3–8). In C. Kenner, A. Brueggemeyer, & L.P. Gunderson (eds.), *Comprehensive neonatal nursing: A physiologic perspective.* Philadelphia: W.B. Saunders.

Harper, R.G., Little, G.A., & Sia, C.G. (1982). The scope of nursing practice in level III neonatal intensive care units. *Pediatrics, 70*(6), 875–878.

27. Answer: (**A**) The active mucosal transport of monosaccharides or simple sugars such as glucose is present even in the fetus and continues to provide a simple mechanism for carbohydrate absorption when other mechanisms fail. Infants with intestinal damage after necrotizing enterocolitis or prolonged ileus with atrophy can be disaccharide intolerant and yet absorb glucose or glucose polymers such as polycose.

REFERENCES

Lebenthal, E. (ed.). (1989). *Textbook of gastroenterology and nutrition in infancy.* New York: Raven Press.

Lefrak-Okikawa, L. & Meier, P.P. (1993). Nutrition: Physiologic basis of metabolism and management of enteral and parenteral nutrition (pp. 414–433). In C. Kenner, A. Brueggemeyer, & L.P. Gunderson (eds.), *Comprehensive neonatal nursing: A physiologic perspective.* Philadelphia: W.B. Saunders.

Tsang, R.E. & Nichols, B.L. (eds.). (1988). *Nutrition during infancy.* Philadelphia: Hanley & Belfus.

28. Answer: (**C**) Nonmaleficence is the obligation to prevent actual or potential harm and to act in a prudent, thoughtful manner. Nonmaleficence focuses on the notions of risk-benefit analysis and detriment-benefit analysis. Beneficence is the process of actively promoting good and preventing or removing harm. Justice is acting justly by giving what is owed to the entitled person.

REFERENCES

Beauchamp, T.L. & Childress, J.F. (1983). *Principles of biomedical ethics.* New York: Oxford University Press.

Cunningham, N. & Hutchinson, S. (1990). Neonatal nurses and issues in research ethics. *Neonatal Network, 8*(5), 29–48.

Fowler, M.D. (1987). Introduction to ethics and ethical theory (pp. 659–670). In M.D. Fowler & J. Levine-Ariff (eds.), *Ethics at the bedside: A source book for the critical care nurse.* New York: McGraw-Hill.

Southwell, S.M., & Archer-Dusté, H. (1993). Ethical aspects of perinatal care (pp. 14–35). In C. Kenner, A. Brueggemeyer, & L.P. Gunderson (eds.), *Comprehensive neonatal nursing: A physiologic perspective.* Philadelphia: W.B. Saunders.

29. Answer: (**C**) Zinc that has been ingested is absorbed in the proximal small bowel. Absorption varies based on the bioavailability of the source and the presence of other minerals in the diet such as iron and copper.

REFERENCES

Lebenthal, E. (ed.). (1989). *Textbook of gastroenterology and nutrition in infancy.* New York: Raven Press.

Lefrak-Okikawa, L. & Meier, P.P. (1993). Nutrition: Physiologic basis of metabolism and management of enteral and parenteral nutrition (pp. 414–433). In C. Kenner, A. Brueggemeyer, & L.P. Gunderson (eds.),

Comprehensive neonatal nursing: A physiologic perspective. Philadelphia: W.B. Saunders.

Tsang, R.E. & Nichols, B.L. (eds.). (1988). *Nutrition during infancy*. Philadelphia: Hanley & Belfus.

30. Answer: (**C**) The main purpose of the review of the literature is to bring together data and theories that pertain to the topic of interest. The relationships between the concepts and the major issues are uncovered and the gaps or potential flaws in the current knowledge also are identified. In essence, the review of the literature provides a logical step toward the formulation of the research.

REFERENCES

Brink, P.J. & Wood, M.J. (eds.) (1989). *Advanced design in nursing research*. Newbury Park, CA: Sage Publications.

Franck, L.S., Gunderson, L.P., & Kenner, C. (1993). Collaborative research in neonatal nursing (pp. 52–66). In C. Kenner, A. Brueggemeyer, & L.P. Gunderson (eds.), *Comprehensive neonatal nursing: A physiologic perspective*. Philadelphia: W.B. Saunders.

31. Answer: (**C**) With Class D diabetic, onset is before age 10 or greater than 10 years' duration or early vascular complications and the condition requires insulin therapy. The following neonatal effects are seen (Creasy & Resnik, 1989; Gilbert & Harmon, 1986): (1) hypoglycemia in the transitional period because of high insulin production but loss of maternal glucose supply; (2) hyperbilirubinemia from increased "sugar"-coated fetal hemoglobin and breakdown of this in the early neonatal period; (3) hypercalcemia, hypokalemia, and other lacerations in electrolytes; (4) increased cesarean birth; (5) increased incidence of traumatic vaginal birth, usually from shoulder dystocias; (6) neonatal respiratory distress syndrome even after 36 weeks. Due to or related to high maternal blood glucose, high placental glucose storage, high placental production of cortisol, low fetal production of cortisol, and low surfactant production lead to low lung maturity at expected gestation.

REFERENCES

Creasy, R. & Resnick, M. (1989). *Maternal fetal medicine: Principles and practice*. Philadelphia: W.B. Saunders.

Gilbert, E. & Harmon, J. (1986). *High risk pregnancy and delivery*. St. Louis: C.V. Mosby.

Harmon, J.S. (1993). High-risk pregnancy (pp. 157–170). In C. Kenner, A. Brueggemeyer, & L.P. Gunderson (eds.), *Comprehensive neonatal nursing: A physiologic perspective*. Philadelphia: W.B. Saunders.

Moore, K. (1989). *The developing human* (4th ed.). Philadelphia: W.B. Saunders.

32. Answer: (**A**) Expanded and extended practice roles have provided a significant clinical renaissance, a quiet revolution within nursing that has helped the profession not only to survive but to keep pace with and to go forward and strengthen itself despite dramatic and far-reaching changes in health care. Nurse practitioners and clinical specialists have advanced neonatal nursing to a complex, highly technological enterprise. These include (1) innovation and refinement of practice, (2) acceptance of control of neonatal nursing practice, and (3) development of a research basis for practice. Recent discussion with the American Nurses' Association suggested that specialist and practitioner roles will be merged. Yet there is within the profession ambivalence, uncertainty, and lack of clarity about specialization and the advanced practice of neonatal nursing. This ambivalence attracts unfavorable attention to the public's image of a neonatal nurse.

REFERENCES

France, M.H. & McDowell, C. (1983). A systematic career development model: An overview. *Canadian Vocational Journal, 19*(1), 31–34.

Harrigan, R.C. & Perez, D. (1993). Neonatal nursing and its role in comprehensive care (pp. 3–8). In C. Kenner, A. Brueggemeyer, & L.P. Gunderson (eds.), *Comprehensive neonatal nursing: A physiologic perspective*. Philadelphia: W.B. Saunders.

Perez, R. (1981). *Protocols for perinatal nursing practice*. St. Louis: C.V. Mosby.

33. Answer: (**B**) The total fluid volume that the infant can safely receive, based on organ maturity and disease state, dictates the concentration of all other nutrients to be delivered.

REFERENCES

Kerner, J.A. (1983). *Manual of pediatric parenteral nutrition* (pp. 63–68, 117–217). New York: Raven Press.

Lefrak-Okikawa, L. & Meier, P.P. (1993). Nutrition: Physiologic basis of metabolism and management of enteral and parenteral nutrition (pp. 414–433). In C.

Kenner, A. Brueggemeyer, & L.P. Gunderson (eds.), *Comprehensive neonatal nursing: A physiologic perspective*. Philadelphia: W.B. Saunders.

34. Answer: (**B**) Quality assurance programs can be thought of as the proactive counterpart of risk management efforts. What implications does quality assurance have for neonatal nursing practice? First, they suggest nurses need to examine their interventions to determine if they improve infant functional outcomes. Second, as data about the relationship of interventions and outcomes are generated, quality assurance programs will generate new standards of care. Health care providers should assist parents in the decision-making process. Unfortunately, they can sometimes be at odds with parental choices. These situations can generate legal action in the form of case law, statutory law, and regulatory law. By law, the responsibility for obtaining informed consent for treatments resides with the physician.

REFERENCES

American Academy of Pediatrics/American College of Obstetrician and Gynecologists. (1992). *Guidelines for perinatal care*. Elk Grove Village, IL: Author.
American Nurses' Association. (1984). *Code for nurse with interpretive statements*. Kansas City: Author.
Driscoll, K.M. (1993). Legal aspects of perinatal care (pp. 36–51). In C. Kenner, A. Brueggemeyer, & L.P. Gunderson (eds.), *Comprehensive neonatal nursing: A physiologic perspective*. Philadelphia: W.B. Saunders.
Pegalis, S.E. & Wachsman, H.F. (1990). *American law of medical malpractice*. (Cum. Suppl.). Rochester, NY: Lawyers Co-Operative Publishing.

35. Answer: (**C**) Metaethics and descriptive ethics are nonnormative; they do not prescribe behaviors (Fowler, 1987). The application of normative ethics to specific issues, cases, or situations is applied ethics. The Code for Nurses is an example of applied ethics. It establishes a normative standard for a specific professional group.

REFERENCES

ANA. (1985). *Code for nurses with interpretive statements*. Kansas City, MO: American Nurses' Association.
Beauchamp, T.L. & Childress, J.F. (1983). *Principles of biomedical ethics*. New York: Oxford University Press.
Fowler, M.D. (1987). Introduction to ethics and ethical theory (pp. 659–670). In M.D. Fowler & J. Levine-Ariff (eds.), *Ethics at the bedside: A source book for the critical care nurse*. New York: McGraw-Hill.
Southwell, S.M. & Archer-Dusté, H. (1993). Ethical aspects of perinatal care (pp. 14–35). In C. Kenner, A. Brueggemeyer, & L.P. Gunderson (eds.), *Comprehensive neonatal nursing: A physiologic perspective*. Philadelphia: W.B. Saunders.

36. Answer: (**C**) Hyperglycemia and hypoglycemia are probably the most common ongoing problems associated with the use of TPN.

REFERENCES

Binder, N.D., Raschko, P.K., Benda, G.I, & Reynolds, J.W. (1989). Insulin infusion with parenteral nutrition in extremely low birth weight infants with hyperglycemia. *Journal of Pediatrics, 114,* 273–280.
Kerner, J.A. (1991). Parenteral nutrition. In W.A. Walker, P. Durie, R. Hamilton, J. Watkins, & J.A. Walker-Smith (eds.), *Pediatric gastrointestinal disease* (Vol. 2). Philadelphia: B.C. Decker.
Lefrak-Okikawa, L. & Meier, P.P. (1993). Nutrition: Physiologic basis of metabolism and management of enteral and parenteral nutrition (pp. 414–433). In C. Kenner, A. Brueggemeyer, & L.P. Gunderson (eds.), *Comprehensive neonatal nursing: A physiologic perspective*. Philadelphia: W.B. Saunders.

37. Answer: (**B**) Implantation is completed during the second week.

REFERENCES

Lott, J.W. (1993). Fetal development: Environmental influences and critical periods (pp. 132–156). In C. Kenner, A. Brueggemeyer, & L.P. Gunderson (eds.), *Comprehensive neonatal nursing: A physiologic perspective*. Philadelphia: W.B. Saunders.
Moore, K.L. (1989). *The developing human* (4th ed.). Philadelphia: W.B. Saunders.
Sadler, T.W. (1985). *Langman's medical embryology* (5th ed.). Baltimore: Williams & Wilkins.

38. Answer: (**B**) Standards should be thought of as general guidelines to practice. But more important is that any nurse be able to defend any action or inaction as reasonable and prudent in relation to care of the neonate.

REFERENCES

American Academy of Pediatrics/American College of Obstetrician and Gynecologists. (1992). *Guidelines for perinatal care*. Elk Grove Village, IL: Author.
American Nurses' Association. (1984). *Code for nurse with interpretive statements*. Kansas City, MO: Author.
Driscoll, K.M. (1993). Legal aspects of perinatal care (pp. 36–51). In C. Kenner, A. Brueggemeyer, & L.P. Gunderson (eds.), *Comprehensive neonatal nursing: A physiologic perspective*. Philadelphia: W.B. Saunders.
Pegalis, S.E. & Wachsman, H.F. (1990). *American law of medical malpractice*. (Cum. Suppl.). Rochester, NY: Lawyers Co-Operative Publishing.

39. Answer: (**A**) Developmental aspects of neonatal nursing roles include ambivalence among neonatal nurses about allowing better educated nurses to be called specialists, the merging of extended and expanded neonatal nursing roles into an advanced practice focus for neonatal nursing, the rights of students and practitioners to understand the basis for credentialing within the specialty, and the education of neonatal nurses for advanced practice. Five groups of neonatal nurses have been identified: *providers* of neonatal nursing care, *communicators* or managers of neonatal nursing practice, *translators* of research data into practice useful information, *generators* of knowledge for neonatal nursing practice, and *shapers* of policy related to neonatal health care.

REFERENCES

France, M.H. & McDowell, C. (1983). A systematic career development model: An overview. *Canadian Vocational Journal, 19*(1), 31–34.

Harrigan, R.C. & Perez, D. (1993). Neonatal nursing and its role in comprehensive care (pp. 3–8). In C. Kenner, A. Brueggemeyer, & L.P. Gunderson (eds.), *Comprehensive neonatal nursing: A physiologic perspective*. Philadelphia: W.B. Saunders.

Perez, R. (1981). *Protocols for perinatal nursing practice*. St. Louis: C.V. Mosby.

40. Answer: (**B**) Research is a formal, systematic inquiry or examination of a given problem. The outcome or goal of research is to discover new information or relationships. In some cases, the purpose is to verify existing knowledge.

REFERENCES

Brink, P.J. & Wood, M.J. (eds.). (1989). *Advanced design in nursing research*. Newbury Park, CA: Sage Publications.

Franck, L.S., Gunderson, L.P., & Kenner, C. (1993). Collaborative research in neonatal nursing (pp. 52–66). In C. Kenner, A. Brueggemeyer, & L.P. Gunderson (eds.), *Comprehensive neonatal nursing: A physiologic perspective*. Philadelphia: W.B. Saunders.

41. Answer: (**A**) Daily weight gains should aim for about 15 to 20 g/kg/day.

REFERENCES

Fenton, T.R., McMillian, D.D., & Sauve, R.S. (1990). Nutrition and growth analysis of very low birth weight infants. *Pediatrics, 86,* 378–383.

Lefrak-Okikawa, L. & Meier, P.P. (1993). Nutrition: Physiologic basis of metabolism and management of enteral and parenteral nutrition (pp. 414–433). In C. Kenner, A. Brueggemeyer, & L.P. Gunderson (eds.), *Comprehensive neonatal nursing: A physiologic perspective*. Philadelphia: W.B. Saunders.

Shaffer, S.G., Quimiro, C., Anderson, J.V., & Hall, R.T. (1987). Postnatal weight changes in low birth weight infants. *Pediatrics, 79,* 702–705.

42. Answer: (**A**) Coughing, choking, and cyanosis (three "Cs") are the common clinical signs of transesophageal fistula. Four of the more common conditions in which lung expansion is impossible despite proper intubations are (1) massive aspiration of meconium that cannot be removed by suctioning, (2) intrauterine pneumonia with organization of exudate, (3) large bilateral diaphragmatic hernias with hypoplastic lungs, and (4) congenital adenomatous cysts of the lung. Condition is usually associated with hydrops and is usually fatal.

REFERENCES

London, M.L. (1993). Resuscitation and stabilization of the neonate (pp. 231–246). In C. Kenner, A. Brueggemeyer, & L.P. Gunderson (eds.), *Comprehensive neonatal nursing: A physiologic perspective*. Philadelphia: W.B. Saunders.

Ringer, S.A. & Stark, A.R. (1989). Management of neonatal emergencies in the delivery room. *Clinics in Perinatology, 16*(1), 23–42.

43. Answer: (**A**) The cephalic area is called the foregut and gives rise to the esophagus, stomach, proximal duodenum (above the bile duct), liver, pancreas, biliary apparatus, and the lower respiratory system.

REFERENCES

Loper, D.L. (1983). Gastrointestinal development: Embryology, congenital anomalies, and impact on feedings. *Neonatal Network, 2*(1), 27–36.

McCollum, L.L. & Thigpen, J.L. (1993). Assessment and management of gastrointestinal dysfunction (pp. 434–479). In C. Kenner, A. Brueggemeyer, & L.P. Gunderson (eds.), *Comprehensive neonatal nursing: A physiologic perspective*. Philadelphia: W.B. Saunders.

Moore, K.L. (1989). *Before we are born: Basic embryology and birth defects* (3rd ed.). Philadelphia: W.B. Saunders.

Sadler, T.W. (1985). *Langman's medical embryology* (5th ed.). Baltimore: Williams & Wilkins.

44. Answer: (**C**) The most commonly observed behaviors among older siblings of a new infant are (1) an increase in aggression and hostility directed toward the mother, newborn, or both,

(2) a regression in functioning (e.g., thumb-sucking and bed-wetting), (3) an increase in efforts to gain the parents' attention, (4) a tendency to anger easily, and (5) difficulty in concentrating in school.

REFERENCES

Baskett, L.M. & Johnson, S.M. (1982). The young child's interactions with parents versus siblings: A behavior analysis. *Child Development, 53,* 643–650.

Craft, M.J. (1979). Help for the family's neglected "other" child. *American Journal of Child Psychology and Psychiatry, 21,* 297–300.

Daniels, M.B. (1983). The birth experience for the sibling: Description/evaluation of a program. *Journal of Nurse Midwifery, 29,* 15–22.

Dunn, J. & Kendrick, D. (1980). The arrival of a sibling: Changes in patterns of interaction between mother and firstborn child. *Journal of Child Psychology and Psychiatry, 21,* 119–132.

Legg, C., Sherick, I., & Wadland, W. (1974). Reaction of preschool children to the birth of a sibling. *Child Psychiatry and Human Development, 5,* 3–39.

Wolterman, M. (1993). Sibling adaptation to the neonate (pp. 80–83). In C. Kenner, A. Brueggemeyer, & L.P. Gunderson (eds.), *Comprehensive neonatal nursing: A physiologic perspective.* Philadelphia: W.B. Saunders.

45. Answer: **(A)** Brief exposure not only provides concrete evidence of the infant's existence but also helps siblings integrate the reality of the experience, prepare for the possible loss of the newborn, and in some cases reverse regressive behavior that had begun before the hospital visit.

REFERENCES

Baskett, L.M. & Johnson, S.M. (1982). The young child's interactions with parents versus siblings: A behavior analysis. *Child Development, 53,* 643–650.

Craft, M.J. (1979). Help for the family's neglected "other" child. *American Journal of Child Psychology and Psychiatry, 21,* 297–300.

Daniels, M.B. (1983). The birth experience for the sibling: Description/evaluation of a program. *Journal of Nurse Midwifery, 29,* 15–22.

Dunn, J. & Kendrick, D. (1980). The arrival of a sibling: Changes in patterns of interaction between mother and firstborn child. *Journal of Child Psychology and Psychiatry, 21,* 119–132.

Flint, N.S. & Walsh, M. (1988). Visiting policies in pediatrics: Parents' perceptions and preferences. *Journal of Pediatric Nursing, 3,* 237–246.

Legg, C., Sherick, I., & Wadland, W. (1974). Reaction of preschool children to the birth of a sibling. *Child Psychiatry and Human Development, 5,* 3–39.

Wolterman, M. (1993). Sibling adaptation to the neonate (pp. 80–83). In C. Kenner, A. Brueggemeyer, & L.P. Gunderson (eds.), *Comprehensive neonatal nursing: A physiologic perspective.* Philadelphia: W.B. Saunders.

46. Answer: **(A)** Positive behaviors are (1) asking the mother to play, (2) coming to the mother for help, (3) hugging the mother, and (4) talking to the mother affectionately about the infant. Several negative behaviors are (1) clinging excessively to the mother, (2) demanding mother's attention, (3) tending not to obey, and (4) wanting to sleep in the mother's bed at night.

REFERENCES

Baskett, L.M. & Johnson, S.M. (1982). The young child's interactions with parents versus siblings: A behavior analysis. *Child Development, 53,* 643–650.

Craft, M.J. (1979). Help for the family's neglected "other" child. *American Journal of Child Psychology and Psychiatry, 21,* 297–300.

Daniels, M.B. (1983). The birth experience for the sibling: Description/evaluation of a program. *Journal of Nurse Midwifery, 29,* 15–22.

Dunn, J. & Kendrick, D. (1980). The arrival of a sibling: Changes in patterns of interaction between mother and firstborn child. *Journal of Child Psychology and Psychiatry, 21,* 119–132.

Flint, N.S. & Walsh, M. (1988). Visiting policies in pediatrics: Parents' perceptions and preferences. *Journal of Pediatric Nursing, 3,* 237–246.

Legg, C., Sherick, I., & Wadland, W. (1974). Reaction of preschool children to the birth of a sibling. *Child Psychiatry and Human Development, 5,* 3–39.

Wolterman, M.C. (1990). Validation of an instrument to study behaviors in siblings following sibling visitation on a neonatal intensive care unit. Unpublished doctoral dissertation. University of Cincinnati, College of Education, Cincinnati, Ohio.

Wolterman, M. (1993). Sibling adaptation to the neonate (pp. 80–83). In C. Kenner, A. Brueggemeyer, & L.P. Gunderson (eds.), *Comprehensive neonatal nursing: A physiologic perspective.* Philadelphia: W.B. Saunders.

47. Answer: **(C)** When siblings visit inside the NICU, their parents usually feel that this helps the older children feel part of a significant family event. It provides opportunities for the siblings to discuss with their parents what is happening to the infant. The sibling usually pays little attention to the environment and more to the new baby.

REFERENCES

Baskett, L.M. & Johnson, S.M. (1982). The young child's interactions with parents versus siblings: A behavior analysis. *Child Development, 53,* 643–650.

Craft, M.J. (1979). Help for the family's neglected "other" child. *American Journal of Child Psychology and Psychiatry, 21,* 297–300.

Daniels, M.B. (1983). The birth experience for the sibling: Description/evaluation of a program. *Journal of Nurse Midwifery, 29,* 15–22.

Dunn, J. & Kendrick, D. (1980). The arrival of a sibling: Changes in patterns of interaction between mother and firstborn child. *Journal of Child Psychology and Psychiatry, 21,* 119–132.
Flint, N.S. & Walsh, M. (1988). Visiting policies in pediatrics: Parents' perceptions and preferences. *Journal of Pediatric Nursing, 3,* 237–246.
Legg, C., Sherick, I., & Wadland, W. (1974). Reaction of preschool children to the birth of a sibling. *Child Psychiatry and Human Development, 5,* 3–39.
Wolterman, M.C. (1990). Validation of an instrument to study behaviors in siblings following sibling visitation on a neonatal intensive care unit. Unpublished doctoral dissertation. University of Cincinnati, College of Education, Cincinnati, Ohio.
Wolterman, M. (1993). Sibling adaptation to the neonate (pp. 80–83). In C. Kenner, A. Brueggemeyer, & L.P. Gunderson (eds.), *Comprehensive neonatal nursing: A physiologic perspective.* Philadelphia: W.B. Saunders.

48. Answer: (**B**) Parents need to be made aware of the impact of the ill infant on the sibling's reaction to the birth. Attention should be directed at how much information is shared with the sibling. Consideration must be given to the developmental stage of the sibling and what the child needs and can understand. Encouraging parents to discuss what is happening at home with the siblings offers the nurse subtle cues about how this event affects each family member.

REFERENCES

Ballard, J., Maloney, M., Shank, M., & Hollister, L. (1984). Sibling visits to a newborn intensive care unit: Implications for siblings, parents and infants. *Child Psychiatry and Human Development, 14,* 203–214.
Baskett, L.M. & Johnson, S.M. (1982). The young child's interactions with parents versus siblings: A behavior analysis. *Child Development, 53,* 643–650.
Craft, M.J. (1979). Help for the family's neglected "other" child. *American Journal of Child Psychology and Psychiatry, 21,* 297–300.
Daniels, M.B. (1983). The birth experience for the sibling: Description/evaluation of a program. *Journal of Nurse Midwifery, 29,* 15–22.
Dunn, J. & Kendrick, D. (1980). The arrival of a sibling: Changes in patterns of interaction between mother and firstborn child. *Journal of Child Psychology and Psychiatry, 21,* 119–132.
Flint, N.S. & Walsh, M. (1988). Visiting policies in pediatrics: Parents' perceptions and preferences. *Journal of Pediatric Nursing, 3,* 237–246.
Legg, C., Sherick, I., & Wadland, W. (1974). Reaction of preschool children to the birth of a sibling. *Child Psychiatry and Human Development, 5,* 3–39.
Newman, C.B. & McSweeney, M.E. (1990). A descriptive study of sibling visitation in the NICU. *Neonatal Network, 9,* 27–31.
Trause, M.A., Voos, D., Rudd, C., Klaus, M., Kennell, J., & Boselt, M. (1981). Separation for childbirth: The effect on the sibling. *Child Psychiatry and Human Development, 12,* 32–39.
Troy, P., Wilkinson-Faulk, D., Smith, A.B., & Alexander, D.A. (1988). Sibling visiting in the NICU. *American Journal of Nursing, 88,* 68–70.
Wolterman, M.C. (1990). Validation of an instrument to study behaviors in siblings following sibling visitation on a neonatal intensive care unit. Unpublished doctoral dissertation. University of Cincinnati, College of Education, Cincinnati, Ohio.
Wolterman, M. (1993). Sibling adaptation to the neonate (pp. 80–83). In C. Kenner, A. Brueggemeyer, & L.P. Gunderson (eds.), *Comprehensive neonatal nursing: A physiologic perspective.* Philadelphia: W.B. Saunders.

49. Answer: (**B**) Normally, humans have 46 chromosomes (23 different pairs) in all cells except mature red blood cells and the mature sex cells (sperm and ova).

REFERENCES

Cohen, F.L. (1984). *Clinical genetics in nursing practice.* Philadelphia: J.B. Lippincott.
Connor, J. & Ferguson-Smith, M. (1987). *Essential medical genetics.* Oxford: Blackwell Scientific.
Cummings, M. (1988). *Human heredity: Principles and issues.* New York: West Publishing.
Thompson, S. & Thompson, M. (1986). *Genetics in medicine* (4th ed.). Philadelphia: W.B. Saunders.
Workman, M.L., Kenner, C., & Hilse, M. (1993). Human genetics (pp. 101–131). In C. Kenner, A. Brueggemeyer, & L.P. Gunderson (eds.), *Comprehensive neonatal nursing: A physiologic perspective.* Philadelphia: W.B. Saunders.

50. Answer: (**B**) Organizational structures that are centralized and hierarchical provide the greatest challenge for collaboration, whereas those that allow for decentralized decision making are the best. Collaboration requires recognition of each individual's ability to contribute to clinical decision making.

REFERENCES

Aradine, C.R. & Hansen, M.F. (1970). Interdisciplinary teamwork in family health care. *Nursing Clinics of North America, 5*(2), 211–222.
Gilles, C. (1991). Nonsurgical management of the infant with gastroesophageal reflux and respiratory problems. *Journal of the American Academy of Nursing Practice, 3*(1), 11–16.
Harrigan, R. & Perez, D. (1993). Collaborative practice in the NICU (pp. 9–13). In C. Kenner, A. Brueggemeyer, & L.P. Gunderson (eds.), *Comprehensive neonatal nursing: A physiologic perspective.* Philadelphia: W.B. Saunders.
Sherwen, L. (1990). Interdisciplinary collaboration in perinatal/neonatal health care. A worthwhile challenge. *Journal of Perinatology, 10*(1), 1–2.

51. Answer: (**A**) Gastrulation is the process by which the bilaminar disk is expanded to a trilaminar embryonic disk, and it is the most important

event that occurs during early fetal formation.

REFERENCES

Lott, J.W. (1993). Fetal development: Environmental influences and critical periods (pp. 132–156). In C. Kenner, A. Brueggemeyer, & L.P. Gunderson (eds.), *Comprehensive neonatal nursing: A physiologic perspective.* Philadelphia: W.B. Saunders.
Moore, K.L. (1989). *The developing human* (4th ed.). Philadelphia: W.B. Saunders.
Sadler, T.W. (1985). *Langman's medical embryology* (5th ed.). Baltimore: Williams & Wilkins.

52. Answer: (**A**) The fetus can be considered at increased risk for asphyxia because it is relatively hypoxic, has high oxygen demands during labor, and is subject to regular interruptions of the gas exchange (placental exchange) during uterine contractions. To meet the challenges of intrauterine existence and the transition to extrauterine life, the fetus has numerous adaptations to hypoxia and compensatory mechanisms that provide for what is called *fetal reserve.* No age group is more susceptible to asphyxia or in more frequent need of resuscitation than the newborn.

REFERENCES

Bloom, R.S. & Cropley, C. & Peckham, G.J. (1983). Principles of neonatal resuscitation (pp. 1–24). In R.A. Polin & F.D. Berg (eds.), *Workbook in practical neonatology.* Philadelphia: W.B. Saunders.
London, M.L. (1993). Resuscitation and stabilization of the neonate (pp. 231–246). In C. Kenner, A. Brueggemeyer, & L.P. Gunderson (eds.), *Comprehensive neonatal nursing: A physiologic perspective.* Philadelphia: W.B. Saunders.

53. Answer: (**A**) Four root principles of ethical decision making have been described by multiple scholars: autonomy, nonmaleficence, beneficence, and justice (Beauchamp & Childress, 1983; Fowler, 1987). From these root principles other ethical rules are derived, including accountability, veracity, integrity, confidentiality, and fidelity. Three issues are related to the principles of autonomy: advocacy, competence, and informed consent.

REFERENCES

Beauchamp, T.L. & Childress, J.F. (1983). *Principles of biomedical ethics.* New York: Oxford University Press.
Fowler, M. D. (1987). Introduction to ethics and ethical theory (pp. 659–670). In M.D. Fowler & J. Levine-Ariff (eds.), *Ethics at the bedside: A source book for the critical care nurse.* New York: McGraw-Hill.
Southwell, S.M. & Archer-Dusté, H. (1993). Ethical aspects of perinatal care (pp. 14–35). In C. Kenner, A. Brueggemeyer, & L.P. Gunderson (eds.), *Comprehensive neonatal nursing: A physiologic perspective.* Philadelphia: W.B. Saunders.

54. Answer: (**C**) Risk factors for BPD include immaturity of the pulmonary parenchyma; surfactant deficiency; exposure to elevated concentrations of inspired oxygen; barotrauma from positive pressure ventilation; systemic-to-pulmonary shunt through a patent ductus arteriosus; pulmonary edema; pulmonary air leak; protease-antiprotease imbalance; family history of reactive airway disease; tissue type HLA-A2; and vitamin A deficiency.

REFERENCES

Boynton, B.R. (1988). Epidemiology of BPD (pp. 19–32). In T.A Merritt, W.H. Northway, Jr., & B.R. Boynton (eds.), *Bronchopulmonary dysplasia.* Boston: Blackwell Scientific.
Southwell, S.M. (1993). Complications of respiratory management (pp. 337–354). In C. Kenner, A. Brueggemeyer, & L.P. Gunderson (eds.), *Comprehensive neonatal nursing: A physiologic perspective.* Philadelphia: W.B. Saunders.

55. Answer: (**C**) The placenta serves four main organ or system functions: (1) fetal lung or respiratory function for exchange of oxygen and carbon dioxide through a process of simple diffusion, dependent on an adequate utero-placental blood flow and moving from the side of greater concentration to the side of lesser; (2) fetal kidney for the metabolic side of acid-base balance, regulating the excretion of wastes and electrolyte balance; (3) fetal gastrointestinal tract for storage and release of nutrients based on fetal need; and (4) fetal skin for temperature control.

REFERENCES

Creasy, R. & Resnick, M. (1989). *Maternal fetal medicine: Principles and practice.* Philadelphia: W.B. Saunders.
Gilbert, E. & Harmon, J. (1986). *High risk pregnancy and delivery.* St. Louis: C.V. Mosby.
Harmon, J.S. (1993). High-risk pregnancy (pp. 157–170). In C. Kenner, A. Brueggemeyer, & L.P. Gunderson (eds.), *Comprehensive neonatal nursing: A physiologic perspective.* Philadelphia: W.B. Saunders.
Moore, K. (1989). *The developing human* (4th ed.). Philadelphia: W.B. Saunders.

56. Answer: (**B**) Internally, the duodenum begins to generate villi between five and six weeks' gestation.

REFERENCES

Loper, D.L. (1983). Gastrointestinal development: Embryology, congenital anomalies, and impact on feedings. *Neonatal Network, 2*(1), 27–36.

McCollum, L.L. & Thigpen, J.L. (1993). Assessment and management of gastrointestinal dysfunction (pp. 434–479). In C. Kenner, A. Brueggemeyer, & L.P. Gunderson (eds.), *Comprehensive neonatal nursing: A physiologic perspective.* Philadelphia: W.B. Saunders.

Moore, K.L. (1989). *Before we are born: Basic embryology and birth defects* (3rd ed.). Philadelphia: W.B. Saunders.

Sadler, T.W. (1985). *Langman's medical embryology* (5th ed.). Baltimore: Williams & Wilkins.

57. Answer: (**C**) The policy purpose of the statutes is to prevent stale claims—that is, claims that have lost their credibility because information bases and persons knowledgeable about events are not available. On the other hand, the time frames set are intended to provide sufficient time for plaintiffs to discover injuries and bring suit while assuring potential defendants they are not at risk forever.

    Actions against nurses in neonatal nursing practice can be brought even beyond the ordinary statutory time limitation because the law has recognized an injustice can occur if parents do not bring an action on behalf of their child during the usual statutory time frame. A common remedy for this potential injustice is to permit individuals to bring actions on their own behalf within the ordinary statutory time frame after they reach the age of majority. For example, a child injured as a result of breach of the standard of care in the neonatal intensive care unit has until age 18 plus the time frame for bringing an action against a physician or hospital. A one-year statute of limitations for physician suits would leave liability open through the child's reaching age 19. A three-year statute of limitations for hospitals would leave liability open through the child's reaching age 21. Statutes of limitations vary from state to state. Nurses in neonatal practice should be aware of the time frames for the states in which they practice.

REFERENCES

American Nurses' Association. (1984). *Code for nurses with interpretive statements.* Kansas City, MO: Author.

Driscoll, K.M. (1993). Legal aspects of perinatal care (pp. 36–51). In C. Kenner, A. Brueggemeyer, & L.P. Gunderson (eds.), *Comprehensive neonatal nursing: A physiologic perspective.* Philadelphia: W.B. Saunders.

Pegalis, S.E. & Wachsman, H.F. (1990). *American law of medical malpractice.* (Cum. Suppl.). Rochester, NY: Lawyers Co-Operative Publishing.

58. Answer: (**C**) Parameters include all except placental grading and chorionic villi sampling. In addition to hypotension, hypertension, and abruptio placentae, *hypertonic contractions* also can be related to decreased maternal perfusion of the placenta. Hypertonic contraction can occur in conjunction with excessive oxytocin administration and precipitous labor. Another factor that can cause or contribute to fetal distress during labor is hemolytic disease of the newborn—*fetal anemia (erythroblastosis fetalis, nonimmune hydrops).* Fetal anemia can occur in relation to Rh incompatibility. In response to the red blood cell destruction, the fetus produces many immature red blood cells—a condition known as erythroblastosis fetalis. In the most severe form of the disease, known as hydrops fetalis, the fetus can become severely anemic. The biophysical profile is a noninvasive assessment system that allows for evaluation of the fetal status based on five or six parameters, with each area receiving a score.

    1. Nonstress test (NST)—This test evaluates the response of the fetal heart rate to fetal activity or stimulation. Normally with activity, the fetus will increase heart rate by at least 15 beats for 15 seconds. This will normally be done by the fetus several times in a 10- to 20-minute period.
    2. Fetal breath movements (FBM)—Done with ultrasound and involves assessing the fetal chest and abdomen for breathing movements.
    3. Fetal movement (FM)—Assesses for movement of the fetal trunk.
    4. Fetal tone—Evaluates the fetus for extension and flexion of the fetal body or extremities.
    5. Amniotic fluid volume (AFV)—Measures the amount of amniotic fluid present. The amniotic sac is

scanned for pockets of fluid that measure at least 2 mm in two different planes.

Placental grading examines the basal and chorionic plates of the placenta. A placenta that is grade 0 is immature, whereas a grade III is significantly aged and may not be functioning optimally. A score of 8 or better indicates a normal infant, with low risk of chronic asphyxia. With a total score of 4 to 7, chronic asphyxia is suspected, and with a score of less than 4, chronic asphyxia is strongly suspected (Manning et al, 1985). Vitzileos et al (1983, 1985) had defined abnormal blood pressure as a score less than 6.

REFERENCES

Gaffney, S.E., Salinger, L. & Venmtzeleos, A.M. (1990). The biophysical profile for fetal surveillance. *The American Journal of Maternal Child Nursery, 15,* 356–360.

Manning, F.A., Morrison, I., Lange, J.D., Harman, C.R., & Chamberlain, M. (1985). Fetal assessment based on fetal biophysical profile scoring: Experience in 12,620 referred high risk pregnancies. *American Journal of Obstetrics and Gynecology, 151*(3), 343–380.

Vintzileos, A.M., Campbell, W.A., Ingradia, C.J., & Nochimson, D.J. (1983). The biophysical profile and its predictive value. *Obstetrics and Gynecology, 62*(3), 271–278.

Vintzileos, A.M., Campbell, W.A., Nochimson, D.J., Cinnolly, M.E., Fuenfer, M.M., & Hochn, G.J. (1985). The fetal biophysical profile in patients with premature rupture of membranes: An early predictor of the fetal infection. *American Journal of Obstetrics and Gynecology, 153*(6), 624–633.

Weitkamp, T.L. & Felblinger, D.M. (1993). Effects of labor on the fetus and neonate (pp. 215–230). In C. Kenner, A. Brueggemeyer, & L.P. Gunderson (eds.), *Comprehensive neonatal nursing: A physiologic perspective.* Philadelphia: W.B. Saunders.

59. Answer: (**C**) During the processes of herniation and return, the intestine has rotated a full 270 degrees.

REFERENCES

Loper, D.L. (1983). Gastrointestinal development: Embryology, congenital anomalies, and impact on feedings. *Neonatal Network, 2*(1), 27–36.

McCollum, L.L. & Thigpen, J.L. (1993). Assessment and management of gastrointestinal dysfunction (pp. 434–479). In C. Kenner, A. Brueggemeyer, & L.P. Gunderson (eds.), *Comprehensive neonatal nursing: A physiologic perspective.* Philadelphia: W.B. Saunders.

Moore, K.L. (1989). *Before we are born: Basic embryology and birth defects* (3rd ed.). Philadelphia: W.B. Saunders.

Sadler, T.W. (1985). *Langman's medical embryology* (5th ed.). Baltimore: Williams & Wilkins.

60. Answer: (**A**) The ductus arteriosus allows blood to flow from the pulmonary artery to the aorta, bypassing the fetal lungs. The ductus venosus permits most blood from the placenta to bypass the liver and enter the inferior vena cava. The foramen ovale is the opening in the interatrial septum that permits a portion of the blood to flow from the right atrium directly to the left atrium.

REFERENCES

Lott, J.W. (1993). Assessment and management of cardiovascular dysfunction (pp. 355–391). In C. Kenner, A. Brueggemeyer, & L.P. Gunderson (eds.), *Comprehensive neonatal nursing: A physiologic perspective.* Philadelphia: W.B. Saunders.

Moller, J.H. (1987). Congenital heart anomalies. Clinical education aid. Columbus, OH: Ross Laboratories.

Park, M.K. (1984). Fetal and perinatal circulation (pp. 87–91). *Pediatric cardiology for practitioners.* Year Book Medical Publishers: Chicago.

61. Answer: (**B**) Secondary prevention includes use of less toxic therapies; exogenous surfactants; high-frequency ventilation; more insightful use of conventional ventilation; antidotes for toxic therapies; antioxidants: vitamin A and E; superoxide dismutase; and corticosteroids.

REFERENCES

Boynton, B.R. (1988). Epidemiology of BPD (pp. 19–32). In T.A. Merritt, W.H. Northway, Jr., & B.R. Boynton (eds.), *Bronchopulmonary dysplasia.* Boston: Blackwell Scientific.

Southwell, S.M. (1993). Complications of respiratory management (pp. 337–354). In C. Kenner, A. Brueggemeyer, & L.P. Gunderson (eds.), *Comprehensive neonatal nursing: A physiologic perspective.* Philadelphia: W.B. Saunders.

62. Answer: (**B**) Clinical manifestations of perinatal asphyxia are (1) loss of beat-to-beat variability that reflects decreased fetal reserve; (2) heart rate greater than 160 beats per minute (bpm) for greater than or equal to 10 minutes (fetal tachycardia); (3) heart rate less than 120 bpm for greater than or equal to 10 minutes (fetal bradycardia); (4) fetal scalp pH less than 7.20 to 7.25; (5) short-term variability, variable decelerations to less than 80 bpm and that are not relieved by repositioning mother to relieve vena caval syndrome; and (6) long-term variability, late decelerations. Inadequate lung expansion, hypoxia,

and acidosis lead to pulmonary arteriolar constriction, increased pulmonary vascular resistance, decreased pulmonary blood flow and perfusion, and persistent right-to-left flow through the ductus arteriosus. Pressures remain high on the right side of the heart, and the foramen ovale remains open. Of the biochemical events that occur due to asphyxia, the conversion from aerobic oxidation of glucose to anaerobic glycolysis is the most significant. This change in metabolism leads to development of metabolic acidosis.

REFERENCES

London, M.L. (1993). Resuscitation and stabilization of the neonate (pp. 231–246). In C. Kenner, A. Brueggemeyer, & L.P. Gunderson (eds.), *Comprehensive neonatal nursing: A physiologic perspective*. Philadelphia: W.B. Saunders.

Woods, J. (1983). Birth asphyxia: Pathophysiologic events and fetal adaptive changes. *Clinics in Perinatology, 10*(2), 473.

63. Answer: (**C**) In the esophagus, the connective tissue layer is covered with peritoneal epithelial cells and is called the serosa.

REFERENCES

Loper, D.L. (1983). Gastrointestinal development: Embryology, congenital anomalies, and impact on feedings. *Neonatal Network, 2*(1), 27–36.

McCollum, L.L. & Thigpen, J.L. (1993). Assessment and management of gastrointestinal dysfunction (pp. 434–479). In C. Kenner, A. Brueggemeyer, & L.P. Gunderson (eds.), *Comprehensive neonatal nursing: A physiologic perspective*. Philadelphia: W.B. Saunders.

Moore, K.L. (1989). *Before we are born: Basic embryology and birth defects* (3rd ed.). Philadelphia: W.B. Saunders.

Sadler, T.W. (1985). *Langman's medical embryology* (5th ed.). Baltimore: Williams & Wilkins.

64. Answer: (**A**) The pedigree is a schematic drawing of a family history, which allows a pictorial representation of patterns of inheritance over many generations. When analyzing a pedigree, the answers to the following specific questions are noted: (1) Is any pattern of inheritance present or does the trait appear sporadic? (2) Is the trait transmitted equally or unequally to males and females? (3) Is the trait present in every generation or does it skip a generation? (4) Do only affected individuals have children affected with the trait or can unaffected individuals also have children who express the trait?

REFERENCES

Cohen, F.L. (1984). *Clinical genetics in nursing practice*. Philadelphia: J.B. Lippincott.

Connor, J. & Ferguson-Smith, M. (1987). *Essential medical genetics*. Oxford: Blackwell Scientific.

Cummings, M. (1988). *Human heredity: Principles and issues*. New York: West Publishing.

Thompson, S. & Thompson, M. (1986). *Genetics in medicine* (4th ed.). Philadelphia: W.B. Saunders.

Workman, M.L., Kenner, C., & Hilse, M. (1993). Human genetics (pp. 101–131). In C. Kenner, A. Brueggemeyer, & L.P. Gunderson (eds.), *Comprehensive neonatal nursing: A physiologic perspective*. Philadelphia: W.B. Saunders.

65. Answer: (**A**) Three cardinal signs point to the possibility of gastrointestinal obstruction, whether it is structural or functional: (1) persistent vomiting, especially if it is bile stained; (2) abdominal distention; and (3) failure to pass meconium within the first 48 hours of birth.

REFERENCES

Chang, J.H.T. (1980). Neonatal surgical emergencies: Part V—Intestinal obstruction. *Perinatology/Neonatology, 4*(2), 34–40.

Ghory, M.J. & Sheldon, C.A. (1985). Newborn surgical emergencies of the gastrointestinal tract. *Surgical Clinics of North America, 65*(5), 1083–1098.

McCollum, L.L. & Thigpen, J.L. (1993). Assessment and management of gastrointestinal dysfunction (pp. 434–479). In C. Kenner, A. Brueggemeyer, & L.P. Gunderson (eds.), *Comprehensive neonatal nursing: A physiologic perspective*. Philadelphia: W.B. Saunders.

66. Answer: (**B**) Coverage for reverse transport is somewhat more difficult to obtain. Insurance companies have a label of "family convenience" that covers many of the reasons that normally apply to the reverse transport of a neonate. Some hospitals are currently building into their budgets funds to cover the reverse transport costs, which may make it easier on families when deciding whether to consent to such a transport.

REFERENCES

Croop, L.H. & Acree, C.M. (1993). Neonatal transport (pp. 1182–212). In C. Kenner, A. Brueggemeyer, & L.P. Gunderson (eds.), *Comprehensive neonatal care: A physiologic perspective*. Philadelphia: W.B. Saunders.

Croop, L. & Kenner, C. (1990). Protocol for reverse neonatal transports. *Neonatal Network, 9*(1), 49–53.

67. Answer: (**A**) Documentation is the legal evidence of professional account-

ability. Assessments, interventions, evaluations, and re-evaluations, and communications not documented are presumed not to have occurred. Without documentation, the nurse who asserts at deposition or trial that an activity occurred can expect a deserved assault on his or her credibility.

REFERENCES

American Academy of Pediatrics/American College of Obstetricians and Gynecologists. (1992). *Guidelines for perinatal care*. Elk Grove Village, IL: Author.

American Nurses' Association. (1984). *Code for nurses with interpretive statements*. Kansas City: Author.

Driscoll, K.M. (1993). Legal aspects of perinatal care (pp. 36–51). In C. Kenner, A. Brueggemeyer, & L.P. Gunderson (eds.), *Comprehensive neonatal nursing: A physiologic perspective*. Philadelphia: W.B. Saunders.

Pegalis, S.E. & Wachsman, H.F. (1990). *American law of medical malpractice*. (Cum. Suppl.). Rochester, NY: Lawyers Co-Operative Publishing.

68. Answer: (**B**) The contractions that strongly sweep over the stomach become more oscillatory in nature in the small intestine, promoting the digestive and absorptive processes that occur there.

REFERENCES

Loper, D.L. (1983). Gastrointestinal development: Embryology, congenital anomalies, and impact on feedings. *Neonatal Network, 2*(1), 27–36.

McCollum, L.L. & Thigpen, J.L. (1993). Assessment and management of gastrointestinal dysfunction (pp. 434–479). In C. Kenner, A. Brueggemeyer, & L.P. Gunderson (eds.), *Comprehensive neonatal nursing: A physiologic perspective*. Philadelphia: W.B. Saunders.

Moore, K.L. (1989). *Before we are born: Basic embryology and birth defects* (3rd ed.). Philadelphia: W.B. Saunders.

Sadler, T.W. (1985). *Langman's medical embryology* (5th ed.). Baltimore: Williams & Wilkins.

69. Answer: (**B**) Size and degree of pulmonary vascular resistance are two main determinants of severity. The location of the VSD is less important than size and degree of pulmonary vascular resistance.

REFERENCES

Avery, G.B. (1987). *Neonatology: Pathophysiology and management of the newborn*. Philadelphia: J.B. Lippincott.

Heymann, M.A. (1989). Fetal and neonatal circulations (pp. 24–35). In F.H. Adams, G.C. Emmanouilides, & T.A. Riemenschneider (eds.), *Heart disease in infants, children, and adolescents*. Baltimore: Williams & Wilkins.

Lott, J.W. (1993). Assessment and management of cardiovascular dysfunction (pp. 355–391). In C. Kenner, A. Brueggemeyer, & L.P. Gunderson (eds.), *Comprehensive neonatal nursing: A physiologic perspective*. Philadelphia: W.B. Saunders.

Park, M.K. (1984). Left-to-right shunts (pp. 125–144). *Pediatric cardiology for practitioners*. Chicago: Year Book Medical Publishers.

70. Answer: (**A**) The most common cause of fetal asphyxia is cord compression (interruption of umbilical blood flow). With severe cord compression, the risk of hypovolemia increases. Placental insufficiency can be caused by natural causes such as pregnancy induced hypertension (PIH), diabetes and primary maternal hypertension, or iatrogenic causes. One iatrogenic cause is regional anesthetic drugs.

REFERENCES

Banagale, R.C. & Donn, S.M. (1986). Asphyxia neonatorum. *The Journal of Family Practice. 22*(6), 539–545.

London, M.L. (1993). Resuscitation and stabilization of the neonate (pp. 231–246). In C. Kenner, A. Brueggemeyer, & L.P. Gunderson (eds.), *Comprehensive neonatal nursing: A physiologic perspective*. Philadelphia: W.B. Saunders.

Woods, J. (1983). Birth asphyxia: Pathophysiologic events and fetal adaptive changes. *Clinics in Perinatology, 10*(2), 473.

71. Answer: (**C**) Indications include all except hypertension. Magnesium sulfate also can be given for the treatment of preeclampsia. The nurse must be aware that $MgSO_4$ has the ability to alter blood pressure due to splanchnic dilatation and that severe maternal hypotension can occur. A decrease in fetal heart rate also can occur when $MgSO_4$ is administered to the mother. There is a possibility of decreased muscle tone and drowsiness in the newborns whose mothers receive $MgSO_4$ for tocolysis. The supine positioning of the mother alters cardiac output via compression of the aorta and the vena cavae, thus adversely affecting the circulatory response of the fetus. Generally, the laboring mother is alternatively placed in the left lateral recumbent position to avoid a hypotensive state.

Alphaprodine (Nisentil) is a synthetic narcotic with similar action to both morphine and meperidine. It has a shorter onset than meperidine, with a duration of only two hours. Fetal monitor pattern may show a sinusoidal pattern due to the drug, not fetal morbidity.

The advantages of opiates are the long-lasting pain relief and minimal effect on the fetus. The major disadvantage of opiates is pruritus and nausea and vomiting. There is also some respiratory depression with these medications. Most often morphine and meperidine are the drugs used.

REFERENCES

Knapp, R.M. & Knapp, C.M.W. (1986). Obstetric anesthesia (pp. 283–302). In D.J. Angelini, C.M.W. Knapp, & R. Gibes (eds.), *Perinatal/neonatal nursing: A clinical handbook.* Boston: Blackwell Scientific.

Pedersen, H. (1990) Analgesia and anesthesia during pregnancy and labor (pp. 425–431). In K. Buckley & N. Kulb (eds.), *High risk maternity nursing manual.* Baltimore: Williams & Wilkins.

Weitkamp, T.L. & Felblinger, D.M. (1993). Effects of labor on the fetus and neonate (pp. 215–230). In C. Kenner, A. Brueggemeyer, & L.P. Gunderson (eds.), *Comprehensive neonatal nursing: A physiologic perspective.* Philadelphia: W.B. Saunders.

72. Answer: (**A**) A typical autosomal dominant pattern of inheritance would have the following criteria: (1) The trait appears in every generation with no skipping. When the trait is a result of a new mutation (de novo), this criterion is demonstrated only in the branch of the pedigree stemming from the person who first exhibited the new mutation. (2) The risk for affected individuals to have affected children is 50% with each pregnancy. (3) Unaffected individuals do not have affected children; therefore, their risk is 0 percent. (4) The trait is found equally in males and females.

REFERENCES

Cohen, F.L. (1984). *Clinical genetics in nursing practice.* Philadelphia: J.B. Lippincott.

Connor, J., & Ferguson-Smith, M. (1987). *Essential medical genetics.* Oxford: Blackwell Scientific.

Cummings, M. (1988). *Human heredity: Principles and issues.* New York: West Publishing.

Thompson, S., & Thompson, M. (1986). *Genetics in medicine* (4th ed.). Philadelphia: W.B. Saunders.

Workman, M.L., Kenner, C., & Hilse, M. (1993). Human genetics (pp. 101–131). In C. Kenner, A. Brueggemeyer, & L.P. Gunderson (eds.), *Comprehensive neonatal nursing: A physiologic perspective.* Philadelphia: W.B. Saunders.

73. Answer: (**A**) The myenteric plexus lies between the longitudinal and circular layers of muscle and is largely motor in function.

REFERENCES

Loper, D.L. (1983). Gastrointestinal development: Embryology, congenital anomalies, and impact on feedings. *Neonatal Network, 2*(1), 27–36.

McCollum, L.L. & Thigpen, J.L. (1993). Assessment and management of gastrointestinal dysfunction (pp. 434–479). In C. Kenner, A. Brueggemeyer, & L.P. Gunderson (eds.), *Comprehensive neonatal nursing: A physiologic perspective.* Philadelphia: W.B. Saunders.

Moore, K.L. (1989). *Before we are born: Basic embryology and birth defects* (3rd ed.). Philadelphia: W.B. Saunders.

Sadler, T.W. (1985). *Langman's medical embryology* (5th ed.). Baltimore: Williams & Wilkins.

74. Answer: (**C**) An infant with pneumothorax presents with tachypnea, retractions, grunting, cyanosis, irritability, and tachycardia or bradycardia. Clinical assessment does not include acrocyanosis. Other signs may be asymmetrical chest movements, shifted heart sounds, and the infant may exhibit signs of decreased cardiac output. On auscultation, decreased breath sounds may be heard on the affected side, although normal breath sounds may be heard because of transmission of normal breath sounds from the contralateral side. The infant may not "pink up" readily even with adequate ventilation. When viewing the infant's chest from the bottom of the bed, there may be an obvious asymmetry of the chest. Transillumination and chest x-ray both are used to confirm the diagnosis. Needle aspiration of the chest is often all that is required.

REFERENCES

London, M.L. (1993). Resuscitation and stabilization of the neonate (pp. 231–246). In C. Kenner, A. Brueggemeyer, & L.P. Gunderson (eds.), *Comprehensive neonatal nursing: A physiologic perspective.* Philadelphia: W.B. Saunders.

Ringer, S.A. & Stark, A.R. (1989). Management of neonatal emergencies in the delivery room. *Clinics in Perinatology, 16*(1), 23–42.

75. Answer: (**B**) The presence of bile further indicates that the point of obstruction is distal to the ampulla of Vater, where bile is emptied from the common bile duct into the duodenum.

REFERENCES

McCollum, L.L. & Thigpen, J.L. (1993). Assessment and management of gastrointestinal dysfunction (pp. 434–479). In C. Kenner, A. Brueggemeyer, & L.P. Gunderson (eds.), *Comprehensive neonatal nursing: A physiologic perspective.* Philadelphia: W.B. Saunders.

Ricketts, R.R. (1984). Workup of neonatal intestinal obstruction. *American Surgeon, 50*(10), 517–521.

76. Answer: (**C**) Attachment models are rooted in the belief that attachment behavior is instinctive and that attachments are essential to human behavior. Cognitive and behavioral models suggest that the bereaved must first relinquish their assumptions about the world and the deceased, and then they must develop a new set of assumptions. Holistic models include the belief that supportive interventions not only facilitate a griever's return to homeostasis but also can promote growth.

REFERENCES

Benfield, D.G., Leib, S.A., & Reuter, J. (1976). Grief response of parents following referral of the critically ill newborn. *New England Journal of Medicine, 294,* 975–978.

Kalish, R.A. (1977). Dying and preparing for death. A view of families. In H. Feifel (ed.), *New meanings of death.* New York: McGraw-Hill.

Kubler-Ross, E. (1969). *On death and dying.* New York: Macmillan.

Nichols, J.A. & Doka, K.J. (1991). No more rosebuds. In K.J. Doka (ed.), *Death and spirituality.* Amityville, NY: Baywood Publishing.

Nichols, J.A. (1993). Bereavement: A state of having suffered a loss (pp. 84–98). In C. Kenner, A. Brueggemeyer, & L.P. Gunderson (eds.), *Comprehensive neonatal nursing: A physiologic perspective.* Philadelphia: W.B. Saunders.

Raphael, B. (1983). *The anatomy of bereavement.* New York: Basic Books.

77. Answer: (**A**) At present, there is only one set of published standards for neonatal transport care for nurses. The National Association of Neonatal Nurses (NANN) published these standards in 1992.

REFERENCES

Croop, L.H. & Acree, C.M. (1993). Neonatal transport (pp. 1182–212), In C. Kenner, A. Brueggemeyer, & L.P. Gunderson (eds.), *Comprehensive neonatal care: A physiologic perspective.* Philadelphia: W.B. Saunders.

National Association of Neonatal Nurses. (1992). *Transport standards & guidelines for neonatal nurses.* Petaluma, CA: NANN.

78. Answer: (**A**) The neurological system of the newborn is quite unstable. If results obtained in this portion of the gestational exam are grossly inconsistent with other findings, the exam may be repeated in 24 hours, or in the case of the Lubchenco evaluation, supplemented by a more detailed "confirmatory" exam on the second postnatal day. A complete physical assessment performed by a physician or nurse practitioner will be on record for legal reasons before discharge. The gestational assessment is a determination of the approximate duration of fetal development and a comparison against standardized norms of neonatal growth versus weeks of gestation to identify those infants unusually too large or small for gestational age. In clinical practice, the gestational assessment tools in common use are generally considered accurate within a range of +2 weeks.

REFERENCES

Battaglia, F.C., & Lubchenco, L.O. (1967). A practical classification of newborn infants by weight and gestational age. *Journal of Pediatrics, 71*(2), 159–163.

Endo, A.S. & Nishioka, E. (1993). Neonatal assessment (pp. 265–293). In C. Kenner, A. Brueggemeyer, & L.P. Gunderson (eds.), *Comprehensive neonatal nursing: A physiologic perspective.* Philadelphia: W.B. Saunders.

Petrucha, R. (1989). Fetal maturity/gestational age evaluation. *Journal of Perinatology, 9*(1), 100–101.

79. Answer: (**A**) Abundant oral secretions or saliva provides an early clue to esophageal atresia, particularly when a history of polyhydramnios has been reported.

REFERENCES

McCollum, L.L. & Thigpen, J.L. (1993). Assessment and management of gastrointestinal dysfunction (pp. 434–479). In C. Kenner, A. Brueggemeyer, & L.P. Gunderson. (eds.), *Comprehensive neonatal nursing: A physiologic perspective.* Philadelphia: W.B. Saunders.

Scanlon, J.W., Nelson, T., Grylack, L.J., & Smith, Y.F. (1979). *A system of newborn physical examination.* Baltimore: University Park Press.

80. Answer: (**C**) Three mechanisms are involved in cold stress. The first mechanism involves the sympathetic nervous system. Peripherally, vasoconstriction occurs to limit the loss of heat. The heart rate increases to compensate for the increased demand of metabolism to maintain heat. The second mechanism involves shivering and posturing. Although infants have limited ability to shiver, some heat can be generated in this manner. Posture changes, chiefly toward a more flexed position, also help the infant re-

tain body heat. The preterm infant has no ability to shiver and an extremely limited ability to change position. The third mechanism involves the stimulation of the pituitary and the release of chemicals to initiate chemical responses to achieve heat energy output.

The cardiorespiratory system has the most obvious symptoms when the infant is cold stressed. As the temperature declines, peripheral vasoconstriction occurs to conserve heat. As central blood volume increases, pulse and blood pressure increase. Once central cooling has occurred, diuresis can result with a decline in pulse and blood pressure leading to decreased cardiac output. Arrhythmias can occur secondary to acidosis as fatty acids break down in an attempt to generate heat.

The central nervous system can be affected by cold stress secondary to cardiovascular changes. As peripheral vasoconstriction occurs, cerebral blood flow diminishes. Decreased blood flow to the brain compromises metabolic activity. Electroencephalographic (EEG) activity can decline. To obtain an accurate EEG, body temperature must be in the normal range. Peripheral nerve conduction also can be delayed. Pupils can become fixed and dilated.

Metabolic response to cold stress encompasses fluid, electrolyte, and glucose aberrations. In the early stages, diuresis occurs. If cold stress continues, further changes occur. With decreased perfusion to the kidneys, glomerular filtration declines with the reabsorption of sodium, water, and glucose. Hypoglycemia results as the consumption of glucose rises with the increase in metabolic rate. Unstable glucose levels can lead to further acidosis and neurologic damage. As the release of nonesterified fatty acid increases, the liver slows metabolism of glucose, inhibiting thermogenesis. As liver function declines, drugs are metabolized and excreted more slowly.

REFERENCES

Dodman, N. (1987). Newborn temperature control. *Neonatal Network, 5*(6), 19–23.

Bruggemeyer, A. (1990). Thermoregulation (pp. 23–38). In L.P. Gunderson & C. Kenner (eds.), *Care of the 24-25 week gestational age infant: Small baby protocol.* Petaluma, CA: Neonatal Network.

Brueggemeyer, A. (1993). Neonatal thermoregulation (pp. 247–262). In C. Kenner, A. Brueggemeyer, & L.P. Gunderson (eds.), *Comprehensive neonatal nursing: A physiologic perspective.* Philadelphia: W.B. Saunders.

81. Answer: (**A**) Using these criteria, the Symposium members identified four diseases that have reliable tests to screen infants on a large scale and that should receive priority in detection: PKU, congenital hypothyroidism, galactosemia, maple syrup urine disease.

REFERENCES

Benson, P.F. (1983). Screening and management of potentially treatable genetic metabolic disorders. Boston: MTP Press abstracts from "proceedings."

Bickel, H., Gutherie, R., & Hammersen, G. (1980). *Neonatal screening for inborn errors of metabolism.* New York: Springer-Verlag.

Crawford, M. d'A., Gibbs, D.A., & Watts, R.W.E. (eds.). (1982). *Advances in the treatment of inborn errors of metabolism.* New York: Wiley.

Scriver, C.R., Beaudet, A.L., Sly, W.S., & Valle, D. (eds.). (1989). *The metabolic basis of inherited disease.* (6th ed.). (Volume I and II). New York: McGraw-Hill.

Theorell, C.J. & Degenhardt, M. (1993). Assessment and management of metabolic dysfunction (pp. 480–526). In C. Kenner, A. Brueggemeyer, & L.P. Gunderson (eds.), *Comprehensive neonatal nursing: A physiologic perspective.* Philadelphia: W.B. Saunders.

82. Answer: (**A**) Suctioning the endotracheal tube has been correlated with significant morbidity, including tracheal injury and hypoxemia. The nurse can decrease adverse reactions associated with suctioning by various means such as suctioning only when the assessment shows a clear patient need, implementing noninvasive oxygenation monitoring during the procedure, measuring suction catheters to only reach the end of the endotracheal tube, increasing the oxygen, and using two-person technique for hypoxemic infants. The primary goal is that suctioning be done only when it benefits the patient. Homeostasis is maintained during the procedure as much as possible, and stress of the procedure is minimized.

REFERENCES

Boynton, B.R. & Jones, B. (1988). Nursing care of the infant with bronchopulmonary dysplasia (pp. 313–330). In T.A. Merritt, W.H. Northway, Jr., & B.R. Boynton (eds.), *Bronchopulmonary dysplasia.* Boston: Blackwell Scientific.

Miller, R.W., Woo, P., Kellman, R.K., & Slagle, T.S. (1987). Tracheobronchial abnormalities in infants

with bronchopulmonary dysplasia. *The Journal of Pediatrics, 111*, 779–782.
Southwell, S.M. (1993). Complications of respiratory management (pp. 337–354). In C. Kenner, A. Brueggemeyer, & L.P. Gunderson (eds.), *Comprehensive neonatal nursing: A physiologic perspective*. Philadelphia: W.B. Saunders.

83. Answer: (**C**). The first effect of an elevated blood glucose is to decrease and eventually arrest glycogen degradation in the liver.

REFERENCES

Ampola, M.G. (1982). *Metabolic disease in pediatric practice*. Boston: Little, Brown.
Burman, D., Holton, J.B., & Pennock, C.A. (eds.). (1978). *Inherited disorders of carbohydrate metabolism*. Baltimore: University Park Press.
Cornblath, M., Wybregt, S.H., & Bacens, G.S. (1963). Studies of carbohydrate metabolism in the newborn infant. *Pediatrics, 32,* 1007.
Theorell, C.J. & Degenhardt, M. (1993). Assessment and management of metabolic dysfunction (pp. 480–526). In C. Kenner, A. Brueggemeyer, & L.P. Gunderson (eds.), *Comprehensive neonatal nursing: A physiologic perspective*. Philadelphia: W.B. Saunders.

84. Answer: (**C**) The attending nurses must be particularly alert during this intervening period for sudden deterioration of the "well" infant. This is demonstrated by increased pallor or duskiness, increasing respiratory rate and retractions, jitteriness, "strange" cry, or other deviations from the expected clinical course. The physician should be notified immediately. Nursing interventions will be consistent with agency policy, physician's orders, and the nurse's clinical judgment, and may include nasopharyngeal suction, estimating blood sugar by Dextrostix, and initiating oxygen therapy via head hood or blowing oxygen to the face.

REFERENCES

Battaglia, F.C., & Lubchenco, L.O. (1967). A practical classification of newborn infants by weight and gestational age. *Journal of Pediatrics, 71*(2), 159–163.
Endo, A.S. & Nishioka, E. (1993). Neonatal assessment (pp. 265–293). In C. Kenner, A. Brueggemeyer, & L.P. Gunderson (eds.), *Comprehensive neonatal nursing: A physiologic perspective*. Philadelphia: W.B. Saunders.
Petrucha, R. (1989). Fetal maturity/gestational age evaluation. *Journal of Perinatology, 9*(1), 100–101.

85. Answer: (**B**) Brink and Wood (1989) suggest that historical research, meta-analysis, epidemiological research, instrument development, and evaluative research are examples of mixed designs.

REFERENCES

Brink, P.J. & Wood, M.J. (eds.) (1989). *Advanced design in nursing research*. Newbury Park, CA: Sage Publications.
Franck, L.S., Gunderson, L.P., & Kenner, C. (1993). Collaborative research in neonatal nursing (pp. 52–66). In C. Kenner, A. Brueggemeyer, & L.P. Gunderson (eds.), *Comprehensive neonatal nursing: A physiologic perspective*. Philadelphia: W.B. Saunders.

86. Answer: (**C**) The timing of the surgery depends on the severity of the circulatory and pulmonary compromise. A grade 2-5/6 systolic regurgitant murmur is typical for a VSD and can be heard without significant decompensation. An enlarged main pulmonary artery segment on x-ray is indicative of an ASD. In VSD, the cardiac enlargement is typically the left atrium, left ventricle, and sometimes the right ventricle.

REFERENCES

Avery, G.B. (1987). *Neonatology: Pathophysiology and management of the newborn*. Philadelphia: J.B. Lippincott.
Graham, T.P., Bender, H.W., & Spach, M.S. (1989). (pp. 189–209). In F.H. Adams, G.C. Emmanouilides, & T.A. Riemenschneider (eds.), *Heart disease in infants, children, and adolescents*. Baltimore: Williams & Wilkins.
Lott, J.W. (1993). Assessment and management of cardiovascular dysfunction (pp. 355–391). In C. Kenner, A. Brueggemeyer, & L.P. Gunderson (eds.), *Comprehensive neonatal nursing: A physiologic perspective*. Philadelphia: W.B. Saunders.
Moller, J.H. (1987). *Congenital heart anomalies. Clinical education aid*. Columbus, OH: Ross Laboratories.

87. Answer: (**C**) The steps to successful role change include identifying the role of the relevant other, identifying expectations of the new role, developing abilities for it, taking on the new role, and modifying it (Hall-Johnson, 1986).

REFERENCES

Berns, S.P., Geiser, R., & Levi, L.A. (1993). The changing family unit (pp. 69–79). In C. Kenner, A. Brueggemeyer, & L.P. Gunderson (eds.), *Comprehensive neonatal nursing: A physiologic perspective*. Philadelphia: W.B. Saunders.
Hall-Johnson, S. (1986). *Nursing assessment and strategies for the family at risk: High-risk parenting*. Philadelphia: J.B. Lippincott.
Hardy, M. & Conway, M.E. (1988). *Role theory: Perspective for health professionals*. (2nd ed.). Norwalk, CT: Appleton & Lange.

88. Answer: (**B**) Crisis is a period of disequilibrium precipitated by an inescapable demand to which the person temporarily is unable to respond adequately (Kaplan & Mason, 1960).

REFERENCES

Berns, S.P., Geiser, R., & Levi, L.A. (1993). The changing family unit (pp. 69–79). In C. Kenner, A. Brueggemeyer, & L.P. Gunderson (eds.), *Comprehensive neonatal nursing: A physiologic perspective*. Philadelphia: W.B. Saunders.

Kaplan, D.N. & Mason, E.A. (1960). Maternal reactions to premature birth viewed as an acute emotional disorder. *American Journal of Orthopsychiatry, 30,* 539–552.

89. Answer: (**B**) One way of defining role is overt and covert goal-directed patterns of behavior that result from individuals interacting with, shaping, and adapting to their social environment. Roles are dynamic, interactional, and reciprocal relationships exist among people.

REFERENCES

Berns, S.P., Geiser, R., & Levi, L.A. (1993). The changing family unit (pp. 69–79). In C. Kenner, A. Brueggemeyer, & L.P. Gunderson (eds.), *Comprehensive neonatal nursing: A physiologic perspective*. Philadelphia: W.B. Saunders.

Thomas, E. & Biddle, B. (1979). Basic concepts for classifying the phenomena of role. In B. Biddle and E. Thomas (eds.), *Role theory: Concepts and research.* New York: Wiley.

90. Answer: (**C**) The major portion of the right ventricular output flows through the lungs, increasing pulmonary vascular resistance to the left atrium. The increasing amount of blood in the lungs and heart causes increased pressure in the left atrium, functionally closing the foramen ovale. Cord occlusion causes a rise in blood pressure and stimulation of aortic baroreceptors and sympathetic nervous system. Onset of respirations and lung expansion cause a decreased pulmonary vascular resistance secondary to direct effect of oxygen and carbon dioxide on blood vessels.

REFERENCES

Heymann, M.A. (1989). Fetal and neonatal circulations (pp. 24–35). In F.H. Adams, G.C. Emmanouilides, & T.A. Riemenschneider (eds.), *Heart disease in infants, children, and adolescents*. Baltimore: Williams & Wilkins.

Heymann, M.A. (1989). Patent ductus arteriosus (pp. 209–223). In F.H. Adams, G.C. Emmanouilides, & T.A. Riemenschneider (eds.), *Heart disease in infants, children, and adolescents*. Baltimore: Williams & Wilkins.

Lott, J.W. (1993). Assessment and management of cardiovascular dysfunction (pp. 355–391). In C. Kenner, A. Brueggemeyer, & L.P. Gunderson (eds.), *Comprehensive neonatal nursing: A physiologic perspective*. Philadelphia: W.B. Saunders.

Moller, J.H. (1987). *Congenital heart anomalies. Clinical education aid.* Columbus, OH: Ross Laboratories.

Sacksteder, S. (1978). Embryology and fetal circulation. *American Journal of Nursing,* (Feb), 262–265.

91. Answer: (**C**) Watery acid diarrhea with excoriated buttocks is the hallmark of carbohydrate intolerance in infants. Fluid losses can be profound and life threatening.

REFERENCES

Ampola, M.G. (1982). *Metabolic disease in pediatric practice*. Boston: Little, Brown.

Burman, D., Holton, J.B., & Pennock, C.A. (eds.). (1978). *Inherited disorders of carbohydrate metabolism*. Baltimore: University Park Press.

Cornblath, M., Wybregt, S.H., & Bacens, G.S. (1963). Studies of carbohydrate metabolism in the newborn infant. *Pediatrics, 32,* 1007.

Theorell, C.J. & Degenhardt, M. (1993). Assessment and management of metabolic dysfunction (pp. 480–526). In C. Kenner, A. Brueggemeyer, & L.P. Gunderson (eds.), *Comprehensive neonatal nursing: A physiologic perspective*. Philadelphia: W.B. Saunders.

Wapnir, R.A. (1985). Congenital metabolic disease diagnosis and treatment. New York: Marcel Dekker.

92. Answer: (**C**) A patient's diagnosis or condition is consideration that must be reviewed when choosing a preferred mode of transportation. Local terrain should be considered when selecting the transport vehicle.

REFERENCES

Croop, L.H. & Acree, C.M. (1993). Neonatal transport (pp. 1182–212). In C. Kenner, A. Brueggemeyer, & L.P. Gunderson (eds.), *Comprehensive neonatal care: A physiologic perspective*. Philadelphia: W.B. Saunders.

Weinger, W. (1987). Setting standards for critical care transport. Fitz-Gibbons' Law revisited. *International Anesthesiology Clinics, 25*(2), 139–159.

93. Answer: (**C**) The tricuspid valve connects the right atrium and right ventricle. The aortic valve (semilunar) connects the left ventricle and the aorta. The mitral valve (A-V) connects the left atrium and the left ventricle.

REFERENCES

Ho, S.Y., Angelini, A., & Moscoso, G. (1990). Developmental cardiac anatomy (pp. 3–16). In W.A. Long (ed.), *Fetal and neonatal cardiology*. Philadelphia: W.B. Saunders.

Lott, J.W. (1993). Assessment and management of cardiovascular dysfunction (pp. 355–391). In C. Kenner, A. Brueggemeyer, & L.P. Gunderson (eds.), *Comprehensive neonatal nursing: A physiologic perspective.* Philadelphia: W.B. Saunders.
Park, M.K. (1984). Valvular heart disease (pp. 245–258). *Pediatric cardiology for practitioners.* Chicago: Year Book Medical Publishers.

94. Answer: (**B**) Although sweat glands are almost nonexistent in the preterm infant, the infant loses enormous amounts of water through the skin's surface. These losses rise dramatically when radiation heating sources are used or the infant is placed under phototherapy lights. Under these circumstances, premature infants can lose as much water as 120 ml/kg/day. Humidification of the environment at the range of 40 percent to 60 percent may protect the premature infant from heat loss due to evaporative losses.

REFERENCES

Brueggemeyer, A. (1993). Neonatal thermoregulation (pp. 247–262). In C. Kenner, A. Brueggemeyer, & L.P. Gunderson (eds.), *Comprehensive neonatal nursing: A physiologic perspective.* Philadelphia: W.B. Saunders.
Dodman, N. (1987). Newborn temperature control. *Neonatal Network, 5*(6), 19–23.
Hammarlund, K., Strömberg, B., & Sedin, G. (1986). Heat loss from the skin of preterm and fullterm newborn infants during the first weeks after birth. *Biology of the Neonate, 50,* 1–10.
Swyer, P. (1978). Heat loss after birth (pp. 91–128). In J. Sinclair (ed.), *Temperature regulation and energy metabolism in the newborn.* New York: Grune & Stratton.

95. Answer: (**B**) Galactokinase deficient individuals are asymptomatic with the exception of cataracts that appear in infancy.

REFERENCES

Ampola, M.G. (1982). *Metabolic disease in pediatric practice.* Boston: Little, Brown.
Burman, D., Holton, J.B., & Pennock, C.A. (eds.), (1978). *Inherited disorders of carbohydrate metabolism.* Baltimore: University Park Press.
Theorell, C.J. & Degenhardt, M. (1993). Assessment and management of metabolic dysfunction (pp. 480–526). In C. Kenner, A. Brueggemeyer, & L.P. Gunderson (eds.), *Comprehensive neonatal nursing: A physiologic perspective.* Philadelphia: W.B. Saunders.
Scriver, C.R., Beaudet, A.L., Sly, W.S., & Valle, D. (eds.). (1989). *The metabolic basis of inherited disease.* (6th ed.). (Volume I and II). New York: McGraw-Hill.

96. Answer: (**A**) Acetylcholine is the active neurotransmitter for the parasympathetic nervous system. Stimulation of the sympathetic nervous system through the ganglionic chain releases norepinephrine and epinephrine, which act on the SA node, AV node, atria, and ventricles.

REFERENCES

Braunwald, E., Sonnenblick, E.H., & Ross, J. (1988). Mechanisms of cardiac contraction and relaxation (pp. 383–425). In E. Braunwald (ed.), *Heart disease: A textbook of cardiovascular medicine.* Philadelphia: W.B. Saunders.
Hazinski, M.F. (1984). Cardiovascular disorders (pp. 63–252). *Nursing care of the critically ill child.* St. Louis: C.V. Mosby.
Lott, J.W. (1993). Assessment and management of cardiovascular dysfunction (pp. 355–391). In C. Kenner, A. Brueggemeyer, & L.P. Gunderson (eds.), *Comprehensive neonatal nursing: A physiologic perspective.* Philadelphia: W.B. Saunders.
Smith, J.J. & Kampine, J.P. (1984). *Circulatory physiology.* Baltimore: Williams & Wilkins.

97. Answer: (**A**) When the mother and father both express type O blood, the alleles for type O blood are recessive. The presumed genotype for this pair is OO, with the expected phenotypes and genotypes of all first-generation offspring to be type O homozygous (OO).

REFERENCES

Cohen, F.L. (1984). *Clinical genetics in nursing practice.* Philadelphia: J.B. Lippincott.
Connor, J. & Ferguson-Smith, M. (1987). *Essential medical genetics.* Oxford: Blackwell Scientific.
Cummings, M. (1988). *Human heredity: Principles and issues.* New York: West Publishing.
Thompson, S. & Thompson, M. (1986). *Genetics in medicine* (4th ed.). Philadelphia: W.B. Saunders.
Workman, M.L., Kenner, C., & Hilse, M. (1993). Human genetics (pp. 101–131). In C. Kenner, A. Brueggemeyer, & L.P. Gunderson (eds.), *Comprehensive neonatal nursing: A physiologic perspective.* Philadelphia: W.B. Saunders.

98. Answer: (**A**) The primary purpose of the gestational assessment is to anticipate problems related to development. Further research has demonstrated that both gestational age and whether the individual's development are appropriate for that age will have considerable influence on outcome.

REFERENCES

Battaglia, F.C. & Lubchenco, L.O. (1967). A practical classification of newborn infants by weight and gestational age. *Journal of Pediatrics, 71*(2), 159–163.
Endo, A.S. & Nishioka, E. (1993). Neonatal assessment (pp. 265–293). In C. Kenner, A. Brueggemeyer, & L.P. Gunderson (eds.), *Comprehensive neonatal nursing: A physiologic perspective.* Philadelphia: W.B. Saunders.

99. Answer: (**A**) Long-term treatment of fructose-1,6-diphosphate deficiency consists of frequent meals and the restriction of fructose or sorbitol.

REFERENCES

Ampola, M.G. (1982). *Metabolic disease in pediatric practice*. Boston: Little, Brown.

Burman, D., Holton, J.B., & Pennock, C.A. (eds.). (1978). *Inherited disorders of carbohydrate metabolism*. Baltimore: University Park Press.

Scriver, C.R., Beaudet, A.L., Sly, W.S., & Valle, D. (eds.). (1989). *The metabolic basis of inherited disease*. (6th ed.). (Volume I and II). New York: McGraw-Hill.

Theorell, C.J. & Degenhardt, M. (1993). Assessment and management of metabolic dysfunction (pp. 480–526). In C. Kenner, A. Brueggemeyer, & L.P. Gunderson. (eds.), *Comprehensive neonatal nursing: A physiologic perspective*. Philadelphia: W.B. Saunders.

100. Answer: (**B**) High-frequency oscillatory ventilation (HFOV) delivers very small frequencies of 300 to 3000 breaths per minute. Expiration is active and is achieved by a piston pump or acoustic speaker. Active expiration decreases the risk of air trapping, and may explain the minimal air trapping with HFOV.

High-frequency jet ventilation (HFJV) delivers tidal volumes that may be less than or greater than anatomic dead space at frequencies of 60 to 600 breaths per minute. HFJV provides constant flow-time-cycled ventilation with passive expiration. Adequate humidification is needed with HFJV to prevent tracheal lesions.

REFERENCES

Boros, S.J., Mammel, M.C., Coleman, J.M., et al. (1985). Neonatal high-frequency jet ventilation: Four years' experience. *Pediatrics, 75,* 657–663.

Carlo, W.A. & Chatburn, R.L. (1988). *Neonatal respiratory care*. Chicago: Year Book Medical Publishers.

Donovan, E.F. & Spangler, L.L. (1993). New technologies applied to the management of respiratory dysfunction. In C. Kenner, A. Brueggemeyer, & L.P. Gunderson (eds.), *Comprehensive neonatal nursing: A physiologic perspective*. Philadelphia: W.B. Saunders.

Gordin, P. (1989). High-frequency jet ventilation for severe respiratory failure. *Pediatric Nursing, 15*(6), 625–629.

HIFI Study Group. (1989). High-frequency oscillatory ventilation compared with conventional mechanical ventilation in the treatment of respiratory failure in preterm infants. *New England Journal of Medicine, 320*(2), 88–93.

Wetzel, R.C. & Gioia, F.R. (1987). Extracorporeal membrane oxygenation: Its use in neonatal respiratory failure. *AORN Journal, 45*(3), 725–739.

101. Answer: (**B**) Cyanosis would be present with 5 grams/dl of deoxygenated hemoglobin. Cyanosis cannot be present with only 2 grams/dl of deoxygenated blood in the circulation and can be severe with 8 gm/dl of deoxygenated hemoglobin.

REFERENCES

Avery, G. B. (1987). *Neonatology: Pathophysiology and management of the newborn*. Philadelphia: J.B. Lippincott.

Lott, J.W. (1993). Assessment and management of cardiovascular dysfunction (pp. 355–391). In C. Kenner, A. Brueggemeyer, & L.P. Gunderson (eds.), *Comprehensive neonatal nursing: A physiologic perspective*. Philadelphia: W.B. Saunders.

Park, M.K. (1984). Pathophysiology of cyanotic congenital heart defects (pp. 108–123). *Pediatric cardiology for practitioners*. Chicago: Year Book Medical Publishers.

102. Answer: (**C**) Conductive heat losses occur when the infant is on a cool surface such as an infant scale.

REFERENCES

Brueggemeyer, A. (1993). Neonatal thermoregulation (pp. 247–262). In C. Kenner, A. Brueggemeyer, & L.P. Gunderson (eds.), *Comprehensive neonatal nursing: A physiologic perspective*. Philadelphia: W.B. Saunders.

Laburn, D.M. & Laburn, H.P. (1985). Pathophysiology of temperature regulation. *The Physiologist, 28*(6), 507–517.

Mestyán, J. (1978). Energy metabolism and substrate utilization in the newborn (pp. 39–74). In J. Sinclair (ed.), *Temperature regulation and energy metabolism in the newborn*. New York : Grune & Stratton.

103. Answer: (**C**) Persistent pulmonary hypertension of the newborn (PPHN), or persistent fetal circulation, is a term applied to the combination of pulmonary hypertension (high pressure in the pulmonary artery), subsequent right-to-left shunting through fetal channels (the foramen ovale and/or ductus arteriosus) away from the pulmonary vascular bed, and a structurally normal heart. The syndrome can be idiopathic or more commonly secondary to another disorder such as meconium aspiration syndrome, congenital diaphragmatic hernia, respiratory distress syndrome, sepsis, hyperviscosity of the blood, or even hypoglycemia.

REFERENCES

Chernick, V. & Kendig, E.L. (1990). *Kendig's disorders of the respiratory tract in children*. Philadelphia: W.B. Saunders Company.

Haywood, J.L., Coghill III, C.H., Carlo, W.A., & Ross, M. (1993). Assessment and management of respiratory dysfunction (pp. 294–312). In C. Kenner, A. Brueggemeyer, & L.P. Gunderson (eds.), *Comprehensive neonatal nursing: A physiologic perspective.* Philadelphia: W.B. Saunders.
Kattwinkel, J. (1977). Neonatal apnea: Pathogenesis and therapy. *Journal of Pediatrics, 90,* 342–347.
Langston, C.J. & Thurlbeck, W. (1986). Conditions altering normal lung growth and development. In D. Thibeault & G. Gregory (eds.), *Neonatal pulmonary care* (2nd ed.). Norwalk, CT: Appleton-Century-Crofts.
Speidel, B.D. & Dunn, P.M. (1976). Use of nasal continuous positive airway pressure to treat severe recurrent apnea in very preterm infants. *Lancet, 2,* 58–660.

104. Answer: (**B**) Cyanotic heart defects typically have left-to-right shunts and decreased pulmonary blood flow.

REFERENCES

Hazinski, M.F. (1983). Congenital heart disease in the neonate (Part III): Congestive heart failure. *Neonatal Network, 1* (6), 8–17.
Hazinski, M.F. (1984). Cardiovascular disorders (pp. 63–252). *Nursing care of the critically ill child.* St. Louis: C.V. Mosby.
Heymann, M.A. (1989). Fetal and neonatal circulations (pp. 24–35). In F.H. Adams, G.C. Emmanouilides, & T.A. Riemenschneider (eds.), *Heart disease in infants, children, and adolescents.* Baltimore: Williams & Wilkins.
Heymann, M.A. (1989). Patent ductus arteriosus (pp. 209–223). In F.H. Adams, G.C. Emmanouilides, & T.A. Riemenschneider (eds.), *Heart disease in infants, children, and adolescents.* Baltimore: Williams & Wilkins.
Lott, J.W. (1993). Assessment and management of cardiovascular dysfunction (pp. 355–391). In C. Kenner, A. Brueggemeyer, & L.P. Gunderson (eds.), *Comprehensive neonatal nursing: A physiologic perspective.* Philadelphia: W.B. Saunders.

105. Answer: (**A**) Serum concentrations of chloride and bicarbonate are inversely correlated, keeping the total anion concentration (chloride + bicarbonate) constant. For this reason, although chloride has no buffer effect, it plays an important part in acid-base regulation. When chloride is retained in the body, serum bicarbonate increases and metabolic alkalosis follows.

REFERENCES

Costarino, A. & Baumgart, S. (1986). Modern fluid and electrolyte management of the critically ill premature infant. *Pediatric Clinics of North America, 33,* 153–158.
DeMarini, S., Tsang, R.C., & Rath, L.L. (1993). Fluids, electrolytes, vitamins, and trace minerals: Basis of ingestion, digestion, elimination, and metabolism (pp. 393–413). In C. Kenner, A. Brueggemeyer, & L.P. Gunderson (eds.), *Comprehensive neonatal nursing: A physiologic perspective.* Philadelphia: W.B. Saunders.
Turnberg, L.A. (1971b). Potassium transport in the human small bowel. *Gut, 12,* 811–818.
Turnberg, L.A., Bieberdort, F.A., Mordowsky, S.G., & Gordtran, J.S. (1970). Interrelations of choloride, bicarbonate, sodium and hydrogen transport in human ileum. *Journal of Clinical Investigation, 49,* 557–567.

106. Answer: (**B**) Neurulation is the process by which the neural plate, neural folds, and neural tube are formed. This begins during the third week of gestation.

REFERENCES

Cohen, F.L. (1984). *Clinical genetics in nursing practice.* Philadelphia: J.B. Lippincott.
Connor, J. & Ferguson-Smith, M. (1987). *Essential medical genetics.* Oxford: Blackwell Scientific.
Cummings, M. (1988). *Human heredity: Principles and issues.* New York: West Publishing.
Lott, J.W. (1993). Fetal development: Environmental influences and critical periods (pp. 132–156). In C. Kenner, A. Brueggemeyer, & L.P. Gunderson (eds.), *Comprehensive neonatal nursing: A physiologic perspective.* Philadelphia: W.B. Saunders.
Moore, K.L. (1989). *The developing human* (4th ed.). Philadelphia: W.B. Saunders.
Sadler, T.W. (1985). *Langman's medical embryology* (5th ed.). Baltimore: Williams & Wilkins.
Thompson, S. & Thompson, M. (1986). *Genetics in medicine* (4th ed.). Philadelphia: W.B. Saunders.

107. Answer: (**C**) The embryonic period lasts from the beginning of week four through the end of week eight.

REFERENCES

Lott, J.W. (1993). Fetal development: Environmental influences and critical periods (pp. 132–156). In C. Kenner, A. Brueggemeyer, & L.P. Gunderson (eds.), *Comprehensive neonatal nursing: A physiologic perspective.* Philadelphia: W.B. Saunders.
Moore, K.L. (1989). *The developing human* (4th ed.). Philadelphia: W.B. Saunders.
Sadler, T.W. (1985). *Langman's medical embryology* (5th ed.). Baltimore: Williams & Wilkins.

108. Answer: (**A**) The neural crest cells give rise to the spinal ganglia, the ganglia of the autonomic nervous system, and a portion of the cranial nerves.

REFERENCES

Lott, J.W. (1993). Fetal development: Environmental influences and critical periods (pp. 132–156). In C. Kenner, A. Brueggemeyer, & L.P. Gunderson (eds.), *Comprehensive neonatal nursing: A physiologic perspective.* Philadelphia: W.B. Saunders.
Moore, K.L. (1989). *The developing human* (4th ed.). Philadelphia: W.B. Saunders.
Sadler, T.W. (1985). *Langman's medical embryology* (5th ed.). Baltimore: Williams & Wilkins.

109. Answer: (**C**) The cavity of the neural tube develops into the ventricles of the brain and the central canal of the spinal column. The neuroepithelial cells lining the neural tube give rise to nerves and glial cells of the central nervous system.

REFERENCES

Lott, J.W. (1993). Fetal development: Environmental influences and critical periods (pp. 132–156). In C. Kenner, A. Brueggemeyer, & L.P. Gunderson (eds.), *Comprehensive neonatal nursing: A physiologic perspective*. Philadelphia: W.B. Saunders.

Moore, K.L. (1989). *The developing human* (4th ed.). Philadelphia: W.B. Saunders.

Sadler, T.W. (1985). *Langman's medical embryology* (5th ed.). Baltimore: Williams & Wilkins.

110. Answer: (**B**) Neonatal ECMO is used in the management of intractable hypoxemia in near-term newborns with meconium aspiration syndrome, respiratory distress syndrome, pneumonia/sepsis, and congenital diaphragmatic hernia. Various criteria are used to determine the point at which the risk of persistent hypoxemia is greater than the risk of ECMO. In a practical sense, most ECMO centers probably use a combination of oxygenation criteria, ventilation criteria, and clinical judgment.

Various contraindications exist to the uses of ECMO. The most important contraindication is prematurity. Early reports of ECMO use in premature infants revealed alarmingly high rates of intracranial hemorrhage. Other contraindications to ECMO use include preexisting intracranial hemorrhage and hypoxemia, which is not potentially reversible such as that seen in patients with cyanotic congenital heart disease.

To avoid permanent carotid artery ligation, two new approaches are currently being evaluated. Several ECMO centers are now attempting to reanastomose the proximal and distal carotid artery segments after removal of the carotid artery catheter. Another approach that avoids carotid artery ligation is the use of veno–venous bypass. With this technique blood is both removed from and returned to the systemic venous circulation. A double-lumen catheter is inserted via the external jugular vein with this specially designed equipment. One lumen opens distally in the right atrium, whereas the more proximal lumen is in the superior vena cava. Blood is removed by gravity from the proximal lumen, and oxygenated blood that has passed through the ECMO circuit is pumped back into the distal lumen. The most important functional limitation of veno–venous bypass using this particular technique is the sufficiency of circuit flow. Because blood is both withdrawn and returned to the same vessel, flow may be inadequate to meet the patient's oxygen utilization rate.

REFERENCES

Donovan, E.F. & Spangler, L.L. (1993). New technologies applied to the management of respiratory dysfunction. In C. Kenner, A. Brueggemeyer, & L.P. Gunderson (eds.), *Comprehensive neonatal nursing: A physiologic perspective*. Philadelphia: W.B. Saunders.

Roberts, P.M. & Jones, M.B. (1990). Extracorporeal membrane oxygenation and indications for cardiopulmonary bypass in the neonate. *JOGNN, 19*(6), 391–399.

Wetzel, R.C. & Gioia, F.R. (1987). Extracorporeal membrane oxygenation: Its use in neonatal respiratory failure. *AORN Journal, 45*(3), 725–739.

111. Answer: (**B**) The endocardial cushion normally contributes to the formation of the primum portion of the atrial septum, the inlet ventricular septum, and the mitral and tricuspid valves. The tricuspid and mitral valves are the atrioventricular or A-V valves.

REFERENCES

Avery, G.B. (1987). *Neonatology: Pathophysiology and management of the newborn*. Philadelphia: J.B. Lippincott.

Friedman, W.F. (1988). Congenital heart disease in infancy and childhood (pp. 896–975). In E. Braunwald (ed.), *Heart disease: A textbook of cardiovascular medicine*. Philadelphia: W.B. Saunders.

Friedman, W.F. (1989). Aortic stenosis (pp. 224–243). In F.H. Adams, G.C. Emmanouilides, & T.A. Riemenschneider (eds.), *Heart disease in infants, children, and adolescents*. Baltimore: Williams & Wilkins.

Lott, J.W. (1993). Assessment and management of cardiovascular dysfunction (pp. 355–391). In C. Kenner, A. Brueggemeyer, & L.P. Gunderson (eds.), *Comprehensive neonatal nursing: A physiologic perspective*. Philadelphia: W.B. Saunders.

112. Answer: (**A**) The most common one found is the simian crease, a palmar crease, associated with trisomy 21 or Down syndrome. As this crease is found in the general population as

well, presence of this crease does not in itself signify that the infant has Down syndrome.

REFERENCES

Battaglia, F.C., & Lubchenco, L.O. (1967). A practical classification of newborn infants by weight and gestational age. *Journal of Pediatrics, 71*(2), 159–163.

Endo, A.S. & Nishioka, E. (1993). Neonatal assessment (pp. 265–293). In C. Kenner, A. Brueggemeyer, & L.P. Gunderson (eds.), *Comprehensive neonatal nursing: A physiologic perspective*. Philadelphia: W.B. Saunders.

Petrucha, R. (1989). Fetal maturity/gestational age evaluation. *Journal of Perinatology, 9*(1), 100–101.

113. Answer: (**A**) Intrapulmonary interstitial emphysema (IIE) is a common air leak in ventilated VLBW neonates. Mechanical ventilation at high pressures causes stress and rupture of alveoli, probably at the bases or ducts. The air then dissects perivascularly and peribronchially, probably along lymphatic channels. The lungs on chest x-ray have a "bubbly" appearance either unilaterally or bilaterally, and the affected lung is usually hyperventilated. Those who survive usually develop significant BPD.

REFERENCES

Southwell, S.M. (1993). Complications of respiratory management (pp. 337–354). In C. Kenner, A. Brueggemeyer, & L.P. Gunderson (eds.), *Comprehensive neonatal nursing: A physiologic perspective*. Philadelphia: W.B. Saunders.

Thiebeault, D.W. (1986). Pulmonary barotrauma: Interstitial emphysema, pneumomediastinum, and pneumothorax (pp. 499–517). In D.W. Thibeault & G.A. Gregory (eds.), *Neonatal pulmonary care* (2nd ed.). Norwalk, CT: Appleton-Century-Crofts.

114. Answer: (**A**) Back transfer strengthens the referral system in the region by promoting communication and mutual trust among hospitals. An efficient back-transfer program helps eliminate an acute shortage of NICU beds. Planning ahead for an infant's return transfer to the community hospital optimizes the management of NICU beds in a shortage crisis. The back transfer of infants also promotes sharing of fiscal responsibility with the region. The community hospital staff can maintain expertise and skills by caring for back-transferred infants. The result is an increase in pride and an investment in accountability in the care of these infants. The local physician can become involved with both the infant and family sooner, which facilitates the transfer of trust from the level III, or tertiary, center to the local community hospital.

REFERENCES

Croop, L. & Kenner, C. (1990). Protocol for reverse neonatal transports. *Neonatal Network, 9*(1), 49–53.

Fickeissen, J.L. (1986). Interhospital perinatal nursing transport conferences. *Neonatal Network, 5*(3), 45–48.

Gates, M. & Shelton, S. (1989). Back-transfer in neonatal care. *The Journal of Perinatal & Neonatal Nursing, 2*(3), 39–50.

Wolfe, L.S. (1993). Regionalization of care (pp. 171–181). In C. Kenner, A. Brueggemeyer, & L.P. Gunderson (eds.), *Comprehensive neonatal care: A physiologic perspective*. Philadelphia: W.B. Saunders.

115. Answer: (**A**) S1 is the sound resulting from closure of the mitral and tricuspid valves after atrial systole. S1 is the beginning of ventricular systole. S2 is the sound created by closure of the aortic and pulmonary valves, which marks the end of systole and the beginning of ventricular diastole.

REFERENCES

Johnson, G.L. (1990). Clinical examination (pp. 223–235). In W.A. Long (ed.), *Fetal and neonatal cardiology*. Philadelphia: W.B. Saunders.

Lott, J.W. (1993). Assessment and management of cardiovascular dysfunction (pp. 355–391). In C. Kenner, A. Brueggemeyer, & L.P. Gunderson (eds.), *Comprehensive neonatal nursing: A physiologic perspective*. Philadelphia: W.B. Saunders.

Park, M.K. (1984). Physical examination (pp. 9–33). *Pediatric cardiology for practitioners*. Chicago: Year Book Medical Publishers.

116. Answer: (**C**) Given the premature infant with RDS requiring respiratory support, the next strategy is to limit the iatrogenic tissue injury in the first few weeks of life that leads to the development of chronic BPD. This strategy includes the prevention of oxygen toxicity injury by limitation of intubation and mechanical ventilation, by the use of extracorporeal membrane oxygenation (ECMO), alternative ventilation techniques, and development enhancement techniques.

REFERENCES

Sinkin, R.A. & Phelps, D.L. (1987). New strategies for the prevention of bronchopulmonary dysplasia. *Clinics in Perinatology, 14*, 599–620.

Southwell, S.M. (1993). Complications of respiratory management (pp. 337–354). In C. Kenner, A. Brueggemeyer, & L.P. Gunderson (eds.), *Comprehensive neonatal nursing: A physiologic perspective*. Philadelphia: W.B. Saunders.

Tepper, R.S. (1988). Assessment of pulmonary function in the post neonatal period (pp. 263–276). In T.A. Merritt, W.H. Northway, Jr., & B.R. Boynton (eds.), *Bronchopulmonary dysplasia*. Boston: Blackwell Scientific.

117. Answer: (**C**) The S2 is heard as a single sound because of the absence of the pulmonic valve in pulmonary atresia or severe stenosis. ASD results in a widely split S2 because the amount of blood ejected by the right ventricle is increased, making the pulmonic valve close later than the aortic valve. PAPVR results in a widely split S2 because the amount of blood ejected by the right ventricle is increased.

REFERENCES

Johnson, G.L. (1990). Clinical examination (pp. 223–235). In W.A. Long (ed.), *Fetal and neonatal cardiology*. Philadelphia: W.B. Saunders.

Lott, J.W. (1993). Assessment and management of cardiovascular dysfunction (pp. 355–391). In C. Kenner, A. Brueggemeyer, & L.P. Gunderson (eds.), *Comprehensive neonatal nursing: A physiologic perspective*. Philadelphia: W.B. Saunders.

Park, M.K. (1984). Physical examination (pp. 9–33). *Pediatric cardiology for practitioners*. Chicago: Year Book Medical Publishers.

118. Answer: (**A**) Coating the alveoli with an agent to decrease surface tension would reduce the effort required to inflate the lungs from low volume. Pulmonary surfactant, a surface tension-reducing phospholipid, is the natural material found in mature alveoli. Surfactant is produced by an alveolar cell known as the type II pneumocyte. Surfactant coats alveoli, preventing alveolar collapse and loss of lung volume during expiration. That is, expiration ensues, elastic recoil works to deflate the lung, and alveolar diameter becomes smaller. Surfactant coating the alveolus reduces surface tension so that collapse is prevented and less pressure is required to reinflate it with the next inspiration.

REFERENCES

Avery, G.B. (1987). *Neonatology: Pathophysiology and management of the newborn*. (3rd ed.). Philadelphia: J.B. Lippincott.

Haywood, J.L., Coghill III, C.H., Carlo, W.A., & Ross, M. (1993). Assessment and management of respiratory dysfunction (pp. 294–312). In C. Kenner, A. Brueggemeyer, & L.P. Gunderson (eds.), *Comprehensive neonatal nursing: A physiologic perspective*. Philadelphia: W.B. Saunders.

119. Answer: (**C**) Folate is essential for the synthesis of nucleic acids and for the metabolism of some amino acids.

REFERENCES

Dallman, P.R. (1988). Nutritional anemia of infancy: Iron, folic acid and vitamin B_{12} (pp. 175–189). In R.C. Tsang & B.L. Nichols (eds.), *Nutrition during infancy*. St. Louis: C.V. Mosby.

DeMarini, S., Tsang, R.C., & Rath, L.L. (1993). Fluids, electrolytes, vitamins, and trace minerals: Basis of ingestion, digestion, elimination, and metabolism (pp. 393–413). In C. Kenner, A. Brueggemeyer, & L.P. Gunderson (eds.), *Comprehensive neonatal nursing: A physiologic perspective*. Philadelphia: W.B. Saunders.

Kalser, M.H. (1985). Absorption of cobalamin (vitamin B_{12}), folate and other water-soluble vitamins (pp. 1553–1566). In J.E. Berk (ed.), *Gastroenterology* (4th ed.). Philadelphia: W.B. Saunders.

120. Answer: (**B**) Aortic or pulmonic valve incompetence causes high-pitched regurgitation murmurs. Aortic regurgitation is present in bicuspid aortic valve, subaortic stenosis, and subarterial infundibular VSD. Pulmonary regurgitation murmurs are present with postoperative tetralogy of Fallot, pulmonary hypertension, postoperative pulmonary valvotomy for pulmonic stenosis, or other deformities of the pulmonic valve.

Mid-diastolic murmurs result from abnormal ventricular filling caused by turbulent blood flow through the tricuspid or mitral valve due to stenosis. Presystolic or late diastolic murmurs result from flow through A-V valves during ventricular diastole as a result of active atrial contraction ejecting blood into the ventricle.

REFERENCES

Johnson, G.L. (1990). Clinical examination (pp. 223–235). In W.A. Long (ed.), Fetal and neonatal cardiology. Philadelphia: W.B. Saunders.

Lott, J.W. (1993). Assessment and management of cardiovascular dysfunction (pp. 355–391). In C. Kenner, A. Brueggemeyer, & L.P. Gunderson (eds.), *Comprehensive neonatal nursing: A physiologic perspective*. Philadelphia: W.B. Saunders.

Park, M.K. (1984). Physical examination (pp. 9–33). *Pediatric cardiology for practitioners*. Chicago: Year Book Medical Publishers.

121. Answer: (**A**) Prevention of heat loss is the first goal in neonatal thermoregulation. The secondary goal is to mini-

mize the energy necessary for the infant to produce heat. The neonate is capable of heat production through three ways: voluntary muscle activity, shivering, and nonshivering or chemical thermogenesis. Of these three, shivering is the most inefficient method of heat production. Although it is the chief method of heat production in the adult, the infant has limited ability to produce heat in this manner. The preterm infant has virtually no ability to generate heat using this method. This activity is generally limited to movement related to positioning in an effort to conserve heat losses. Term infants are capable of assuming a flexed position, unless impeded, to conserve heat loss from exposed surfaces. The main source of heat production, then, is chemical thermogenesis. Stimulated by norepinephrine, brown fat metabolism takes place.

REFERENCES

Brueggemeyer, A. (1993). Neonatal thermoregulation (pp. 247–262). In C. Kenner, A. Brueggemeyer, & L.P. Gunderson (eds.), *Comprehensive neonatal nursing: A physiologic perspective*. Philadelphia: W.B. Saunders.

Nalepka, C.D. (1976). Understanding thermoregulation in newborns. *Journal of Obstetrical, Gynecological and Neonatal Nursing, 5*(6), 17–19.

Ringer, S.A. & Stark, A.R. (1990). Management of neonatal emergencies in the delivery room. *Clinics in Perinatology, 16*(1), 23–41.

122. Answer: **(C)** Passive and active high-frequency ventilators differ in two important ways. First, the very high driving pressure required during the inspiratory phase of passive HFV creates very high, although brief, inspiratory flow rates. Maintaining adequate humidification at these flow rates requires specially designed humidification systems. In contrast, active HFV requires conventional gas flows and therefore humidification can be achieved with the same humidifiers as used in conventional mechanical ventilation. Another difference between passive and active HFV is that very high rates (greater than 300 breaths per minute) cannot be used with passive HFV because of hyperinflation. Active HFV, on the other hand, allows the use of ventilator rates at 1800 breaths per minute.

REFERENCES

Boros, S.J., Mammel, M.C., Coleman, J.M., et al. (1985). Neonatal high-frequency jet ventilation: Four years' experience. *Pediatrics, 75,* 657–663.

Carlo, W.A. & Chatburn, R.L. (1988). *Neonatal respiratory care*. Chicago: Year Book Medical Publishers, Inc.

Donovan, E.F. & Spangler, L.L. (1993). New technologies applied to the management of respiratory dysfunction. In C. Kenner, A. Brueggemeyer, & L.P. Gunderson (eds.), *Comprehensive neonatal nursing: A physiologic perspective*. Philadelphia: W.B. Saunders.

Gordin, P. (1989). High-frequency jet ventilation for severe respiratory failure. *Pediatric Nursing, 15*(6), 625–629.

HIFI Study Group. (1989). High-frequency oscillatory ventilation compared with conventional mechanical ventilation in the treatment of respiratory failure in preterm infants. *New England Journal of Medicine, 320*(2), 88–93.

Nugent, J. (1991). *Acute respiratory care of the neonate*. Petaluma, CA: NICU, INK.

123. Answer: **(A)** Neonatal pyridoxine-dependent seizures are due to a congenital abnormality of vitamin B_6 metabolism, and pharmacologic doses of vitamin B_6 are needed.

REFERENCES

DeMarini, S., Tsang, R.C., & Rath, L.L. (1993). Fluids, electrolytes, vitamins, and trace minerals: Basis of ingestion, digestion, elimination, and metabolism (pp. 393–413). In C. Kenner, A. Brueggemeyer, & L.P. Gunderson (eds.), *Comprehensive neonatal nursing: A physiologic perspective*. Philadelphia: W.B. Saunders.

Schanler, R.J. (1988). Water-soluble vitamins: C, B_1, B_2, B_6, niacin, biotin and pantothenic acid (pp. 236–252). In R.C. Tsang & B.L. Nichols (eds.), *Nutrition during infancy*. St. Louis: C.V. Mosby.

124. Answer: **(C)** VSD is the most common congenital heart defect; it accounts for 20 to 25 percent of all CHDs. ASD accounts for 5 to 10 percent of all CHDs. PDA accounts for 5 to 10 percent of all CHDs.

REFERENCES

Lott, J.W. (1993). Assessment and management of cardiovascular dysfunction (pp. 355–391). In C. Kenner, A. Brueggemeyer, & L.P. Gunderson (eds.), *Comprehensive neonatal nursing: A physiologic perspective*. Philadelphia: W.B. Saunders.

Moller, J.H. (1987). *Congenital heart anomalies. Clinical education aid*. Columbus, OH: Ross Laboratories.

Park, M.K. (1984). Left-to-right shunts (pp. 125–144). *Pediatric cardiology for practitioners*. Chicago: Year Book Medical Publishers.

125. Answer: **(A)** Jaundice is considered physiologic if it occurs after day two and is resolving by days five to seven.

In the premature infant, this jaundice may peak slightly later, usually around day five. Breast milk jaundice normally appears just as the physiologic jaundice is beginning to subside.

REFERENCES

Battaglia, F.C., & Lubchenco, L.O. (1967). A practical classification of newborn infants by weight and gestational age. *Journal of Pediatrics, 71*(2), 159–163.

Endo, A.S. & Nishioka, E. (1993). Neonatal assessment (pp. 265–293). In C. Kenner, A. Brueggemeyer, & L.P. Gunderson (eds.), *Comprehensive neonatal nursing: A physiologic perspective.* Philadelphia: W.B. Saunders.

Petrucha, R. (1989). Fetal maturity/gestational age evaluation. *Journal of Perinatology, 9*(1), 100–101.

126. Answer: (**B**) Chloride is the main inorganic anion in the extracellular fluid and with sodium is essential for maintenance of plasma volume.

REFERENCES

Arieff, A., & Guisado, R. (1976). Effects on the central nervous system of hypernatremic and hyponatremic states. *Kidney International, 10,* 104–116.

Bell, E.F., Warburton, D., Stonestreet, B.S., & Oh, W. (1980). Effect of fluid administration on the development of symptomatic patent ductus arteriosus and congestive heart failure in premature infants. *New England Journal of Medicine, 302,* 598–604.

Costarino, A. & Baumgart, S. (1986). Modern fluid and electrolyte management of the critically ill premature infant. *Pediatric Clinics of North America, 33,* 153–158.

DeMarini, S., Tsang, R.C., & Rath, L.L. (1993). Fluids, electrolytes, vitamins, and trace minerals: Basis of ingestion, digestion, elimination, and metabolism (pp. 393–413). In C. Kenner, A. Brueggemeyer, & L.P. Gunderson (eds.), *Comprehensive neonatal nursing: A physiologic perspective.* Philadelphia: W.B. Saunders.

Papile, L., Burstein, J., Burstein, R., Koffler, H., & Koops, B. (1978). Relationship of intravenous sodium bicarbonate infusions and cerebral intraventricular hemorrhage. *Journal of Pediatrics, 93,* 834–836.

Spahr, R.C., Klein, A.M., Brown, D.R., Holzman, I.R., & MacDonald, H.M. (1980). Fluid administration and bronchopulmonary dysplasia. *American Journal of Diseases of Childhood, 134,* 958–960.

127. Answer: (**B**) HLHS, TOF, and TGA do usually present with cyanosis; however other defects also can present with cyanosis. ASD, VSD, and ECD generally do not produce cyanosis. TAPVR, TA, PS, and COA must also be considered, as well as multiple cardiac anomalies. TAPVR and TA are cyanotic heart defects.

REFERENCES

Lott, J.W. (1993). Assessment and management of cardiovascular dysfunction (pp. 355–391). In C. Kenner, A. Brueggemeyer, & L.P. Gunderson (eds.), *Comprehensive neonatal nursing: A physiologic perspective.* Philadelphia: W.B. Saunders.

Park, M.K. (1984). Cyanotic congenital heart defects (pp. 157–196). *Pediatric cardiology for practitioners.* Chicago: Year Book Medical Publishers.

128. Answer: *Improvement of oxygenation* is the most critical need. Endotracheal intubation and mechanical ventilation should be performed immediately. *Correction of acidosis* is also critical. Administration of bicarbonate in conjunction with mechanical ventilation should be performed. *Correction of hypoglycemia* through parenteral glucose administration is required. *Correction of hypocalcemia* through addition of calcium to parenteral fluids is required. A rapid assessment of whether the heart defect is one that is ductal-dependent is crucial. *If the CHD is ductal-dependent, then administration of* PGE_1 *is critical.* Ordering *further evaluation* tests as needed should be done stat.

REFERENCES

Castaneda, A.R. & Stark, J. (1990). Neonatal repair of transposition of the great arteries (pp. 789–795). In W.A. Long (ed.), *Fetal and neonatal cardiology.* Philadelphia: W.B. Saunders.

Lott, J.W. (1993). Assessment and management of cardiovascular dysfunction (pp. 355–391). In C. Kenner, A. Brueggemeyer, & L.P. Gunderson (eds.), *Comprehensive neonatal nursing: A physiologic perspective.* Philadelphia: W.B. Saunders.

Norwood, W.I., Lang, P., & Hansen, D.D. (1983). Physiologic repair of aortic atresia—Hypoplastic left heart syndrome. *New England Journal of Medicine, 308,* 23–26.

Park, M.K. (1984). Cyanotic congenital heart defects (pp. 157–196). *Pediatric cardiology for practitioners.* Chicago: Year Book Medical Publishers.

Paul, M.H. (1989). Complete transposition of the great arteries (pp. 371–423). In F.H. Adams, G.C. Emmanouilides, & T.A. Riemenschneider (eds.), *Heart disease in infants, children, and adolescents.* Baltimore: Williams & Wilkins.

129. Answer: (**C**) The aorta normally arises from the left ventricle, and the pulmonary artery arises from the right ventricle. Thus, this represents D-TGA with an associated VSD and PDA. The VSD allows mixing of deoxygenated and oxygenated blood at the ventricular level. The small PDA indicates that little mixing of blood is occurring at the ductal level. TOF consists of large VSD, pulmonic stenosis, over-riding aorta, and right ventricu-

lar hypertrophy. HLHS consists of a small aorta, aortic and mitral valve stenosis or atresia, and a small left atrium and ventricle.

REFERENCES

Castaneda, A.R. & Stark, J. (1990). Neonatal repair of transposition of the great arteries (pp. 789–795). In W.A. Long (ed.), *Fetal and neonatal cardiology*. Philadelphia: W.B. Saunders.

Lott, J.W. (1993). Assessment and management of cardiovascular dysfunction (pp. 355–391). In C. Kenner, A. Brueggemeyer, & L.P. Gunderson (eds.), *Comprehensive neonatal nursing: A physiologic perspective*. Philadelphia: W.B. Saunders.

Norwood, W.I., Lang, P., & Hansen, D.D. (1983). Physiologic repair of aortic atresia—Hypoplastic left heart syndrome. *New England Journal of Medicine, 308*, 23–26.

Park, M.K. (1984). Cyanotic congenital heart defects (pp. 157–196). *Pediatric cardiology for practitioners*. Chicago: Year Book Medical Publishers.

Paul, M.H. (1989). Complete transposition of the great arteries (pp. 371–423). In F.H. Adams, G.C. Emmanouilides, & T.A. Riemenschneider (eds.), *Heart disease in infants, children, and adolescents*. Baltimore: Williams & Wilkins.

130. Answer: (**A**) The most common adverse effect to PGE_1 infusion is apnea. Ventilatory status must be monitored during the initial phases of PGE_1 administration. Because the infant is already being mechanically ventilated, this is not a major problem. Other effects include flush, fever, hypotension, decreased heart rate, and seizure-like activity. The other symptoms occur less frequently but require careful monitoring.

REFERENCES

Kirklin, J.W., Colvin, E.V., McConnell, M.E., & Bargeron, L.M. (1990). Complete transposition of the great arteries. Treatment in the current era. *Pediatric Clinics of North America, 37*, 171–178.

Lott, J.W. (1993). Assessment and management of cardiovascular dysfunction (pp. 355–391). In C. Kenner, A. Brueggemeyer, & L.P. Gunderson (eds.), *Comprehensive neonatal nursing: A physiologic perspective*. Philadelphia: W.B. Saunders.

Park, M.K. (1984). Cardiac problems of the newborn (pp. 292–306). *Pediatric cardiology for practitioners*. Chicago: Year Book Medical Publishers.

Paul, M.H. (1989). Complete transposition of the great arteries (pp. 371–423). In F.H. Adams, G.C. Emmanouilides, & T.A. Riemenschneider (eds.), *Heart disease in infants, children, and adolescents*. Baltimore: Williams & Wilkins.

131. Answer: (**B**) The balloon atrial septostomy can be performed during cardiac catheterization to improve mixing of blood. Blalock-Hanlon procedure is the surgical creation of an ASD. It is rarely used except in presence of complex TGA or mitral valve atresia and single ventricle. It requires cardiopulmonary bypass. The Mustard procedure is a surgical procedure in which pericardial or synthetic baffle is placed in the atria to shunt blood in appropriate direction. (Venous blood: Right atrium–left ventricle–pulmonary artery; Systemic blood: Left atrium–right ventricle–aorta.) The Mustard procedure also requires cardiopulmonary bypass.

REFERENCES

Kirklin, J.W., Colvin, E.V., McConnell, M.E., & Bargeron, L.M. (1990). Complete transposition of the great arteries: Treatment in the current era. *Pediatric Clinics of North America, 37*, 171–178.

Lott, J.W. (1993). Assessment and management of cardiovascular dysfunction (pp. 355–391). In C. Kenner, A. Brueggemeyer, & L.P. Gunderson (eds.), *Comprehensive neonatal nursing: A physiologic perspective*. Philadelphia: W.B. Saunders.

Park, M.K. (1984). Cyanotic congenital heart defects (pp. 157–196). *Pediatric cardiology for practitioners*. Chicago: Year Book Medical Publishers.

Paul, M.H. (1989). Complete transposition of the great arteries (pp. 371–423). In F.H. Adams, G.C. Emmanouilides, & T.A. Riemenschneider (eds.), *Heart disease in infants, children, and adolescents*. Baltimore: Williams & Wilkins.

132. Answer: (**B**) The Jatene procedure involves switching at the artery level. Jatene's procedure is newer and seems to have fewer postoperative complications. Rastelli's procedure switches the circulations at the ventricular level. Senning's or Mustard's procedure involves switching at the atrial level.

REFERENCES

Kirklin, J.W., Colvin, E.V., McConnell, M.E., & Bargeron, L.M. (1990). Complete transposition of the great arteries: Treatment in the current era. *Pediatric Clinics of North America, 37*, 171–178.

Lott, J.W. (1993). Assessment and management of cardiovascular dysfunction (pp. 355–391). In C. Kenner, A. Brueggemeyer, & L.P. Gunderson (eds.), *Comprehensive neonatal nursing: A physiologic perspective*. Philadelphia: W.B. Saunders.

Park, M.K. (1984). Cyanotic congenital heart defects (pp. 157–196). *Pediatric cardiology for practitioners*. Chicago: Year Book Medical Publishers.

Paul, M.H. (1989). Complete transposition of the great arteries (pp. 371–423). In F.H. Adams, G.C. Emmanouilides, & T.A. Riemenschneider (eds.), *Heart disease in infants, children, and adolescents*. Baltimore: Williams & Wilkins.

133. Answer: (**A**) The risk of pneumothorax is high, and the symmetry of breath sounds must be verified regularly. The patient receiving nasal CPAP must be kept calm, as a crying infant loses airway pressure when the mouth is open. The intubated infant must be monitored for appropriate endotracheal tube position and patency. Suctioning of the airway should be done carefully. The suction catheter should be passed only as far as the end of the endotracheal tube, as overzealous suctioning can denude the tracheal endothelium. Lung volume can be lost during prolonged disconnection from the ventilator. Any sudden decompensation should alert the nurse to investigate for ventilator failure, pneumothorax, or tracheal tube plugging. These infants often have invasive catheters, and the nurse should be adept at their care.

A too-frequent complication of RDS in the tiny premature infant is chronic lung disease, or bronchopulmonary dysplasia (BPD). BPD is variously defined by authors in the field, but the definition always includes bronchiolar metaplasia, emphysema and interstitial edema. A working definition includes those infants who continue to require oxygen supplementation at 28 days of age.

REFERENCES

Bancalari, E. (1985). Bronchopulmonary dysplasia. In A.D. Milder & R.J. Martin (eds.), *Neonatal and pediatric respiratory medicine*. London: Butterworths.

Haywood, J.L., Coghill III, C.H., Carlo, W.A., & Ross, M. (1993). Assessment and management of respiratory dysfunction (pp. 294–312). In C. Kenner, A. Brueggemeyer, & L.P. Gunderson (eds.), *Comprehensive neonatal nursing: A physiologic perspective*. Philadelphia: W.B. Saunders.

134. Answer: (**B**) The osmolality of intracellular and extracellular spaces is therefore equal, although the composition of ICW and ECW is different.

REFERENCES

Costarino, A.T. & Baumgart, S. (1988). Controversies in fluid and electrolyte therapy for the premature infant. *Clinics in Perinatology, 15,* 863–878.

DeMarini, S., Tsang, R.C., & Rath, L.L. (1993). Fluids, electrolytes, vitamins, and trace minerals: Basis of ingestion, digestion, elimination, and metabolism (pp. 393–413). In C. Kenner, A. Brueggemeyer, & L.P. Gunderson (eds.), *Comprehensive neonatal nursing: A physiologic perspective*. Philadelphia: W.B. Saunders.

135. Answer: (**B**) If there are any abnormalities associated with the neonate, they should be pointed out to the parents, because the defects are usually not as severe as the parents had imagined them to be during pregnancy or at the time of delivery. Positive features also can be pointed out at this time to encourage the parents to look at the whole infant as opposed to only the defects.

REFERENCES

Croop, L.H. & Acree, C.M. (1993). Neonatal transport (pp. 1182–1212). In C. Kenner, A. Brueggemeyer, & L.P. Gunderson (eds.), *Comprehensive neonatal care: A physiologic perspective*. Philadelphia: W.B. Saunders.

Kenner, C. & Gunderson, L.P. (1988). Parent care: Anticipatory guidance for the neonate and family. In C. Kenner, J. Harjo, & A. Brueggemeyer (eds.), *Neonatal surgery: A nursing perspective*. Orlando: Grune & Stratton.

136. Answer: (**C**) Cocci in chains is usually *Streptococcus*.

REFERENCES

Lott, J.W. & Kilb, J.R. (1992). Selection of antimicrobial agents for treatment of neonatal sepsis: Which drug kills which bug. *Neonatal Pharmacology, 1*(1), 19–29, 1992.

Sweet, A.Y. (1991). Bacterial infections (pp. 84–167). In A.Y. Sweet & E.G. Brown (eds.), *Fetal and neonatal effects of maternal disease*. St. Louis: Mosby-Year Book.

137. Answer: (**C**) A combination of ampicillin and gentamicin will provide adequate coverage for most gram-positive and gram-negative organisms. Ampicillin and gentamicin provide antibacterial coverage against *Streptococci, Listeria monocytogenes,* and gram-negative enteric rods.

REFERENCES

Lott, J.W. & Kilb, J.R. (1992). Selection of antimicrobial agents for treatment of neonatal sepsis: Which drug kills which bug. *Neonatal Pharmacology, 1*(1), 19–29, 1992.

Lott, J.W., Nelson, K., Fahrner, R., & Kenner, C. (1993). Assessment and management of immunologic dysfunction (pp. 553–581). In C. Kenner, A. Brueggemeyer, & L.P. Gunderson (eds.), *Comprehensive neonatal nursing: A physiologic perspective*. Philadelphia: W.B. Saunders.

Sweet, A.Y. (1991). Bacterial infections (pp. 84–167). In A.Y. Sweet & E.G. Brown (eds.), *Fetal and neonatal effects of maternal disease*. St. Louis: Mosby-Year Book.

138. Answer: (**B**) Microorganisms that are coagulase positive and are cocci found

in clusters are usually *Staphylococcus*. In this case, *Staphylococcus aureus*.

REFERENCES

Lott, J.W. & Kilb, J.R. (1992). Selection of antimicrobial agents for treatment of neonatal sepsis: Which drug kills which bug. *Neonatal Pharmacology, 1*(1), 19–29, 1992.

Lott, J.W., Nelson, K., Fahrner, R., & Kenner, C. (1993). Assessment and management of immunologic dysfunction (pp. 553–581). In C. Kenner, A. Brueggemeyer, & L.P. Gunderson (eds.), *Comprehensive neonatal nursing: A physiologic perspective*. Philadelphia: W.B. Saunders.

Sweet, A.Y. (1991). Bacterial infections (pp. 84–167). In A.Y. Sweet & E.G. Brown (eds.), *Fetal and neonatal effects of maternal disease*. St. Louis: Mosby-Year Book.

139. Answer: (**B**) Nafcillin is very effective against gram-positive microorganisms, especially *Staphylococcus aureus*. Gentamicin can be used in conjunction with Nafcillin to provide broad-spectrum coverage.

REFERENCES

Lott, J.W. & Kilb, J.R. (1992). Selection of antimicrobial agents for treatment of neonatal sepsis: Which drug kills which bug. *Neonatal Pharmacology, 1*(1), 19–29, 1992.

Lott, J.W., Nelson, K., Fahrner, R., & Kenner, C. (1993). Assessment and management of immunologic dysfunction (pp. 553–581). In C. Kenner, A. Brueggemeyer, & L.P. Gunderson (eds.), *Comprehensive neonatal nursing: A physiologic perspective*. Philadelphia: W.B. Saunders.

Sweet, A.Y. (1991). Bacterial infections (pp. 84–167). In A.Y. Sweet & E.G. Brown (eds.), *Fetal and neonatal effects of maternal disease*. St. Louis: Mosby-Year Book.

140. Answer: (**A**) According to the classic definition of maintenance fluids, 100 ml of water is needed for each 100 kcal of energy expended.

REFERENCES

Costarino, A.T. & Baumgart, S. (1988). Controversies in fluid and electrolyte therapy for the premature infant. *Clinics in Perinatology, 15*, 863–878.

DeMarini, S., Tsang, R.C., & Rath, L.L. (1993). Fluids, electrolytes, vitamins, and trace minerals: Basis of ingestion, digestion, elimination, and metabolism (pp. 393–413). In C. Kenner, A. Brueggemeyer, & L.P. Gunderson (eds.), *Comprehensive neonatal nursing: A physiologic perspective*. Philadelphia: W.B. Saunders.

Winters, R.W. (1973). Maintenance fluid therapy. In *The body fluids in pediatrics* (pp. 113–133). Boston: Little, Brown.

141. Answer: (**B**) During the last three months of gestation, the bone marrow is the chief source of blood cell production, with extramedullary sources of hematopoiesis generally ceasing by the first postnatal month.

REFERENCES

Oski, F. & Naiman, J. (1982c). Normal blood values in the newborn period (pp. 1–31). In F. Oski & J. Naiman (eds.), *Hematologic problems in the newborn. Vol IV. Major problems in clinical pediatrics* (3rd ed.). Philadelphia: W.B. Saunders.

Shaw, N. (1993). Assessment and management of hematologic dysfunction (pp. 582–634). In C. Kenner, A. Brueggemeyer, & L.P. Gunderson (eds.), *Comprehensive neonatal nursing: A physiologic perspective*. Philadelphia: W.B. Saunders.

142. Answer: (**A**) Transcutaneous Po_2 ($TcPo_2$) is measured, indirectly, by an electrode applied to the warmed skin under the electrode. Therefore, it depends on local skin perfusion. The reading can become unreliable as the hyperthermic skin changes. Therefore, the electrode site should be changed every four hours. A review of the maternal/perinatal history and a complete physical examination, combined with a limited laboratory and radiologic evaluation, will lead to a timely diagnosis in most circumstances.

REFERENCES

Haywood, J.L., Coghill III, C.H., Carlo, W.A., & Ross, M. (1993). Assessment and management of respiratory dysfunction (pp. 294–312). In C. Kenner, A. Brueggemeyer, & L.P. Gunderson (eds.), *Comprehensive neonatal nursing: A physiologic perspective*. Philadelphia: W.B. Saunders.

Pollitzer, M.J., Whitehead, M.D., Reynolds, E.O.R., et al. (1980). Effect of electrode temperature and in vivo calibration on accuracy of transcutaneous estimation of arterial oxygen tension in infants. *Pediatrics, 65*, 515.

143. Answer: (**B**) Because immature RBC still maintain their nuclei and are relatively high in number during the newborn period for the first four days of life, they can be incorrectly counted in the total WBC count.

REFERENCES

Polin, R.A. & Fox, W.W. (1992). *Fetal and neonatal physiology* (pp. 1339–1342). Philadelphia: W.B. Saunders.

Shaw, N. (1993). Assessment and management of hematologic dysfunction (pp. 582–634). In C. Kenner, A. Brueggemeyer, & L.P. Gunderson (eds.), *Comprehensive neonatal nursing: A physiologic perspective*. Philadelphia: W.B. Saunders.

144. Answer: (**B**) Apnea is a problem associated with temperature changes, especially in the premature infant. Sudden or dramatic infant temperature

changes can lead to apnea. Overheating can be a cause of an increase in apneic spells in premature infants. Special attention must be paid to the infant during rewarming to prevent complications from rapid temperature changes. Sudden increases in ambient temperature also can lead to an increase in apnea spells, as well as rapid rewarming of the cold-stressed infant.

Overheating can often be differentiated from febrile episodes by determining the differences in core or rectal temperature from the skin temperatures of the central body and distal extremities. When core temperatures are elevated in febrile conditions, the skin temperature of the distal extremities remains cool in comparison to the skin temperature of the trunk. This difference also can be evident in very low birth weight infants if thermoregulation has not been satisfactorily achieved. Overheating can lead to various responses in the infant. Infants tend to be less active as the environmental temperature increases.

REFERENCES

Brueggemeyer, A. (1993). Neonatal thermoregulation (pp. 247–262). In C. Kenner, A. Brueggemeyer, & L.P. Gunderson (eds.), *Comprehensive neonatal nursing: A physiologic perspective.* Philadelphia: W.B. Saunders.

Fanaroff, A.A. & Martin, R.J. (1992). *Neonatal-perinatal medicine: Diseases of the fetus and newborn* (5th ed.). St. Louis: C.V. Mosby.

Harpin, V.A., Chellappah, G., & Nutter, N. (1983). Responses of the newborn infant to overheating. *Biology of the Neonate, 44,* 65–75.

Perlstein, P.H., Edwards, N.K., & Sutherland, J.M. (1970). Apnea in premature infants and incubator-air-temperature changes. *New England Journal of Medicine, 282*(9), 461–466.

145. Answer: (**C**) Sodium is absorbed in both the small intestine and the colon, the largest amount being absorbed in the jejunum.

REFERENCES

Bell, E.F., Warburton, D., Stonestreet, B.S., & Oh, W. (1980). Effect of fluid administration on the development of symptomatic patent ductus arteriosus and congestive heart failure in premature infants. *New England Journal of Medicine, 302,* 598–604.

DeMarini, S., Tsang, R.C., & Rath, L.L. (1993). Fluids, electrolytes, vitamins, and trace minerals: Basis of ingestion, digestion, elimination, and metabolism (pp. 393–413). In C. Kenner, A. Brueggemeyer, & L.P. Gunderson (eds.), *Comprehensive neonatal nursing: A physiologic perspective.* Philadelphia: W.B. Saunders.

Spitzer, A. (1982). The role of the kidney in sodium homeostasis during maturation. *Kidney International, 21,* 539–545.

Turnberg, L.A. (1971a). Abnormalities in intestinal electrolyte transport in congenital chloridorrhea. *Gut, 12,* 544–551.

Turnberg, L.A. (1971b). Potassium transport in the human small bowel. *Gut, 12,* 811–818.

Turnberg, L.A., Bieberdort, F.A., Mordowsky, S.G., & Gordtran, J.S. (1970). Interrelations of chloride, bicarbonate, sodium and hydrogen transport in human ileum. *Journal of Clinical Investigation, 49,* 557–567.

146. Answer: (**B**) The perinatal caregiver's first line of defense for the prevention or treatment of hypoxemia is to provide an increased inspired oxygen concentration. For the hypoxemic newborn, the response to an increased inspired oxygen concentration depends on the etiology of the hypoxemia. A second mainstay of current management of the newborn at risk for hypoxemia is the maintenance of an adequate oxygen-carrying capacity by intermittent blood transfusion.

REFERENCES

Carlo, W.A. & Chatburn, R.L. (1988). *Neonatal respiratory care.* Chicago: Year Book Medical Publishers.

Donovan, E.F. & Spangler, L.L. (1993). New technologies applied to the management of respiratory dysfunction. In C. Kenner, A. Brueggemeyer, & L.P. Gunderson (eds.), *Comprehensive neonatal nursing: A physiologic perspective.* Philadelphia: W.B. Saunders.

Merenstein, G.B. & Gardner, S.L. (1989). *Handbook of neonatal intensive care.* St. Louis: C.V. Mosby.

147. Answer: (**A**) Stridor is common in neonates with upper airway and laryngeal lesions. Inspiratory stridor occurs most frequently with upper airway and laryngeal lesions, whereas expiratory stridor commonly accompanies lower airway disorders. Hoarseness is a common sign of laryngeal involvement, whereas expiratory wheezes suggest a lower airway disease.

Pallor and poor perfusion can indicate anemia, hypotension, and/or hypovolemia. Polycythemia with plethora also can cause respiratory distress. Cardiovascular signs of congestive failure (e.g., hyperactive precordium, tachycardia, hepatomegaly), poor cardiac output, pathologic murmurs, decreased femoral pulses, and nonsinus rhythm suggest a primary cardiac etiology for the respiratory distress.

Methemoglobinemia also can cause

respiratory distress in the neonate. Radiographic examination is often the most useful part of the laboratory evaluation and serves to narrow the differential diagnosis. An anteroposterior view is usually sufficient, but lateral chest radiograph can be useful if fluid, masses, or free air are present. Considerable skill is required in sampling both venous and arterial blood from small patients who are at substantial risk for iatrogenic anemia and vascular damage.

REFERENCES

Avery, M.E., Fletcher, B.D., & Williams, R.G. (1981). *The lung and its disorders in the newborn infant* (4th ed.). Philadelphia: W.B. Saunders.

Haywood, J.L., Coghill III, C.H., Carlo, W.A., & Ross, M. (1993). Assessment and management of respiratory dysfunction (pp. 294–312). In C. Kenner, A. Brueggemeyer, & L.P. Gunderson (eds.), *Comprehensive neonatal nursing: A physiologic perspective.* Philadelphia: W.B. Saunders.

148. Answer: (**A**) Decreased cardiac output stimulates the sympathetic nervous system causing tachycardia, increased contractility, increased vasomotor tone, peripheral vasoconstriction, and diaphoresis. Decreased renal perfusion stimulates the renin-angiotensin/aldosterone mechanism to cause water and sodium retention. Pulmonary venous engorgement results in decreased tidal volume, decreased lung compliance, early closure of small airways with air trapping, and increased work of breathing with signs/symptoms of increased respiratory effort, grunting, and rales/rhonchi.

REFERENCES

Bull, C. (1990). Total anomalous pulmonary venous drainage (pp. 439–451). In W.A. Long (ed.), *Fetal and neonatal cardiology.* Philadelphia: W.B. Saunders.

Lott, J.W. (1993). Assessment and management of cardiovascular dysfunction (pp. 355–391). In C. Kenner, A. Brueggemeyer, & L.P. Gunderson (eds.), *Comprehensive neonatal nursing: A physiologic perspective.* Philadelphia: W.B. Saunders.

Lucas, R.V. & Krabill, K.A. (1990). Anomalous venous connections, pulmonary and systemic. *Pediatric Clinics of North America, 37,* 580–616.

149. Answer: (**C**) Caput succedaneum, subcutaneous edema of the soft tissues of the scalp, extending across suture lines, is caused by pressure on the head during labor and delivery in the vertex presentation. Similarly, edema or bruising can be noted in other areas such as the buttocks or extremities in the case of abnormal presentations. Caput is evident at birth and is gradually reabsorbed and disappears within a few days. Cephalohematoma, a collection of blood from ruptured blood vessels that forms between the skull and the periosteum, also can be caused by trauma to the head during the birth process. The hematoma does not cross suture lines. The cephalohematoma increases in size within 24 to 48 hours and may not be obvious at the time of birth.

REFERENCES

Battaglia, F.C., & Lubchenco, L.O. (1967). A practical classification of newborn infants by weight and gestational age. *Journal of Pediatrics, 71*(2), 159–163.

Endo, A.S. & Nishioka, E. (1993). Neonatal assessment (pp. 265–293). In C. Kenner, A. Brueggemeyer, & L.P. Gunderson (eds.), *Comprehensive neonatal nursing: A physiologic perspective.* Philadelphia: W.B. Saunders.

Petrucha, R. (1989). Fetal maturity/gestational age evaluation. *Journal of Perinatology, 9*(1), 100–101.

150. Answer: (**C**) The main factors involved in the regulation of sodium reabsorption are the oncotic and hydrostatic pressure in the peritubular capillaries and the action of the hormone aldosterone, which increases the absorption of sodium in exchange with potassium or hydrogen. Although it does not affect sodium excretion directly, antidiuretic hormone can influence serum sodium concentration indirectly because it regulates the excretion or the reabsorption of free water.

REFERENCES

Bell, E.F., Warburton, D., Stonestreet, B.S., & Oh, W. (1980). Effect of fluid administration on the development of symptomatic patent ductus arteriosus and congestive heart failure in premature infants. *New England Journal of Medicine, 302,* 598–604.

DeMarini, S., Tsang, R.C., & Rath, L.L. (1993). Fluids, electrolytes, vitamins, and trace minerals: Basis of ingestion, digestion, elimination, and metabolism (pp. 393–413). In C. Kenner, A. Brueggemeyer, & L.P. Gunderson (eds.), *Comprehensive neonatal nursing: A physiologic perspective.* Philadelphia: W.B. Saunders.

Spitzer, A. (1982). The role of the kidney in sodium homeostasis during maturation. *Kidney International, 21,* 539–545.

Turnberg, L.A. (1971a). Abnormalities in intestinal electrolyte transport in congenital chloridorrhea. *Gut, 12,* 544–551.

Turnberg, L.A. (1971b). Potassium transport in the human small bowel. *Gut, 12,* 811–818.
Turnberg, L.A., Bieberdort, F.A., Mordowsky, S.G., & Gordtran, J.S. (1970). Interrelations of chloride, bicarbonate, sodium and hydrogen transport in human ileum. *Journal of Clinical Investigation, 49,* 557–567.
Weinberg, J., Weitzman, R., Zakauddin, S., & Leake, R. (1977). Inappropriate secretion of antidiuretic hormone in a premature infant. *Journal of Pediatrics, 90,* 111–114.

151. Answer: **(C)** The most effective drug for treatment of *C. albicans* is amphotericin B.

REFERENCES

Lott, J.W., Nelson, K., Fahrner, R., & Kenner, C. (1993). Assessment and management of immunologic dysfunction (pp. 553–581). In C. Kenner, A. Brueggemeyer, & L.P. Gunderson (eds.), *Comprehensive neonatal nursing: A physiologic perspective.* Philadelphia: W.B. Saunders.
Sweet, A.Y. (1991). Fungal infections (pp. 170–182). In A.Y. Sweet & E.G. Brown (eds.), *Fetal and neonatal effects of maternal disease.* St. Louis: Mosby-Year Book.
Xanthou, M. (1987). Neonatal immunity. In L. Stern & P. Vert (eds.), *Neonatal medicine* (pp. 555–586). New York: Masson Publishing.

152. Answer: **(B)** Dopamine has both direct and indirect β-adrenergic effects that are dose-dependent. Low doses (2–5 mcg/kg/min) have increased renal blood flow but have minimal effect on heart rate, blood pressure, or contractility. Moderate doses (5–10 mcg/kg/min) increase renal blood flow, heart rate, blood pressure, and contractility. High doses (10–20 mcg/kg/min) cause alpha effects, resulting in peripheral vasoconstriction, increased rate, and contractility. Dobutamine has decreased effects on the heart rate and causes less peripheral vasoconstriction. Isoproterenol has β-1 and β-2 adrenergic effects. Its usefulness in the neonate is limited because it causes increased heart rate, arrhythmias, and decreased systemic vascular resistance, making hypotension worse.

REFERENCES

Hazinski, M.F. (1983). Congenital heart disease in the neonate (Part III): Congestive heart failure. *Neonatal Network, 1*(6), 8–17.
Lott, J.W. (1993). Assessment and management of cardiovascular dysfunction (pp. 355–391). In C. Kenner, A. Brueggemeyer, & L.P. Gunderson (eds.), *Comprehensive neonatal nursing: A physiologic perspective.* Philadelphia: W.B. Saunders.
Talner, N.S. (1989). Heart failure (pp. 890–911). In F.H. Adams, G.C. Emmanouilides, & T.A. Riemenschneider (eds.), *Heart disease in infants, children, and adolescents.* Baltimore: Williams & Wilkins.

153. Answer: **(C)** Magnesium is absorbed by passive diffusion throughout the small intestine. Absorption is related to intake, and approximately 50–70 percent of the dietary magnesium is absorbed. It is involved in energy production, cell membrane function, mitochondrial function, and protein synthesis.

REFERENCES

DeMarini, S., Tsang, R.C., & Rath, L.L. (1993). Fluids, electrolytes, vitamins, and trace minerals: Basis of ingestion, digestion, elimination, and metabolism (pp. 393–413). In C. Kenner, A. Brueggemeyer, & L.P. Gunderson (eds.), *Comprehensive neonatal nursing: A physiologic perspective.* Philadelphia: W.B. Saunders.
Moya, M. & Domenech, E. (1982). Role of calcium phosphate ratio of milk formulae on calcium balance in low birth weight infants during the first three days of life. *Pediatric Research, 16,* 675–681.
Okamoto, E., Muttart, C., Zucker, C., & Heird, W. (1982). Use of medium-chain triglycerides in feeding the low birthweight infant. *American Journal of Disease of Childhood, 136,* 428–431.

154. Answer: **(C)** The American Academy of Pediatrics recommends that under all but emergency circumstances, surfactant only be administered in nurseries able to sustain long-term mechanical ventilation. Exogenous surfactant is probably used in all tertiary NICUs in the U.S.

REFERENCES

Donovan, E.F. & Spangler, L.L. (1993). New technologies applied to the management of respiratory dysfunction. In C. Kenner, A. Brueggemeyer, & L.P. Gunderson (eds.), *Comprehensive neonatal nursing: A physiologic perspective.* Philadelphia: W.B. Saunders.
Merenstein, G.B. & Gardner, S.L. (1989). *Handbook of neonatal intensive care.* St. Louis: C.V. Mosby.

155. Answer: **(A)** Hypermagnesemia does not cause hypocalcemia in the neonatal period and appears to be associated only with hypotonia.

REFERENCES

DeMarini, S., Tsang, R.C., & Rath, L.L. (1993). Fluids, electrolytes, vitamins, and trace minerals: Basis of ingestion, digestion, elimination, and metabolism (pp. 393–413). In C. Kenner, A. Brueggemeyer, & L.P. Gunderson (eds.), *Comprehensive neonatal nursing: A physiologic perspective.* Philadelphia: W.B. Saunders.
Paunier, L., Ingeborg, C.R., Kooh, S.Y., Cohen, P.E., & Fraser, D. (1968). Primary hypomagnesemia with

secondary hypocalcemia in an infant. *Pediatrics, 41,* 385–402.

156. Answer: (**C**) In hypoplastic left heart syndrome, the only cardiac output occurs with a PDA in which blood is shunted from the pulmonary artery into the aorta. When the PDA begins to close, HLHS leads to decreased systemic circulation, cardiac output, and aortic pressure with metabolic acidosis and shock. HLHS complications are the leading cause of death from CHDs in the first month of life. Although infants with congenital heart defects are at increased risk for development of subacute bacterial endocarditis secondary to turbulent blood flow, it is not the leading cause of death in the neonatal period. Congestive heart failure is a frequent complication of congenital heart defects, but in many cases it can be managed medically or surgically except in severe defects.

REFERENCES

Bull, C. (1990). Total anomalous pulmonary venous drainage (pp. 439–451). In W.A. Long (ed.), *Fetal and neonatal cardiology.* Philadelphia: W.B. Saunders.

Lott, J.W. (1993). Assessment and management of cardiovascular dysfunction (pp. 355–391). In C. Kenner, A. Brueggemeyer, & L.P. Gunderson (eds.), *Comprehensive neonatal nursing: A physiologic perspective.* Philadelphia: W.B. Saunders.

Lucas, R.V. & Krabill, K.A. (1990). Anomalous venous connections, pulmonary and systemic. *Pediatric Clinics of North America, 37,* 580–616.

157. Answer: (**B**) Phosphorus is absorbed mainly in the jejunum by both active and passive diffusion. Absorption depends mainly on the absolute amount of P in the diet, on the relative concentrations of calcium and phosphorus (an excessive amount of either one can reduce the absorption of the other), and on the presence of substances that bind to phosphorus and make it unavailable for absorption (phytates in soy-based formulas).

REFERENCES

DeMarini, S., Tsang, R.C., & Rath, L.L. (1993). Fluids, electrolytes, vitamins, and trace minerals: Basis of ingestion, digestion, elimination, and metabolism (pp. 393–413). In C. Kenner, A. Brueggemeyer, & L.P. Gunderson (eds.), *Comprehensive neonatal nursing: A physiologic perspective.* Philadelphia: W.B. Saunders.

Greer, F.R. & Tsang, R.C. (1985). Calcium, phosphorus, magnesium and vitamin D requirements for the preterm infant (pp. 99–136). In R.C. Tsang (ed.), *Vitamin and mineral requirements in preterm infants.* New York: Marcel Dekker.

Koo, W.W.K. & Tsang, R.C. (1988). Calcium, magnesium and phosphorus (pp. 175–189). In R.C. Tsang & B.L. Nichols (eds.), *Nutrition during infancy.* St. Louis: C.V. Mosby.

158. Answer: (**A**) Hypocalcemia develops within the first three days of life and is seen primarily in the infant of the insulin-dependent diabetic mother. It is thought that hypocalcemia may be secondary to decreased hypoparathyroid functioning resulting from hypomagnesemia.

REFERENCES

Cowett, R.M. & Schwartz, R. (1982). The infant of the diabetic mother. *Pediatric Clinics of North America, 29,* 1213–1231.

Gamblien, V., Bivens, K., Burton, K.S., Kissler, C.H., Kleeman, T.A., Freije, M. & Prows, C. (1993). Assessment and management of endocrine dysfunction (pp. 527–552). In C. Kenner, A. Brueggemeyer, & L.P. Gunderson (eds.), *Comprehensive neonatal nursing: A physiologic perspective.* Philadelphia: W.B. Saunders.

Goetzman, B.W. & Wenneberg, R.P. (1991). *Neonatal intensive care handbook* (2nd ed.). St. Louis: Mosby-Year Book.

Perlman, R.H. (1983). The infant of the diabetic mother. *Primary Care, 10,* 751–760.

159. Answer: (**B**) The embryonic component of lung development is marked by sequential branching of the lung bud that appears at about four weeks and is complete by the sixth week. The next 10 weeks are marked by the formation of conducting airways by branching of the aforementioned lung buds. This phase, the pseudoglandular phase, continues through week 16, and ends with completion of the conducting airways. The canalicular phase follows through week 28, when gas exchange units, known as acini, develop. Type II alveolar cells, the surfactant producing cells, begin to form during the latter part of this phase. Mature, vascularized gas-exchange sites form during the saccular phase that spans the 29th through the 35th weeks. During this phase, the interstitial space between alveoli thins, tightly opposing the alveolar wall with the developing capillaries. The alveolar development phase, marked by expansion of gas-exchange surface area, arbitrarily begins at 36 weeks

and extends into the distant postnatal period. The alveolar wall and interstitial spaces become very thin, and the single capillary network comes into closest proximity with the alveolar membrane. There are no firm boundaries separating these phases.

REFERENCES

Haywood, J.L., Coghill III, C.H., Carlo, W.A., & Ross, M. (1993). Assessment and management of respiratory dysfunction (pp. 294–312). In C. Kenner, A. Brueggemeyer, & L.P. Gunderson (eds.), *Comprehensive neonatal nursing: A physiologic perspective.* Philadelphia: W.B. Saunders.

Thibeault, D.W. & Gregory, G.A. (1986). *Neonatal pulmonary care* (2nd ed.). Norwalk, CT: Appleton-Century-Crofts.

160. Answer: (**C**) In infancy, hypophosphatemias can occur in various forms. The first type is vitamin D-resistant rickets, caused by a deficient activity of renal-α-hydroxylase, a major enzyme that converts 25-hydroxyvitamin D to the active hormone 1,25-dihydroxyvitamin D. Low concentrations of serum 1,25-dihydroxyvitamin D result in decreased intestinal calcium absorption, with secondary hyperparathyroidism and hypophosphatemia. Treatment is with 1,25-dihydroxyvitamin D at physiologic doses. The second type is X-linked hypophosphatemia, in which the primary disorder is a phosphate "leak" in the kidney and an impaired intestinal absorption of phosphorus. Treatment includes phosphate salts and large doses of vitamin D or near physiologic doses of 1,25-dihydroxy-vitamin D. The third type is represented by several disorders of renal tubular reabsorption grouped under the term Fanconi's syndrome (which result in phosphate losses in urine). Treatment also consists of phosphate and large doses of vitamin D. Severe hypophosphatemia (serum phosphorus <1.0 mg/dl, or <0.32 mmol/L) is uncommon and may occur only in newborns on parenteral alimentation with inadequate phosphorus administration. Respiratory failure, decreased myocardial performance, and neurologic abnormalities have been described as possible consequences of severe hypophosphatemia in adults.

REFERENCES

DeMarini, S., Tsang, R.C., & Rath, L.L. (1993). Fluids, electrolytes, vitamins, and trace minerals: Basis of ingestion, digestion, elimination, and metabolism (pp. 393–413). In C. Kenner, A. Brueggemeyer, & L.P. Gunderson (eds.), *Comprehensive neonatal nursing: A physiologic perspective.* Philadelphia: W.B. Saunders.

Lentz, R.D., Brown, D.M., & Kjellstrand, C.M. (1978). Treatment of severe hypophosphatemia. *Annals of Internal Medicine, 89,* 941–944.

161. Answer: (**C**) Pulmonary vascular resistance is high at birth so pulmonary and systemic flows are initially relatively equal. Pulmonary vascular resistance gradually decreases, causing increased pulmonary blood flow.

Systemic vessels do not dilate in response to hypoxia. Ventricular hypertrophy can occur as a compensatory mechanism, and the overall heart size will appear increased, but atrial hypertrophy alone does not occur. The pressure in both ventricles is equal. The amount of blood flow depends on the resistance of the pulmonary and systemic circulations.

REFERENCES

Lott, J.W. (1993). Assessment and management of cardiovascular dysfunction (pp. 355–391). In C. Kenner, A. Brueggemeyer, & L.P. Gunderson (eds.), *Comprehensive neonatal nursing: A physiologic perspective.* Philadelphia: W.B. Saunders.

Mair, D.D., Edwards, W.D., Julsrud, P.R., Sewards, J.B., & Danielson, G.K. (1989). Truncus arteriosus (pp. 504–515). In F.H. Adams, G.C. Emmanouilides, & T.A. Riemenschneider (eds.), *Heart disease in infants, children, and adolescents.* Baltimore: Williams & Wilkins.

Park, M.K. (1984). Cyanotic congenital heart defects (pp. 157–196). *Pediatric cardiology for practitioners.* Chicago: Year Book Medical Publishers.

162. Answer: (**C**) Another critical factor that affects the delivery of oxygen to the tissues is the adequacy of organ blood flow. Organ blood flow may be globally decreased due to decreased cardiac output, thus increasing the risk of tissue hypoxia. Methods commonly employed for maintenance of adequate cardiac output include volume expansion of the hypovolemic newborn and inotropic drugs to stimulate the poorly contractile myocardium. Clinical evaluation, including determination of the rate of capillary refill; determination of the presence or absence of acrocyanosis, skin mottling,

or relative coolness of the extremities; and determination of pulse strength and blood pressure are often used to estimate cardiac output.

REFERENCES

Carlo, W.A. & Chatburn, R.L. (1988). *Neonatal respiratory care*. Chicago: Year Book Medical Publishers.

Donovan, E.F. & Spangler, L.L. (1993). New technologies applied to the management of respiratory dysfunction. In C. Kenner, A. Brueggemeyer, & L.P. Gunderson (eds.), *Comprehensive neonatal nursing: A physiologic perspective*. Philadelphia: W.B. Saunders.

Merenstein, G.B. & Gardner, S.L. (1989). *Handbook of neonatal intensive care*. St. Louis: C.V. Mosby.

163. Answer: (**A**) Because potassium is involved in the regulation of cell membrane potential, variations in serum potassium concentrations have important effects. The effects on myocardial cells are the most prominent and severe.

REFERENCES

DeMarini, S., Tsang, R.C., & Rath, L.L. (1993). Fluids, electrolytes, vitamins, and trace minerals: Basis of ingestion, digestion, elimination, and metabolism (pp. 393–413). In C. Kenner, A. Brueggemeyer, & L.P. Gunderson (eds.), *Comprehensive neonatal nursing: A physiologic perspective*. Philadelphia: W.B. Saunders.

Spitzer, A. (1982). The role of the kidney in sodium homeostasis during maturation. *Kidney International, 21,* 539–545.

Turnberg, L.A. (1971b). Potassium transport in the human small bowel. *Gut, 12,* 811–818.

Turnberg, L.A., Bieberdort, F.A., Mordowsky, S.G., & Gordtran, J.S. (1970). Interrelations of chloride, bicarbonate, sodium and hydrogen transport in human ileum. *Journal of Clinical Investigation, 49,* 557–567.

164. Answer: (**A**) Splenic rupture is associated with severe erythroblastosis fetalis and should be suspected at the time of exchange transfusion when the CVP is low rather than elevated.

REFERENCES

Gomella, T.L. (1992). *Neonatology* (2nd ed.). Norwalk, CT: Appleton & Lange.

Polin, R.A. & Fox, W.W. (1992). *Fetal and neonatal physiology*. Philadelphia: W.B. Saunders.

Shaw, N. (1993). Assessment and management of hematologic dysfunction (pp. 582–634). In C. Kenner, A. Brueggemeyer, & L.P. Gunderson (eds.), *Comprehensive neonatal nursing: A physiologic perspective*. Philadelphia: W.B. Saunders.

165. Answer: (**B**) Although encephaloceles can occur in any region, approximately 75 percent occur in the occipital region.

REFERENCES

Blackburn, S.T. (1993). Assessment and management of neurologic dysfunction (pp. 635–689). In C. Kenner, A. Brueggemeyer, & L.P. Gunderson (eds.), *Comprehensive neonatal nursing: A physiologic perspective*. Philadelphia: W.B. Saunders.

Gomella, T.L. (1992). *Neonatology* (2nd ed.). Norwalk, CT: Appleton & Lange.

Polin, R.A., & Fox, W.W. (1992). *Fetal and neonatal physiology* (p. 1492). Philadelphia: W.B. Saunders.

166. Answer: (**A**) In light of all the controversy surrounding transfusions, evidence of impaired tissue oxygenation remains the ultimate criteria for the use of blood products.

REFERENCES

Gomella, T.L. (1992). *Neonatology* (2nd ed.). Norwalk, CT: Appleton & Lange.

Polin, R.A. & Fox, W.W. (1992). *Fetal and neonatal physiology*. Philadelphia: W.B. Saunders.

Shaw, N. (1993). Assessment and management of hematologic dysfunction (pp. 582–634). In C. Kenner, A. Brueggemeyer, & L.P. Gunderson (eds.), *Comprehensive neonatal nursing: A physiologic perspective*. Philadelphia: W.B. Saunders.

167. Answer: (**A**) The VSD causes equalization of pressures in the ventricles. Unsaturated blood flows through the VSD into the aorta because of the obstacle to blood flow from the right ventricle into the artery. With a large VSD (without TOF), blood is shunted from the left to right ventricle. The larger the VSD, the greater is the shunt and the higher is the pressure in the right ventricle and pulmonary artery. Pulmonic stenosis results in obstruction to blood flow from the right ventricle to the pulmonary artery. The right ventricle hypertrophies in response to the increased pressure caused by the obstruction to outflow.

REFERENCES

Graham, T.P., Bender, H.W., & Spach, M.S. (1989). (pp. 189–209). In F.H. Adams, G.C. Emmanouilides, & T.A. Riemenschneider (eds.), *Heart disease in infants, children, and adolescents*. Baltimore: Williams & Wilkins.

Hazinski, M.F. (1983). Congenital heart disease in the neonate (Part III): Congestive heart failure. *Neonatal Network, 1*(6), 8–17.

Hazinski, M.F. (1984). Cardiovascular disorders (pp. 63–252). *Nursing care of the critically ill child*. St. Louis: C.V. Mosby.

Lott, J.W. (1993). Assessment and management of cardiovascular dysfunction (pp. 355–391). In C. Kenner, A. Brueggemeyer, & L.P. Gunderson (eds.), *Comprehensive neonatal nursing: A physiologic perspective*. Philadelphia: W.B. Saunders.

Pinsky, W.W. & Arciniegas, E. (1990). Tetralogy of Fallot. *Pediatric Clinics of North America, 37*(1), 179–192.

Rocchini, A.P. & Emmanouilides, G.C. (1989). Pulmonic stenosis (pp. 308–338). In F.H. Adams, G.C. Emmanouilides, & T.A. Riemenschneider (eds.), *Heart disease in infants, children, and adolescents.* Baltimore: Williams & Wilkins.

168. Answer: (**B**) The loss of potassium leads to decreased chloride reabsorption (hypochloremia). Hypochloremia results in an increased aldosterone production and increased bicarbonate resulting in a metabolic alkalosis.

REFERENCES

Hazinski, M.F. (1983). Congenital heart disease in the neonate (Part III): Congestive heart failure. *Neonatal Network, 1*(6), 8–17.

Lott, J.W. (1993). Assessment and management of cardiovascular dysfunction (pp. 355–391). In C. Kenner, A. Brueggemeyer, & L.P. Gunderson (eds.), *Comprehensive neonatal nursing: A physiologic perspective.* Philadelphia: W.B. Saunders.

Talner, N.S. (1989). Heart failure (pp. 890–911). In F.H. Adams, G.C. Emmanouilides, & T.A. Riemenschneider (eds.), *Heart disease in infants, children, and adolescents.* Baltimore: Williams & Wilkins.

169. Answer: (**B**) The treatment of choice is fluid restriction, which decreases the availability of free water. Exceptions are if the serum sodium is less than approximately 120 mEq/L or if neurologic signs such as seizures are present.

REFERENCES

Gamblien, V., Bivens, K., Burton, K.S., Kissler, C.H., Kleeman, T.A., Freije, M. & Prows, C. (1993). Assessment and management of endocrine dysfunction (pp. 527–552). In C. Kenner, A. Brueggemeyer, & L.P. Gunderson (eds.), *Comprehensive neonatal nursing: A physiologic perspective.* Philadelphia: W.B. Saunders.

Kinzie, B.J. (1987). Management of the syndrome of inappropriate secretion of antidiuretic hormone. *Clinical Pharmacy, 6,* 625–633.

Klaus, M.H. & Fanaroff, A.A. (1986). *Care of the high-risk neonate* (3rd ed.). Philadelphia: W.B. Saunders.

170. Answer: (**A**) The head usually grows a maximum of 0.5 cm/week in term infants or 0.5 to 1 cm/week in preterm infants during the first weeks after birth.

REFERENCES

Amiel-Tison, C. & Larroche, J.C. (1988). Brain development and neurological survey during the neonatal period (pp. 245–267). In L. Stern & P. Vert (eds.), *Neonatal medicine.* New York: Masson Publishing.

Blackburn, S.T. (1993). Assessment and management of neurologic dysfunction (pp. 635–689). In C. Kenner, A. Brueggemeyer, & L.P. Gunderson (eds.), *Comprehensive neonatal nursing: A physiologic perspective.* Philadelphia: W.B. Saunders.

171. Answer: (**A**) Because of high urinary loss of sodium, VLBW infants (<1500 grams) can temporarily require up to 4–8 mEq/kg/day (4–8 mmol/kg/day) in the first week of life.

REFERENCES

American Academy of Pediatrics, Committee on Nutrition. (1985). Nutritional needs of low-birth-weight infants. *Pediatrics, 75,* 976–986.

Bell, E.F., Warburton, D., Stonestreet, B.S., & Oh, W. (1980). Effect of fluid administration on the development of symptomatic patent ductus arteriosus and congestive heart failure in premature infants. *New England Journal of Medicine, 302,* 598–604.

DeMarini, S., Tsang, R.C., & Rath, L.L. (1993). Fluids, electrolytes, vitamins, and trace minerals: Basis of ingestion, digestion, elimination, and metabolism (pp. 393–413). In C. Kenner, A. Brueggemeyer, & L.P. Gunderson (eds.), *Comprehensive neonatal nursing: A physiologic perspective.* Philadelphia: W.B. Saunders.

172. Answer: (**C**) Subtle seizures are the most common type of seizure seen in neonates, particularly among preterm infants.

REFERENCES

Blackburn, S.T. (1993). Assessment and management of neurologic dysfunction (pp. 635–689). In C. Kenner, A. Brueggemeyer, & L.P. Gunderson (eds.), *Comprehensive neonatal nursing: A physiologic perspective.* Philadelphia: W.B. Saunders.

Gomella, T.L. (1992). *Neonatology* (2nd ed.). Norwalk, CT: Appleton & Lange.

Polin, R.A. & Fox, W.W. (1992). *Fetal and neonatal physiology.* Philadelphia: W.B. Saunders.

173. Answer: (**C**) Thyroid extracts contain 0.21 iodide. Synthetic hormones are available as a sodium salt of L-thyroxine (L-T_4) and L-triiodothyronine (L-T_3). Methimazole and carbimazole are used for hyperthyroidism. Propranolol is given to the severely hyperthyroid infant to reduce heart rate and to lessen tremors.

REFERENCES

Gamblien, V., Bivens, K., Burton, K.S., Kissler, C.H., Kleeman, T.A., Freije, M. & Prows, C. (1993). Assessment and management of endocrine dysfunction (pp. 527–552). In C. Kenner, A. Brueggemeyer, & L.P. Gunderson (eds.), *Comprehensive neonatal nursing: A physiologic perspective.* Philadelphia: W.B. Saunders.

Goetzman, B.W. & Wenneberg, R.P. (1991). *Neonatal*

intensive care handbook (2nd ed.). St. Louis: Mosby-Year Book.
Walfish, P.G. & Tseng, K.H. (1989). Thyroid physiology and pathology (pp. 367–375). In R.J. Duchame & H. Guyda (eds.), *Pediatric endocrinology*. New York: Raven Press.

174. Answer: (**C**) Late hypocalcemia typically occurs by the end of the first week of life and is caused by increased dietary phosphate load. It was relatively common with the use of evaporated cow's milk formulas, which have a phosphate content greatly exceeding that of human milk. With modern "adapted" formulas, whose P content is closer to that of human milk, late neonatal hypocalcemia has become much less frequent but has not disappeared. Maternal vitamin D deficiency can represent a predisposing factor.

REFERENCES

DeMarini, S., Tsang, R.C., & Rath, L.L. (1993). Fluids, electrolytes, vitamins, and trace minerals: Basis of ingestion, digestion, elimination, and metabolism (pp. 393–413). In C. Kenner, A. Brueggemeyer, & L.P. Gunderson (eds.), *Comprehensive neonatal nursing: A physiologic perspective*. Philadelphia: W.B. Saunders.
Roberts, S.A., Cohen, M.D., & Fortar, J.O. (1973). Antenatal factors associated with neonatal hypocalcemic convulsions. *Lancet, 2,* 809–811.
Venkatamaran, P.S., Tsang, R.C., Greer, F.R., Noguchi, A., Larskazewski, P., & Steichen, J.J. (1985). Late infantile tetany and secondary hyperparathyroidism in infants fed humanized cow milk formula. *American Journal of Diseases of Childhood, 139,* 664–668.

175. Answer: (**B**) Nursing systems toward effective parenting-preterm (NSTEP-P) is an example of one type of parent-focused home follow-up intervention program designed specifically to address the problems of parenting a preterm infant.

REFERENCES

Barnard, K.E. (1985). *Nursing systems toward effective parenting-preterm*. Final report supported by Maternal and Child Health Training. Grant #MCH-009035, Bureau of HCDA, HRSA, PHS, DHHS.
Johnson-Crowley, N. & Sumner, G.A. (1987a). *Concept manual: Nursing systems toward effective parenting-preterm*. Seattle, WA: NCAST Publications.
Johnson-Crowley, N. & Sumner, G.A. (1987b). *Protocol manual: Nursing systems toward effective parenting-preterm*. Seattle, WA: NCAST Publications.
Johnson-Crowley, N. (1993). Systematic assessment and home follow-up: A basis for monitoring the neonate's integration into the family unit (pp. 1055–1076). In C. Kenner, A. Brueggemeyer, & L.P. Gunderson (eds.), *Comprehensive neonatal care: A physiologic perspective*. Philadelphia: W.B. Saunders.

176. Answer: (**A**) Signs and symptoms associated with SIADH secretion are indicative of water retention or edema. The most classic signs are a low serum osmolality and hyponatremia accompanied by a high urine osmolality.

REFERENCES

Gamblien, V., Bivens, K., Burton, K.S., Kissler, C.H., Kleeman, T.A., Freije, M. & Prows, C. (1993). Assessment and management of endocrine dysfunction (pp. 527–552). In C. Kenner, A. Brueggemeyer, & L.P. Gunderson (eds.), *Comprehensive neonatal nursing: A physiologic perspective*. Philadelphia: W.B. Saunders.
Kinzie, B.J. (1987). Management of the syndrome of inappropriate secretion of antidiuretic hormone. *Clinical Pharmacy, 6,* 625–633.
Klaus, M.H. & Fanaroff, A.A. (1986). *Care of the high-risk neonate* (3rd ed.). Philadelphia: W.B. Saunders.

177. Answer: (**A**) In infants <28 weeks the hemorrhage generally arises from the subependymal germinal matrix at the head of the caudate nucleus near the foramen of Monro.

REFERENCES

Blackburn, S.T. (1993). Assessment and management of neurologic dysfunction (pp. 635–689). In C. Kenner, A. Brueggemeyer, & L.P. Gunderson (eds.), *Comprehensive neonatal nursing: A physiologic perspective*. Philadelphia: W.B. Saunders.
Gomella, T.L. (1992). *Neonatology* (2nd ed.). Norwalk, CT: Appleton & Lange.
Polin, R.A. & Fox, W.W. (1992). *Fetal and neonatal physiology*. Philadelphia: W.B. Saunders.
Volpe, J.J. (1987). *Neurology of the newborn* (2nd ed.). Philadelphia: W.B. Saunders.

178. Answer: (**C**) The single greatest factor responsible for hyperbilirubinemia is prematurity, with the severity of jaundice directly correlated to decreasing gestational age.

REFERENCES

Gomella, T.L. (1992). *Neonatology* (2nd ed.). Norwalk, CT: Appleton & Lange.
Polin, R.A. & Fox, W.W. (1992). *Fetal and neonatal physiology*. Philadelphia: W.B. Saunders.
Shaw, N. (1993). Assessment and management of hematologic dysfunction (pp. 582–634). In C. Kenner, A. Brueggemeyer, & L.P. Gunderson (eds.), *Comprehensive neonatal nursing: A physiologic perspective*. Philadelphia: W.B. Saunders.

179. Answer: (**A**) During the initial cytotoxic edema, management is directed toward decreasing localized increases

in pressure with fluid restriction and decreasing energy requirements.

REFERENCES

Blackburn, S.T. (1993). Assessment and management of neurologic dysfunction (pp. 635–689). In C. Kenner, A. Brueggemeyer, & L.P. Gunderson (eds.), *Comprehensive neonatal nursing: A physiologic perspective.* Philadelphia: W.B. Saunders.

Gomella, T.L. (1992). *Neonatology* (2nd ed.). Norwalk, CT: Appleton & Lange.

180. Answer: (**C**) Toxic effects have not been reported.

REFERENCES

DeMarini, S., Tsang, R.C., & Rath, L.L. (1993). Fluids, electrolytes, vitamins, and trace minerals: Basis of ingestion, digestion, elimination, and metabolism (pp. 393–413). In C. Kenner, A. Brueggemeyer, & L.P. Gunderson (eds.), *Comprehensive neonatal nursing: A physiologic perspective.* Philadelphia: W.B. Saunders.

Moran, J.R. & Greene, H.L. (1979). The B vitamins and vitamin C in human nutrition. I. General considerations and "obligatory" B vitamins. *American Journal of Diseases of Childhood, 133,* 192–199.

181. Answer: (**A**) Hypoxia plays a large role in the development of the acute prerenal type of renal failure.

REFERENCES

Kenner, C. & Brueggemeyer, A. (1993). Assessment and management of genitourinary dysfunction (pp. 706–741). In C. Kenner, A. Brueggemeyer, & L.P. Gunderson (eds.), *Comprehensive neonatal nursing: A physiologic perspective.* Philadelphia: W.B. Saunders.

Vander, A.J. (1985). Renal physiology (3rd ed.). New York: McGraw-Hill.

182. Answer: (**C**) It is this free portion of unconjugated bilirubin that can migrate into brain cells, causing damage known as kernicterus.

REFERENCES

Mollison, P. (1984). *Blood transfusion in clinical medicine* (7th ed.). (pp. 675). Oxford: Blackwell Scientific.

Gomella, T.L. (1992). *Neonatology* (2nd ed.). Norwalk, CT: Appleton & Lange.

Polin, R.A. & Fox, W.W. (1992). *Fetal and neonatal physiology* (pp. 1161–1162). Philadelphia: W.B. Saunders.

Shaw, N. (1993). Assessment and management of hematologic dysfunction (pp. 582–634). In C. Kenner, A. Brueggemeyer, & L.P. Gunderson (eds.), *Comprehensive neonatal nursing: A physiologic perspective.* Philadelphia: W.B. Saunders.

183. Answer: (**C**) The usual finding with Wilms' tumor is a smooth, solid abdominal or flank mass that is actually a renal mass. It is accompanied by hypertension owing to the possibility of renal artery stenosis. Fever is another common symptom with Wilms' tumor.

REFERENCES

Kenner, C. & Brueggemeyer, A. (1993). Assessment and management of genitourinary dysfunction (pp. 706–741). In C. Kenner, A. Brueggemeyer, & L.P. Gunderson (eds.), *Comprehensive neonatal nursing: A physiologic perspective.* Philadelphia: W.B. Saunders.

Vander, A.J. (1985). *Renal physiology* (3rd ed.). New York: McGraw-Hill.

184. Answer: (**A**) Hypoglycemia is the most common and most severe in infants with Type I glycogen storage disease due to debranching enzyme deficiency.

REFERENCES

Ampola, M.G. (1982). *Metabolic disease in pediatric practice.* Boston: Little, Brown.

Burman, D., Holton, J.B., & Pennock, C.A. (eds.). (1978). *Inherited disorders of carbohydrate metabolism.* Baltimore: University Park Press.

Scriver, C.R., Beaudet, A.L., Sly, W.S., & Valle, D. (eds.). (1989). *The metabolic basis of inherited disease.* (6th ed.). (Volumes I and II). New York: McGraw-Hill.

Theorell, C.J. & Degenhardt, M. (1993). Assessment and management of metabolic dysfunction (pp. 480–526). In C. Kenner, A. Brueggemeyer, & L.P. Gunderson (eds.), *Comprehensive neonatal nursing: A physiologic perspective.* Philadelphia: W.B. Saunders.

185. Answer: (**A**) Dermatoglyphics is the study of the pattern of epidermal ridges.

REFERENCES

Kuller, J.M. & Lund, C.H. (1993). Assessment and management of integumentary dysfunction (pp. 742–781). In C. Kenner, A. Brueggemeyer, & L.P. Gunderson (eds.), *Comprehensive neonatal nursing: A physiologic perspective.* Philadelphia: W.B. Saunders.

Moore, K. (1988). The developing human (4th ed.). Philadelphia: W.B. Saunders.

186. Answer: (**C**) Prevention of hyperkalemia is most important in the management of renal failure, thus monitoring of potassium is essential.

REFERENCES

Gomella, T.L. (1992). *Neonatology* (2nd ed.). Norwalk, CT: Appleton & Lange.

Kenner, C. & Brueggemeyer, A. (1993). Assessment and management of genitourinary dysfunction (pp. 706–741). In C. Kenner, A. Brueggemeyer, & L.P. Gunderson (eds.), *Comprehensive neonatal nursing: A physiologic perspective.* Philadelphia: W.B. Saunders.

Vander, A.J. (1985). *Renal physiology* (3rd ed.). New York: McGraw-Hill.

187. Answer: (**C**) A conductive hearing loss exists when there is a dysfunction in the outer or middle ear, disrupting the normal sequence of sound localization and vibration.

REFERENCES

Beachy, P. & Deacon, J. (eds.) (1993). *Core curriculum for neonatal intensive care.* Philadelphia: W.B. Saunders.
Haubrich, K. (1993). Assessment and management of auditory dysfunction (pp. 782–808). In C. Kenner, A. Brueggemeyer, & L.P. Gunderson (eds.), *Comprehensive neonatal nursing: A physiologic perspective.* Philadelphia: W.B. Saunders.
Hoekelman, R.A., Friedman, S.B., Nelson, N.M., & Seidel, H.M. (1992). *Primary pediatric care* (2nd ed.). St. Louis: C.V. Mosby.

188. Answer: (**C**) Respiratory or ventilatory management of the severely affected achondroplastic dwarf is the primary concern. It can be challenging to try and support positive pulmonary functioning due to the reduced lung volume capacity within the narrow thorax. Mildly affected infants may be able to compensate for decreased lung volume with a mild to moderate increase in the work of breathing. As the infant grows, this compensation becomes more difficult.

Compensatory mechanisms such as increased work of breathing in the mildly affected achondroplastic dwarf require meticulous attention to nutrition to support the increased energy being used. There is a need for increased caloric intake in an infant exhibiting tachypnea or retractions if positive growth is to occur. However, if growth is allowed to occur too rapidly, the infant's body mass can exceed the pulmonary capacity and decompensation can occur. For this reason, nutritionists may provide additional insights in daily management as to how to provide calories but not add to the work of the infant.

REFERENCES

Butler, J. (1993). Assessment and management of musculoskeletal dysfunction (pp. 690–705). In C. Kenner, A. Brueggemeyer, & L.P. Gunderson (eds.), *Comprehensive neonatal nursing: A physiologic perspective.* Philadelphia: W.B. Saunders.
Fanaroff, A.A. & Martin, R.J. (1992). *Neonatal-perinatal medicine* (5th ed.). St. Louis: C.V. Mosby.
Polin, R.A. & Fox, W.W. (1992). *Fetal and neonatal physiology.* Philadelphia: W.B. Saunders.

189. Answer: (**A**) Growth hormone is one of at least seven hormones secreted from the anterior portion of the pituitary gland. Specifically, growth hormone (somatotropin) is secreted from somatotroph cells.

REFERENCES

Gamblien, V., Bivens, K., Burton, K.S., Kissler, C.H., Kleeman, T.A., Freije, M. & Prows, C. (1993). Assessment and management of endocrine dysfunction (pp. 527–552). In C. Kenner, A. Brueggemeyer, & L.P. Gunderson (eds.), *Comprehensive neonatal nursing: A physiologic perspective.* Philadelphia: W.B. Saunders.
Rimoin, D.L. (1990). Genetic disorders of the pituitary gland (pp. 1461–1488). In A.E. Emery & D.L. Rimoin (eds.), *Principles and practice of medical genetics* (Vol. 2).
Wallis, M. (1988). The molecular basis of growth hormone deficiency. *Molecular aspects of medicine, 10,* 431–509.

190. Answer: (**A**) Notwithstanding the inherent problems associated with omphaloceles, gastroschisis, encephaloceles, clubfeet, syndactyly, and facial clefts, the clinician must be attuned to the unique complications of constricting bands. Constricting bands are usually associated with edema distal to the band. The resulting edema and vascular compromise contribute to complications such as skin breakdown, necrosis, and thromboemboli formation due to venostasis and infection. Care should include frequent vascular checks to assess perfusion. Trauma and tissue breakdown are discouraged through positioning and skin care. Observation for localized areas of necrosis is stressed.

REFERENCES

Butler, J. (1993). Assessment and management of musculoskeletal dysfunction (pp. 690–705). In C. Kenner, A. Brueggemeyer, & L.P. Gunderson (eds.), *Comprehensive neonatal nursing: A physiologic perspective.* Philadelphia: W.B. Saunders.
Gomella, T.L. (1992). *Neonatology* (2nd ed.). Norwalk, CT: Appleton & Lange.

191. Answer: (**B**) Otitis media, an infection of the middle ear, is the most common cause of conductive hearing loss. In this instance, fluid accumulates in the middle ear, preventing the tympanic membrane and ossicular chain from vibrating normally.

REFERENCES

Beachy, P. & Deacon, J. (eds.) (1993). *Core curriculum for neonatal intensive care.* Philadelphia: W.B. Saunders.

Haubrich, K. (1993). Assessment and management of auditory dysfunction (pp. 782–808). In C. Kenner, A. Brueggemeyer, & L.P. Gunderson (eds.), *Comprehensive neonatal nursing: A physiologic perspective.* Philadelphia: W.B. Saunders.

Hoekelman, R.A., Friedman, S.B., Nelson, N.M., & Seidel, H.M. (1992). *Primary pediatric care* (2nd ed.). St. Louis: C.V. Mosby.

192. Answer: (**A**) The direct Coombs is a measurement of the presence of antibody on the RBC surface, whereas the indirect Coombs is a measurement of antibody in the serum.

REFERENCES

Mollison, P. (1984). *Blood transfusion in clinical medicine* (7th ed.) (pp. 675). Oxford: Blackwell Scientific.

Gomella, T.L. (1992). *Neonatology* (2nd ed.). Norwalk, CT: Appleton & Lange.

Shaw, N. (1993). Assessment and management of hematologic dysfunction (pp. 582–634). In C. Kenner, A. Brueggemeyer, & L.P. Gunderson (eds.), *Comprehensive neonatal nursing: A physiologic perspective.* Philadelphia: W.B. Saunders.

193. Answer: (**B**) Overt reactions include arousal, gross body movements, orienting behavior, turning of the head, flexes, facial grimaces, displacement of a single digit, crying or cessation of crying, and acceleration or deceleration of the heart rate. Preterm infants have been shown to have changes in heart rate and various types of body movements in response to sound.

REFERENCES

Haubrich, K. (1993). Assessment and management of auditory dysfunction (pp. 782–808). In C. Kenner, A. Brueggemeyer, & L.P. Gunderson (eds.), *Comprehensive neonatal nursing: A physiologic perspective.* Philadelphia: W.B. Saunders.

Mencher, G.T., Mencher, L.S., & Rohland, S.L. (1985). Maturation of behavioral response. *Ear and Hearing, 6*(1), 10–14.

194. Answer: (**B**) Congenital muscular torticollis, with an incidence of 0.4 percent of all live births, is another musculosketetal deformity with unknown pathogenesis (Coventry & Harris, 1959). It is known to be primarily a disorder of the sternocleidomastoid muscle.

REFERENCES

Butler, J. (1993). Assessment and management of musculoskeletal dysfunction (pp. 690–705). In C. Kenner, A. Brueggemeyer, & L.P. Gunderson (eds.), *Comprehensive neonatal nursing: A physiologic perspective.* Philadelphia: W.B. Saunders.

Coventry, M.B. & Harris, I.E. (1959). Congenital muscular torticollis in infancy. *Journal of Bone and Joint Surgery, 41,* 815.

195. Answer: (**A**) Vulnerable child syndrome (VCS) has been associated with preterm infants. In this phenomenon, parents continue to see their infant as vulnerable (susceptibility to a negative outcome) despite evidence to the contrary that the infant is physically and developmentally normal. This results in maladaptive behavior both on the part of the parent (usually the mother) and the infant.

REFERENCES

Culley, B.S., Perrin, E.C., & Chaberski, M.J. (1989). Parental perception of vulnerability of formerly premature infants. *Journal of Pediatric Health Care, 3,* 237–245.

Johnson-Crowley, N. (1993). Systematic assessment and home follow-up: A basis for monitoring the neonate's integration into the family unit (pp. 1055–1076). In C. Kenner, A. Brueggemeyer, & L.P. Gunderson (eds.), *Comprehensive neonatal care: A physiologic perspective.* Philadelphia: W.B. Saunders.

Macey, T.J., Harmon, R.J., & Easterbrooks, M.A. (1987). Impact of premature birth on the development of the infant in the family. *Journal of Consulting and Clinical Psychology, 55*(6), 846–852.

McCormick, M.C., Shapiro, S., & Starfield, B. (1982). Factors associated with maternal opinion of infant development-clues to the vulnerable child? *Pediatrics, 69,* 537–543.

Perrin, E.C., West, P.S., & Culley, B.S. (1989). Is my child normal yet? Correlates of vulnerability. *Pediatrics, 83,* 355–363.

196. Answer: (**B**) Immunoglobulin M (IgM) makes up about 10 percent of the immunoglobulin pool. It is confined primarily to the intravascular pool. IgM is the predominant early antibody; it is frequently directed against antigenetically complex infectious organisms. IgM is produced by the fetus in response to intrauterine infection.

REFERENCES

Lott, J.W., Nelson, K., Fahrner, R., & Kenner, C. (1993). Assessment and management of immunologic dysfunction (pp. 553–581). In C. Kenner, A. Brueggemeyer, & L.P. Gunderson (eds.), *Comprehensive neonatal nursing: A physiologic perspective.* Philadelphia: W.B. Saunders.

Xanthou, M. (1987). Neonatal immunity (pp. 555–586). In L. Stern & P. Vert (eds.), *Neonatal medicine.* New York: Masson Publishing.

197. Answer: (**B**) The enzyme-linked immunoassay test (ELISA) will detect the

presence of antibodies to a viral agent. These may be maternally or fetally derived antibodies.

REFERENCES

Gomella, T.L. (1992). *Neonatology* (2nd ed.). Norwalk, CT: Appleton & Lange.
Lott, J.W., Nelson, K., Fahrner, R., & Kenner, C. (1993). Assessment and management of immunologic dysfunction (pp. 553–581). In C. Kenner, A. Brueggemeyer, & L.P. Gunderson (eds.), *Comprehensive neonatal nursing: A physiologic perspective.* Philadelphia: W.B. Saunders.
Xanthou, M. (1987). Neonatal immunity (pp. 555–586). In L. Stern & P. Vert (eds.), *Neonatal medicine.* New York: Masson Publishing.

198. Answer: (**C**) A urine latex is used to detect *Group B streptococcus.*

REFERENCES

Gomella, T.L. (1992). *Neonatology* (2nd ed.). Norwalk, CT: Appleton & Lange.
Lott, J.W., Nelson, K., Fahrner, R., & Kenner, C. (1993). Assessment and management of immunologic dysfunction (pp. 553–581). In C. Kenner, A. Brueggemeyer, & L.P. Gunderson (eds.), *Comprehensive neonatal nursing: A physiologic perspective.* Philadelphia: W.B. Saunders.
Xanthou, M. (1987). Neonatal immunity (pp. 555–586). In L. Stern & P. Vert (eds.), *Neonatal medicine.* New York: Masson Publishing.

199. Answer: (**C**) A mother with a fever or who has been ill before delivery can pass the infection to the infant. If a maternal temperature of 101°F is noted at delivery, a septic workup is indicated. Maternal cervical or amniotic fluid cultures can be necessary to determine the causative agent of elevated temperature. If the maternal illness suggests viral infection, neonatal viral cultures should be drawn.

REFERENCES

Lott, J.W., Nelson, K., Fahrner, R., & Kenner, C. (1993). Assessment and management of immunologic dysfunction (pp. 553–581). In C. Kenner, A. Brueggemeyer, & L.P. Gunderson (eds.), *Comprehensive neonatal nursing: A physiologic perspective.* Philadelphia: W.B. Saunders.
Sweet, A.Y. (1991). Bacterial infections (pp. 84–167). In A.Y. Sweet & E.G. Brown (eds.), *Fetal and neonatal effects of maternal disease.* St. Louis: Mosby-Year Book.
Xanthou, M. (1987). Neonatal immunity (pp. 555–586). In L. Stern & P. Vert (eds.), *Neonatal medicine.* New York: Masson Publishing.

200. Answer: (**A**) The introduction of broad-spectrum antimicrobials dramatically improved the prognosis of infection. They need to be started pending culture results as even with aggressive therapy, the mortality of early-onset group B streptococcal infection is very high.

REFERENCES

Lott, J.W., Nelson, K., Fahrner, R., & Kenner, C. (1993). Assessment and management of immunologic dysfunction (pp. 553–581). In C. Kenner, A. Brueggemeyer, & L.P. Gunderson (eds.), *Comprehensive neonatal nursing: A physiologic perspective.* Philadelphia: W.B. Saunders.
Sweet, A.Y. (1991). Bacterial infections (pp. 84–167). In A.Y. Sweet & E.G. Brown (eds.), *Fetal and neonatal effects of maternal disease.* St. Louis: Mosby-Year Book.
Xanthou, M. (1987). Neonatal immunity (pp. 555–586). In L. Stern & P. Vert (eds.), *Neonatal medicine.* New York: Masson Publishing.

201. Answer: (**B**) Streptococcus is a gram-positive diplococcus with an ultrastructure similar to other gram-positive cocci.

REFERENCES

Lott, J.W., Nelson, K., Fahrner, R., & Kenner, C. (1993). Assessment and management of immunologic dysfunction (pp. 553–581). In C. Kenner, A. Brueggemeyer, & L.P. Gunderson (eds.), *Comprehensive neonatal nursing: A physiologic perspective.* Philadelphia: W.B. Saunders.
Sweet, A.Y. (1991). Bacterial infections (pp. 84–167). In A.Y. Sweet & E.G. Brown (eds.), *Fetal and neonatal effects of maternal disease.* St. Louis: Mosby-Year Book.
Xanthou, M. (1987). Neonatal immunity (pp. 555–586). In L. Stern & P. Vert (eds.), *Neonatal medicine.* New York: Masson Publishing.

202. Answer: (**B**) Preterm birth associated with meconium staining should always be considered suspicious for listeriosis.

REFERENCES

Lott, J.W., Nelson, K., Fahrner, R., & Kenner, C. (1993). Assessment and management of immunologic dysfunction (pp. 553–581). In C. Kenner, A. Brueggemeyer, & L.P. Gunderson (eds.), *Comprehensive neonatal nursing: A physiologic perspective.* Philadelphia: W.B. Saunders.
Sweet, A.Y. (1991). Bacterial infections (pp. 84–167). In A.Y. Sweet & E.G. Brown (eds.), *Fetal and neonatal effects of maternal disease.* St. Louis: Mosby-Year Book.
Xanthou, M. (1987). Neonatal immunity (pp. 555–586). In L. Stern & P. Vert (eds.), *Neonatal medicine.* New York: Masson Publishing.

203. Answer: (**B**) Use of a transparent dressing such as Op-Site to serve as a "second skin" may be preferred to treat skin disruptions. But Op-Site is contraindicated over monilial rash.

REFERENCES

Kuller, J. & Tobin, C. (1990). Skin care management of the low-birthweight infant. In L. Gunderson & C. Kenner (eds.), *Care of the 24-25 week gestational age infant*. Petaluma, CA: Neonatal Network.

Kuller, J.M. & Lund, C.H. (1993). Assessment and management of integumentary dysfunction (pp. 742–781). In C. Kenner, A. Brueggemeyer, & L.P. Gunderson (eds.), *Comprehensive neonatal nursing: A physiologic perspective*. Philadelphia: W.B. Saunders.

204. Answer: (**A**) Ritodrine hydrochloride is a β-adrenergic antagonist that readily crosses the placenta, can cause depression in the fetal glomerular perfusion and glomerular filtration rate (GFR).

REFERENCES

Kenner, C. & Brueggemeyer, A. (1993). Assessment and management of genitourinary dysfunction (pp. 706–741). In C. Kenner, A. Brueggemeyer, & L.P. Gunderson (eds.), *Comprehensive neonatal nursing: A physiologic perspective*. Philadelphia: W.B. Saunders.

Smith, F.G. & Robillard, J.E. (1989). Pathophysiology of fetal renal disease. *Seminars in Perinatology, 20*(2), 186–187.

205. Answer: (**B**) Ritodrine hydrochloride is a β-adrenergic antagonist that readily crosses the placenta, can cause depression in the fetal glomerular perfusion and glomerular filtration rate (GFR).

REFERENCES

Kenner, C. & Brueggemeyer, A. (1993). Assessment and management of genitourinary dysfunction (pp. 706–741). In C. Kenner, A. Brueggemeyer, & L.P. Gunderson (eds.), *Comprehensive neonatal nursing: A physiologic perspective*. Philadelphia: W.B. Saunders.

Smith, F.G. & Robillard, J.E. (1989). Pathophysiology of fetal renal disease. *Seminars in Perinatology, 20*(2), 186–187.

206. Answer: (**C**) Initially the clinical manifestations are those of spinal cord shock with hypotonia, weakness, flaccid extremities, sensory deficits, relaxed abdominal muscles, diaphragmatic breathing, Horner's syndrome (ipsilateral ptosis, anhidrosis and miosis), and a distended bladder.

REFERENCES

Blackburn, S.T. (1993). Assessment and management of neurologic dysfunction (pp. 635–689). In C. Kenner, A. Brueggemeyer, & L.P. Gunderson (eds.), *Comprehensive neonatal nursing: A physiologic perspective*. Philadelphia: W.B. Saunders.

Gomella, T.L. (1992). *Neonatology* (2nd ed.). Norwalk, CT: Appleton & Lange.

Merenstein, G.B. & Gardner, S.L. (1993). *Handbook of neonatal intensive care* (2nd ed.). St. Louis: C.V. Mosby.

207. Answer: (**C**) The clinical manifestations of zinc deficiency include lethargy, growth retardation, skin lesions, alopecia, diarrhea. The striking sign of zinc deficiency, however, is some form of skin lesion. Common sites of involvement are the groin and perianal area, the neck folds, and the face, particularly the angles of the mouth and the cheeks. Lesions also have been noted at sites of trauma, such as endotracheal and cardiac monitor tape sites.

REFERENCES

Esterly, N. & Spraker, M. (1985). Neonatal skin problems (pp. 1882–1903). In S. Moschella & H. Hurley (eds.), *Dermatology* (2nd ed.). (Vol. 2). Philadelphia: W.B. Saunders.

Kuller, J.M. & Lund, C.H. (1993). Assessment and management of integumentary dysfunction (pp. 742–781). In C. Kenner, A. Brueggemeyer, & L.P. Gunderson (eds.), *Comprehensive neonatal nursing: A physiologic perspective*. Philadelphia: W.B. Saunders.

208. Answer: (**C**) Several factors that can potentially enhance the risk of ototoxicity include increased drug serum levels, decreased renal function, the use of more than one ototoxic drug simultaneously or in increased dose or for an extended time, age, health, heredity, and concurrent noise.

REFERENCES

Haubrich, K. (1993). Assessment and management of auditory dysfunction (pp. 782–808). In C. Kenner, A. Brueggemeyer, & L.P. Gunderson (eds.), *Comprehensive neonatal nursing: A physiologic perspective*. Philadelphia: W.B. Saunders.

Hoekelman, R.A., Friedman, S.B., Nelson, N.M., & Seidel, H.M. (1992). *Primary pediatric care* (2nd ed.). St. Louis: C.V. Mosby.

209. Answer: (**A**) Renal vein thrombosis is usually secondary to umbilical or arterial line placement, birth trauma, hypoxia, dehydration, or hypotension or as a complication of maternal diabetes.

REFERENCES

Kenner, C. & Brueggemeyer, A. (1993). Assessment and management of genitourinary dysfunction (pp. 706–741). In C. Kenner, A. Brueggemeyer, & L.P. Gunderson (eds.), *Comprehensive neonatal nursing: A physiologic perspective*. Philadelphia: W.B. Saunders.

Gomella, T.L. (1992). *Neonatology* (2nd ed.). Norwalk, CT: Appleton & Lange.

Vander, A.J. (1985). *Renal physiology* (3rd ed.). New York: McGraw-Hill.

210. Answer: (**A**) The A and B antigens on the fetal and neonatal RBC are not well developed so only a small amount of antibodies will actually attach to the antigen. Other body tissues also have antigen sites to which some circulating antibodies can adhere, thereby decreasing the potential for RBC destruction. The resulting small amounts of IgG in the plasma will not stimulate activation of the complement system so hemolysis is minimal. This may explain why 15 to 20 percent of infants are ABO incompatible with their mothers (Bowman, 1988) but only 3 percent become symptomatic.

REFERENCES

Bowman, J. (1988). Alloimmune hemolytic disease of the neonate (pp. 223–248). In J. Stockman & C. Pochedly (eds.), *Developmental and neonatal hematology*. New York: Raven Press.
Mollison, P. (1984). *Blood transfusion in clinical medicine* (pp. 675). (7th ed.). Oxford: Blackwell Scientific.
Gomella, T.L. (1992). *Neonatology* (2nd ed.). Norwalk, CT: Appleton & Lange.
Shaw, N. (1993). Assessment and management of hematologic dysfunction (pp. 582–634). In C. Kenner, A. Brueggemeyer, & L.P. Gunderson (eds.), *Comprehensive neonatal nursing: A physiologic perspective*. Philadelphia: W.B. Saunders.

211. Answer: (**A**) Cerebrospinal fluid is produced in the choroid plexus at a rate of approximately 0.37 ml/minute. CSF then circulates from the lateral ventricles through the foramen of Monro to the third ventricle and via the aqueduct of Sylvius to the fourth ventricle.

REFERENCES

Blackburn, S.T. (1993). Assessment and management of neurologic dysfunction (pp. 635–689). In C. Kenner, A. Brueggemeyer, & L.P. Gunderson (eds.), *Comprehensive neonatal nursing: A physiologic perspective*. Philadelphia: W.B. Saunders.
Brann, A.W. & Schwartz, J.F. (1987). Central nervous system disturbances (pp. 495–553). In A.A. Fanaroff & R.J. Martin (eds.), *Neonatal-perinatal medicine*. St Louis: C.V. Mosby.
Polin, R.A. & Fox, W.W. (1992). *Fetal and neonatal physiology*. Philadelphia: W.B. Saunders.

212. Answer: (**B**) The hearing loss associated with cleft lip or palate is generally conductive in nature; however, there have been reports of sensorineural and/or mixed losses.

REFERENCES

Bergstrom, L. & Hemenway, W.G. (1971). Otologic problems in submucous cleft palate. *Southern Medical Journal, 64*(10), 1172–1177.
Haubrich, K. (1993). Assessment and management of auditory dysfunction (pp. 782–808). In C. Kenner, A. Brueggemeyer, & L.P. Gunderson (eds.), *Comprehensive neonatal nursing: A physiologic perspective*. Philadelphia: W.B. Saunders.

213. Answer: (**B**) Large hemangiomas can trap platelets and lead to a bleeding dysfunction, cause heart failure, ulcerate and lead to a bacterial infection, or interfere with feeding or visual development depending on its location.

REFERENCES

Kuller, J.M. & Lund, C.H. (1993). Assessment and management of integumentary dysfunction (pp. 742–781). In C. Kenner, A. Brueggemeyer, & L.P. Gunderson (eds.), *Comprehensive neonatal nursing: A physiologic perspective*. Philadelphia: W.B. Saunders.
Rosen, T., Lanning, M., & Hill, M. (1983). The nurses' atlas to dermatology (pp. 97–129). Boston: Little, Brown.

214. Answer: (**B**) If Wilms' tumor is suspected, palpation should *not* be performed because this may break the tumor into small fragments, leading to tumor seeding.

REFERENCES

Gomella, T.L. (1992). *Neonatology* (2nd ed.). Norwalk, CT: Appleton & Lange.
Kenner, C. & Brueggemeyer, A. (1993). Assessment and management of genitourinary dysfunction (pp. 706–741). In C. Kenner, A. Brueggemeyer, & L.P. Gunderson (eds.), *Comprehensive neonatal nursing: A physiologic perspective*. Philadelphia: W.B. Saunders.
Vander, A.J. (1985). Renal physiology (3rd ed.). New York: McGraw-Hill.

215. Answer: (**C**) *Staphylococcus aureus* can result in a severe bullous eruption called scalded skin syndrome.

REFERENCES

Kuller, J.M. & Lund, C.H. (1993). Assessment and management of integumentary dysfunction (pp. 742–781). In C. Kenner, A. Brueggemeyer, & L.P. Gunderson (eds.), *Comprehensive neonatal nursing: A physiologic perspective*. Philadelphia: W.B. Saunders.
Solmon, L. & Esterly, N. (1987). The skin (pp. 1172–1199). In A.A. Fanaroff & R.J. Martin (eds.), *Neonatal-perinatal medicine: Diseases of the fetus and infant* (4th ed.). St. Louis: C.V. Mosby.

216. Answer: (**B**) It is believed that fetal testosterone stimulates this growth.

REFERENCES

Gomella, T.L. (1992). *Neonatology* (2nd ed.). Norwalk, CT: Appleton & Lange.

Kenner, C. & Brueggemeyer, A. (1993). Assessment and management of genitourinary dysfunction (pp. 706–741). In C. Kenner, A. Brueggemeyer, & L.P. Gunderson (eds.), *Comprehensive neonatal nursing: A physiologic perspective*. Philadelphia: W.B. Saunders.

Moore, K. (1988). *The developing human: Clinically oriented embryology* (4th ed.). Philadelphia: W.B. Saunders.

Polin, R.A. & Fox, W.W. (1992). *Fetal and neonatal physiology*. Philadelphia: W.B. Saunders.

Vander, A.J. (1985). *Renal physiology* (3rd ed.). New York: McGraw-Hill.

217. Answer: (**C**) Sodium filtration depends on the glomerular filtration rate.

REFERENCES

Kenner, C. & Brueggemeyer, A. (1993). Assessment and management of genitourinary dysfunction (pp. 706–741). In C. Kenner, A. Brueggemeyer, & L.P. Gunderson (eds.), *Comprehensive neonatal nursing: A physiologic perspective*. Philadelphia: W.B. Saunders.

Wodniak, C. & Szwed, J. (1986). Fluid and electrolytes. In L. Abels (ed.), *Critical care nursing: A physiologic approach*. St. Louis: C.V. Mosby.

218. Answer: (**C**) Hypopigmentation presenting as a diffuse or localized loss of pigment in the neonate can be the result of metabolic (phenylketonuria), endocrine (Addison's disease), genetic (vitiligo, piebaldism, tuberous sclerosis, albinism), traumatic, or postinflammatory causes.

REFERENCES

Avery, G. (1987). *Neonatology* (3rd ed.). Philadelphia: J.B. Lippincott.

Kuller, J.M. & Lund, C.H. (1993). Assessment and management of integumentary dysfunction (pp. 742–781). In C. Kenner, A. Brueggemeyer, & L.P. Gunderson (eds.), *Comprehensive neonatal nursing: A physiologic perspective*. Philadelphia: W.B. Saunders.

219. Answer: (**B**) Meningitis is acquired in most cases postnatally and is the most common cause of hearing loss in infants.

REFERENCES

Haubrich, K. (1993). Assessment and management of auditory dysfunction (pp. 782–808). In C. Kenner, A. Brueggemeyer, & L.P. Gunderson (eds.), *Comprehensive neonatal nursing: A physiologic perspective*. Philadelphia: W.B. Saunders.

Pappas, D.G. (1985). *Diagnosis and treatment of hearing impairment in children*. San Diego: College-Hill Press.

220. Answer: (**C**) Valgus refers to a deformity in which a body part is bent outward and away from the body's midline; a part which is in abduction. Varus implies a body part positioned inward, toward the midline of the body; a part which is in adduction. Talipes refers to any one of various foot deformities. Reduction is the restoration to a normal position. The upper limbs develop more quickly than the lower limbs. There is actually a lapse of several days between the development of the upper limbs compared with the lower limb development.

REFERENCES

Butler, J. (1993). Assessment and management of musculoskeletal dysfunction (pp. 690–705). In C. Kenner, A. Brueggemeyer, & L.P. Gunderson (eds.), *Comprehensive neonatal nursing: A physiologic perspective*. Philadelphia: W.B. Saunders.

Moore, K.L. (1989). *The developing human* (4th ed.). Philadelphia: W.B. Saunders.

221. Answer: (**B**) Osteogenesis imperfecta type I is an autosomal dominant disorder. Fractures are most abundant in the arms, legs, clavicles, and ribs. As the infant ages, the lower extremities are affected more frequently as a result of increased weight-bearing trauma.

REFERENCES

Butler, J. (1993). Assessment and management of musculoskeletal dysfunction (pp. 690–705). In C. Kenner, A. Brueggemeyer, & L.P. Gunderson (eds.), *Comprehensive neonatal nursing: A physiologic perspective*. Philadelphia: W.B. Saunders.

Fanaroff, A.A. & Martin, R.J. (1992). *Neonatal-perinatal medicine* (5th ed.). St. Louis: C.V. Mosby.

Moore, K.L. (1989). *The developing human* (4th ed.). Philadelphia: W.B. Saunders.

222. Answer: (**C**) Neonates affected with this disorder are typically small for gestational age and present with dwarf-like appearance. The extremities are deformed and short as a result of multiple fractures and crumbling of the long bones. Chest radiograms exhibit beaded ribs with numerous fractures, both old and new. Blue sclera are characteristic features in both types I and II. However, blue sclera can be a normal finding in neonates and cannot serve as a diagnostic criterion for this age group.

REFERENCES

Butler, J. (1993). Assessment and management of musculoskeletal dysfunction (pp. 690–705). In C. Kenner, A. Brueggemeyer, & L.P. Gunderson (eds.), *Comprehensive neonatal nursing: A physiologic perspective*. Philadelphia: W.B. Saunders.

Fanaroff, A.A. & Martin, R.J. (1992). *Neonatal-perinatal medicine* (5th ed.). St. Louis: C.V. Mosby.

Gertner, J.M. & Root, L. (1990). Osteogenesis imperfecta. *The Orthopedic Clinics of North America, 21*(1), 151–162.

223. Answer: (**A**) Therapeutic success or failure is not determined by drug concentrations but by the physiologic or biochemical changes (pharmacodynamics) produced by that specific drug in the concentrations achieved at the target site (Kauffman, 1981). The circulation is rarely the target site, but it is often the route used to deliver drugs to the target site within a tissue to exert its action.

REFERENCES

Kauffman, R.E. (1981). The clinical interpretation and application of drug concentration data. *Pediatric Clinics of North America, 28,* 35–45.

Ward, R.M. (1993). Neonatal pharmacology (pp. 926–939). In C. Kenner, A. Brueggemeyer, & L.P. Gunderson (eds.), *Comprehensive neonatal care: A physiologic perspective*. Philadelphia: W.B. Saunders.

224. Answer: (**A**) A developmental variation of infant skin resides in the functional capacity of the skin to form a surface pH less than 5.0, the acid mantle. A skin surface pH of less than 5 is ordinarily seen in both children and adults.

REFERENCES

Behrendt, H. & Green, M. (1971). *Patterns of skin pH from birth through adolescence*. Springfield, IL: Charles C Thomas.

Kuller, J.M. & Lund, C.H. (1993). Assessment and management of integumentary dysfunction (pp. 742–781). In C. Kenner, A. Brueggemeyer, & L.P. Gunderson (eds.), *Comprehensive neonatal nursing: A physiologic perspective*. Philadelphia: W. B. Saunders.

225. Answer: (**C**) The premature newborn, especially the extremely premature newborn born at ≤28 weeks' gestation, is often viewed as unable to metabolize drugs. Studies have shown close correlations between creatinine clearance and gentamicin clearance and gentamicin half-life and birth weight. Thus, gentamicin dosing intervals increase as gestational age decreases. Initial gentamicin dosing intervals must be lengthened up to 24 hours in the most immature newborns and often need to be adjusted empirically thereafter based on measurements of drug concentrations.

REFERENCES

Charlton, C.K., Needelman, H., Thomas, R.W., & Kortas, K. (1986). Gentamicin dosage recommendations for neonates based on half-life predictions from birth weight. *American Journal of Perinatology, 3,* 28–32.

Kildoo C., Modanlou, H.D., Komatsu, G., Harralson, A., & Hodding, J. (1984). Developmental pattern of gentamicin kinetics in very low birth weight (VLBW) sick infants. *Developmental Pharmacologic Therapy 7,* 345–356.

Pelkonen, O., Kaltiala, E.H., Larmi, T.K.I. & Karki, N.T. (1973). Comparison of activities of drug-metabolizing enzymes in human fetal and adult livers. *Clinical Pharmacology Therapeutics, 14,* 840–846.

Ward, R.M. (1993). Neonatal pharmacology (pp. 926–939). In C. Kenner, A. Brueggemeyer, & L.P. Gunderson (eds.), *Comprehensive neonatal care: A physiologic perspective*. Philadelphia: W.B. Saunders.

226. Answer: (**C**) Constriction of the vessels leading into the glomerular capillary and increased resistance to blood flow into the capillary result in a lower hydraulic pressure at the level of the glomerular capillary, thus reducing the glomerular filtration rate.

REFERENCES

Kenner, C. & Brueggemeyer, A. (1993). Assessment and management of genitourinary dysfunction (pp. 706–741). In C. Kenner, A. Brueggemeyer, & L.P. Gunderson (eds.), *Comprehensive neonatal nursing: A physiologic perspective*. Philadelphia: W.B. Saunders.

Vander, A.J. (1985). *Renal physiology* (3rd ed.). New York: McGraw-Hill.

227. Answer: (**B**) This finding has implications for the long-term auditory development of the neonate and supports the need for visualization of the middle ear as part of the septic workup of all neonates.

REFERENCES

Haubrich, K. (1993). Assessment and management of auditory dysfunction (pp. 782–808). In C. Kenner, A. Brueggemeyer, & L.P. Gunderson (eds.), *Comprehensive neonatal nursing: A physiologic perspective*. Philadelphia: W.B. Saunders.

Shurin, P.A. (1976). Antibacterial therapy and middle ear effusions. *Annals of Otology, Rhinology, and Laryngology, 85*(2 Suppl 25 Pt 2), 250–253.

228. Answer: (**A**) Several problems common in neonates can alter enteral drug

absorption. Most GI drug absorption occurs outside the stomach across the large surface of the intestine. Delayed gastric emptying or delayed intestinal peristalsis delays distribution of drug along the intestine and decreases drug absorption. By like manner, rapid intestinal transit due to diarrhea can prevent complete absorption.

REFERENCES

Boreus, L.O. (1982). *Principles of pediatric pharmacology*. New York: Churchill Livingstone.

Peterson, R.G., Simmons, M.A., Rumack, B.H., Levine, R.L., & Brooks, J.G. (1980). Pharmacology of furosemide in the premature newborn infant. *Journal of Pediatrics, 97,* 139–143.

Ward, R.M. (1993). Neonatal pharmacology (pp. 926–939). In C. Kenner, A. Brueggemeyer, & L.P. Gunderson (eds.), *Comprehensive neonatal care: A physiologic perspective*. Philadelphia: W.B. Saunders.

229. Answer: (**B**) Liberal use of povidone-iodine as a prepping agent before invasive procedures has been associated with high iodine levels, iodine goiter, and hypothyroidism in the newborn.

REFERENCES

Chabrolle, J. & Rossier, A. (1978). Goiter and hypothyroidism in the newborn after cutaneous absorption of iodine. *Archives of Disease in Childhood, 53,* 495–498.

Jackson, H. & Sutherland, R. (1981). Effect of povidine-iodine on neonatal thyroid function. *Lancet, 2,* 992.

Kuller, J.M. & Lund, C.H. (1993). Assessment and management of integumentary dysfunction (pp. 742–781). In C. Kenner, A. Brueggemeyer, & L.P. Gunderson (eds.), *Comprehensive neonatal nursing: A physiologic perspective*. Philadelphia: W.B. Saunders.

Pyati, S., Ramamurthy, R., Krauss, M.T., & Pildes, R. (1977). Absorption of iodine in the neonate following topical use of povidone-iodine. *Journal of Pediatrics, 91*(5), 825–828.

230. Answer: (**B**) White shadows of the ossicles can usually be seen through the membrane. Complications of otitis media are not uncommon. Otitis media with middle ear effusion can cause hearing loss, perforation of the tympanic membrane, and potential intracranial complications including meningitis, encephalitis, and brain abscess. Shurin (1976) demonstrated that middle ear effusion occurs in both outpatient and inpatient populations of neonates.

REFERENCES

Haubrich, K. (1993). Assessment and management of auditory dysfunction (pp. 782–808). In C. Kenner, A. Brueggemeyer, & L.P. Gunderson (eds.), *Comprehensive neonatal nursing: A physiologic perspective*. Philadelphia: W.B. Saunders.

Shurin, P.A. (1976). Antibacterial therapy and middle ear effusions. *Annals of Otology, Rhinology, and Laryngology, 85*(2 Suppl 25 Pt 2), 250–253.

231. Answer: (**A**) The goal of drug therapy is to produce an effective concentration of free or unbound drug at a specific site to achieve the desired therapeutic effect. Due to lower concentrations of serum proteins, premature neonates may have circulating *unbound* drug concentrations in the therapeutic, or even the toxic, range when their total drug concentrations are less than the lower limits of the recommended range for adults. Caregivers for neonates must watch for symptoms and signs of drug toxicity in neonates, although total drug concentrations may be within a range considered nontoxic.

REFERENCES

Boreus, L.O. (1982). *Principles of pediatric pharmacology* (pp. 56–61) New York: Churchill Livingstone.

Sheiner, L.B. & Tozer, T.N. (1978). Clinical pharmacokinetics: The use of plasma concentrations of drugs (pp. 71–109). In K.L. Melmon & H.F. Morelli (eds.), *Clinical pharmacology: Basic principles in therapeutics* (2nd ed.). New York: Macmillan.

Ward, R.M. (1993). Neonatal pharmacology (pp. 926–939). In C. Kenner, A. Brueggemeyer, & L.P. Gunderson (eds.), *Comprehensive neonatal care: A physiologic perspective*. Philadelphia: W.B. Saunders.

232. Answer: (**A**) The newborn's sympathetic response to pain, because it is immature, is less predictable than that of the adult. The mobilization of endocrine and metabolic resources results in changes in blood pressure (which can be either increased or decreased), skin color, and temperature. The immature cerebral vascular bed is particularly vulnerable to injury owing to lack of autoregulation, and any stimulus that increases cerebral vascular congestion or results in hypocalcemia, such as crying, can increase the risk for intraventricular hemorrhage.

REFERENCES

Brazy, J.A. (1988). Effects of crying on cerebral blood flow and cytochromosome aa3. *Journal of Pediatrics, 112,* 457–461.

Franck, L.S. (1993). Identification, management, and prevention of pain in the neonate (pp. 913–925). In C. Kenner, A. Brueggemeyer, & L.P. Gunderson (eds.), *Comprehensive neonatal nursing: A physiologic perspective*. Philadelphia: W.B. Saunders.

233. Answer: (**B**) Data about drug toxicities in adults and children are not necessarily relevant to the premature neonate. Premature and extremely premature neonates have immature organ systems that can be more susceptible or even more resistant to specific drug toxicities. Due to immaturity of the renal and liver systems, many drugs have prolonged half-lives in neonates.

REFERENCES

Kauffman, R.E. (1981). The clinical interpretation and application of drug concentration data. *Pediatric Clinics of North America, 28*, 35–45.

Sheiner, L.B. & Tozer, T.N. (1978). Clinical pharmacokinetics: The use of plasma concentrations of drugs (pp. 71–109). In K.L. Melmon, & H.F. Morelli. (eds.), *Clinical pharmacology: Basic principles in therapeutics* (2nd ed.). New York: Macmillan.

Ward, R.M. (1993). Neonatal pharmacology (pp. 926–939). In C. Kenner, A. Brueggemeyer, & L.P. Gunderson (eds.), *Comprehensive neonatal care: A physiologic perspective.* Philadelphia: W.B. Saunders.

234. Answer: (**A**) The gonads should be shielded whenever they are within 5 cm of the primary x-ray beam.

REFERENCES

Kirks, D.R. (1984). *Practical pediatric imaging.* Boston: Little, Brown.

Theorell, C.J. (1993). Diagnostic imaging (pp. 846–871). In C. Kenner, A. Brueggemeyer, & L.P. Gunderson (eds.), *Comprehensive neonatal nursing: A physiologic perspective.* Philadelphia: W.B. Saunders.

235. Answer: (**A**) Some individuals may get AIDS related complex (ARC). ARC is a term that was previously used to describe certain clusters of symptoms. The reason the term ARC is no longer used is due to the confusion that surrounds the term from a public health perspective. A more appropriate label is HIV-positive.

REFERENCES

Gunderson, L.P. & Gumm, B. (1993). Neonatal acquired immunodeficiency syndrome: Human immunodeficiency virus infection and acquired immunodeficiency syndrome in the infant (pp. 940–967). In C. Kenner, A. Brueggemeyer, & L.P. Gunderson (eds.), *Comprehensive neonatal care: A physiologic perspective.* Philadelphia: W.B. Saunders.

Institute of Medicine/National Academy of Sciences. (1988). Confronting AIDS: Update: 1988. *Journal of Acquired Immune Deficiency Syndromes, 1*(2), 173–186.

236. Answer: (**A**) Evaluation for localized bleeding or signs of hypotension resulting in changes in heart rate and blood pressure is essential. Assessment of the insertion site and affected extremity for bleeding, color, peripheral pulses, temperature, and capillary refill should continue for at least 24 hours after the procedure. Complications of the catheterization procedure include hypovolemia (as a result of bleeding or fluid loss during the procedure), infection, thrombosis, and tissue necrosis.

REFERENCES

Harjo, J. & Jones, M.A. (1993). Diagnostic tests and laboratory values (pp. 872–884). In C. Kenner, A. Brueggemeyer, & L.P. Gunderson (eds.), *Comprehensive neonatal nursing: A physiologic perspective.* Philadelphia: W.B. Saunders.

Long, W.A. (1990). *Fetal and neonatal cardiology.* Philadelphia: W.B. Saunders.

237. Answer: (**C**) Pain causes adverse physiologic effects in all major organ systems that can be life threatening in the acutely ill patient.

REFERENCES

Franck, L.S. (1993). Identification, management, and prevention of pain in the neonate (pp. 913–925). In C. Kenner, A. Brueggemeyer, & L.P. Gunderson (eds.), *Comprehensive neonatal nursing: A physiologic perspective.* Philadelphia: W.B. Saunders.

Kehlet, H. (1986). Pain relief and modification of the stress response (pp. 49–75). In M.J. Cousins & G.D. Phillips (eds.), *Acute pain management.* New York: Churchill Livingstone.

238. Answer: (**A**) HIV-exposed newborns in the delivery room do not differ from those neonates that are not HIV exposed. The recommendations for the management of the exposed neonate are the same as those that apply for all neonates. The amount of negative pressure for the mechanical device should be low to avoid tissue trauma that can break skin integrity.

REFERENCES

Gunderson, L.P. & Gumm, B. (1993). Neonatal acquired immunodeficiency syndrome: Human immunodeficiency virus infection and acquired immunodeficiency syndrome in the infant (pp. 940–967). In C. Kenner, A. Brueggemeyer, & L.P. Gunderson (eds.), *Comprehensive neonatal care: A physiologic perspective.* Philadelphia: W.B. Saunders.

Mendez, H. & Jule, J.E. (1990). Care of the infant born exposed to human immunodeficiency virus. *Obstetrics and Gynecology Clinics of North America,* 17(3), 637–649.

239. Answer: (**A**) To evaluate the position of the eyes, bring a noisy toy attached to a bright source of light near the

infant's face. Then note the location of the light reflex on the cornea. The light reflex should be near the center of the cornea in both eyes. This test is called the Hirschberg method (Pilliteri, 1981).

REFERENCES

Avery, G.B. (1987). *Neonatology: Pathophysiology and management of the newborn* (3rd ed.). Philadelphia: J.B. Lippincott.

Isenberg, S.J. (1989). How to examine the eyes of the neonate. *Focal Points: 1989: Clinical Modules for Ophthalmology, 7*(1), 1–6.

Pilliteri, A. (1981). *Maternal-newborn nursing*. Boston: Little, Brown.

Werner, R.B. & Werner, R. (1993). Assessment and management of ophthalmic dysfunction (pp. 809–820). In C. Kenner, A. Brueggemeyer, & L.P. Gunderson (eds.), *Comprehensive neonatal nursing: A physiologic perspective*. Philadelphia: W.B. Saunders.

240. Answer: (**C**) Great care must be taken in selecting dilating drops in these low-weight neonates. Systemic absorption of the eye drops, which is unavoidable to some extent, can cause severe reactions and even death. Excess eye drops that do not remain within the eyelids are easily absorbed through the porous skin of the newborn. The problem can be compounded by absorption of the drop from the nasolacrimal system and the nose. The safest combination for drops to dilate the pupil is the sympathomimetic drop of one percent phenylephrine hydrochloride and the parasympatholytic agent cyclopentolate hydrochloride 0.25 percent (Isenberg, 1989).

REFERENCES

Cohen, K.W. & Bryne, S.M. (1989). The role of the nurse in assisting with eye examinations on the premature infant. *Neonatal Network, 8*(2), 31–35.

Isenberg, S.J. (1989). How to examine the eyes of the neonate. *Focal Points: 1989: Clinical Modules for Ophthalmology, 7*(1), 1–6.

Werner, R.B. & Werner, R. (1993). Assessment and management of ophthalmic dysfunction (pp. 809–820). In C. Kenner, A. Brueggemeyer, & L.P. Gunderson (eds.), *Comprehensive neonatal nursing: A physiologic perspective*. Philadelphia: W.B. Saunders.

241. Answer: (**B**) Leukocoria is the descriptive term for a whitish-appearing pupil.

REFERENCES

Avery, G.B. (1987). *Neonatology: Pathophysiology and management of the newborn* (3rd ed.). Philadelphia: J.B. Lippincott.

Duane, T.D. & Jaeger, E.A. (1988). *Clinical ophthalmology* (Vols. 1, 2, 4, 5). Philadelphia: J.B. Lippincott.

Werner, R.B. & Werner, R. (1993). Assessment and management of ophthalmic dysfunction (pp. 809–820). In C. Kenner, A. Brueggemeyer, & L.P. Gunderson (eds.), *Comprehensive neonatal nursing: A physiologic perspective*. Philadelphia: W.B. Saunders.

242. Answer: (**B**) Leukocoria is the descriptive term for a whitish-appearing pupil. A differential diagnosis for the cause of leukocoria includes retinopathy of prematurity (ROP).

REFERENCES

Avery, G.B. (1987). *Neonatology: Pathophysiology and management of the newborn* (3rd ed.). Philadelphia: J.B. Lippincott.

Duane, T.D. & Jaeger, E.A. (1988). *Clinical ophthalmology* (Vols. 1, 2, 4, 5). Philadelphia: J.B. Lippincott.

Werner, R.B. & Werner, R. (1993). Assessment and management of ophthalmic dysfunction (pp. 809–820). In C. Kenner, A. Brueggemeyer, & L.P. Gunderson (eds.), *Comprehensive neonatal nursing: A physiologic perspective*. Philadelphia: W.B. Saunders.

243. Answer: (**C**) Development of ROP has been correlated with low birth weight, intraventricular hemorrhage, sepsis, and infants of multiple births as well as exposure to oxygen and prematurity. In rare cases, infants who have been exposed to supplemental oxygen have developed ROP (Hittner, 1981).

REFERENCES

Duane, T.D. & Jaeger, E.A. (1988). *Clinical ophthalmology* (Vols. 1, 2, 4, 5). Philadelphia: J.B. Lippincott.

Hittner, H. (1981). Retrolental fibroplasia: Efficacy of vitamin E in a double-blind clinical study of preterm infants. *New England Journal of Medicine, 305*, 1365–1371.

Long, C. (1989). Cryotherapy: A new treatment for retinopathy of prematurity. *Pediatric Nursing, 15*(3), 269–272.

Werner, R.B. & Werner, R. (1993). Assessment and management of ophthalmic dysfunction (pp. 809–820). In C. Kenner, A. Brueggemeyer, & L.P. Gunderson (eds.), *Comprehensive neonatal nursing: A physiologic perspective*. Philadelphia: W.B. Saunders.

244. Answer: (**A**) Infants with a birth weight of 2000 grams or less should receive a dilated fundus examination by an ophthalmologist four to five weeks after birth. Weekly examinations should follow this evaluation. All other low birth weight newborns and those who have been exposed to supplemental oxygen should receive a complete ophthalmic examination

eight weeks after birth (Isenberg, 1989).

REFERENCES

Duane, T.D. & Jaeger, E.A. (1988). *Clinical ophthalmology* (Vols. 1, 2, 4, 5). Philadelphia: J.B. Lippincott.

Isenberg, S.J. (1989). How to examine the eyes of the neonate. *Focal Points: 1989: Clinical Modules for Ophthalmology, 7*(1), 1–6.

Long, C. (1989). Cryotherapy: A new treatment for retinopathy of prematurity. *Pediatric Nursing, 15*(3), 269–272.

Werner, R.B. & Werner, R. (1993). Assessment and management of ophthalmic dysfunction (pp. 809–820). In C. Kenner, A. Brueggemeyer, & L.P. Gunderson (eds.), *Comprehensive neonatal nursing: A physiologic perspective.* Philadelphia: W.B. Saunders.

245. Answer: (**A**) Recent studies have shown that cryotherapy can have a beneficial effect on the reversal of abnormal blood vessel formation (Long, 1989). A probe cooled with liquid nitrogen is applied to the sclera externally over the area of abnormal blood vessels. The resultant scarring causes regression of the disease process. Retinal detachment surgery can be performed during the cicatricial stage of the disease. The results are not usually significant as far as visual improvement is concerned, and most of these eyes are blind.

REFERENCES

Duane, T.D. & Jaeger, E.A. (1988). *Clinical ophthalmology* (Vols. 1, 2, 4, 5). Philadelphia: J.B. Lippincott.

George, D.S., Stephen, S. Fellows, R.R., & Bremer, D.L. (1988). The latest on retinopathy of prematurity. *MCH, American Journal of Maternal Child Nursing, 13*(4), 254–258.

Heveston, E.M. & Ellis, F.D. (1980). *Pediatric ophthalmology practice.* St. Louis: C.V. Mosby.

Long, C. (1989). Cryotherapy: A new treatment for retinopathy of prematurity. *Pediatric Nursing, 15*(3), 269–272.

Werner, R.B. & Werner, R. (1993). Assessment and management of ophthalmic dysfunction (pp. 809–820). In C. Kenner, A. Brueggemeyer, & L.P. Gunderson (eds.), *Comprehensive neonatal nursing: A physiologic perspective.* Philadelphia: W.B. Saunders.

246. Answer: (**C**) A barium enema is used to evaluate the structure and function of the large intestine. The diagnosis of disorders such as Hirschsprung's disease and meconium plug syndrome can easily be supported by using this procedure. Evaluation of the bowel is essential after this procedure to prevent constipation or obstruction. Assessment of bowel elimination is an important nursing concern after barium enema.

REFERENCES

Gomella, T.L., Cunningham, M.D., & Eyal, F.G. (1992). *Neonatology: Management, procedures, on-call problems, diseases, drugs.* Norwalk, CT: Appleton & Lange.

Harjo, J. & Jones, M.A. (1993). Diagnostic tests and laboratory values (pp. 872–884). In C. Kenner, A. Brueggemeyer, & L.P. Gunderson (eds.), *Comprehensive neonatal nursing: A physiologic perspective.* Philadelphia: W.B. Saunders.

Streeter, N.S. (1986). *High risk neonatal care.* Gaithersburg, MD: Aspen Publishers.

247. Answer (**B**) At birth infants possess a well-developed pituitary–adrenal axis and can mount a fight-or-flight stress response with production of catecholamines just as the adult human.

REFERENCES

Anand, K.J.S. & Carr, D.B. (1989). The neuroanatomy, neurophysiology, and neurochemistry of pain, stress, and analgesia in newborns and children. *Pediatric Clinics of North America, 36,* 795–822.

Franck, L.S. (1991). *Pain control in critical care nursing.* Gaithersburg, MD: Aspen Publishers.

Franck, L.S. (1993). Identification, management, and prevention of pain in the neonate (pp. 913–925). In C. Kenner, A. Brueggemeyer, & L.P. Gunderson (eds.), *Comprehensive neonatal nursing: A physiologic perspective.* Philadelphia: W.B. Saunders.

248. Answer: (**A**) Fluoroscopic imaging is a radiologic technique used to evaluate the motion of an organ system.

REFERENCES

Fanaroff, A.A. & Martin, R.J. (eds.), (1992). *Neonatal-perinatal medicine* (5th ed.). St. Louis: C.V. Mosby.

Gyll, C. & Blake, N. (1986). *Pediatric diagnostic imaging.* London: William Heinemann Medical Books.

Haller, J.O. & Slovis, T.L. (1984). *Introduction to radiology in clinical pediatrics.* Chicago: Year Book Medical Publishers.

Kirks, D.R. (1984). *Practical pediatric imaging.* Boston: Little, Brown.

Swischuk, L.E. (1984). *Imaging of the newborn, infant, and young child* (3rd ed.). Baltimore: Williams & Wilkins.

Theorell, C.J. (1993). Diagnostic imaging (pp. 846–871). In C. Kenner, A. Brueggemeyer, & L.P. Gunderson (eds.), *Comprehensive neonatal nursing: A physiologic perspective.* Philadelphia: W.B. Saunders.

249. Answer: (**B**) A ground wire will not protect from excessive current flow through the body if the patient or caretaker completes an electrical connection between both conductors of a high-voltage supply line. Current flow through the body depends on the volt-

age source and the resistance of the body.

REFERENCES

Donnelly, M.M. (1993). Monitoring neonatal biophysical parameters (pp. 823–845). In C. Kenner, A. Brueggemeyer, & L.P. Gunderson (eds.), *Comprehensive neonatal nursing: A physiologic perspective*. Philadelphia: W.B. Saunders.

Gomella, T.L., Cunningham, M.D., & Eyal, F.G. (1992). *Neonatology: Management, procedures, on-call problems, diseases, drugs*. Norwalk, CT: Appleton & Lange.

250. Answer: (**B**) Core temperature is one of the most important indicators of the health status of newborns. Rectal temperature measurement using mercury-in-glass thermometers is gradually being replaced by electronic thermometers, which are inexpensive and prevent cross-contamination.

REFERENCES

Donnelly, M.M. (1993). Monitoring neonatal biophysical parameters (pp. 823–845). In C. Kenner, A. Brueggemeyer, & L.P. Gunderson (eds.), *Comprehensive neonatal nursing: A physiologic perspective*. Philadelphia: W.B. Saunders.

Gomella, T.L., Cunningham, M.D., & Eyal, F.G. (1992). *Neonatology: Management, procedures, on-call problems, diseases, drugs*. Norwalk, CT: Appleton & Lange.

251. Answer: (**B**) The selection of a particular imaging examination should be based on the inherent patient risk, the likelihood that the examination will establish or refute the diagnosis, the potential benefit to the patient, and the risk of liability if the examination is requested or if the examination is not requested.

REFERENCES

Haller, J.O. & Slovis, T.L. (1984). *Introduction to radiology in clinical pediatrics*. Chicago: Year Book Medical Publishers.

Juhl, J.H. & Crummy, A.B. (eds.). (1987). *Paul and Juhl's essentials of radiologic imaging* (5th ed.). Philadelphia: J.B. Lippincott.

Kirks, D.R. (1984). *Practical pediatric imaging*. Boston: Little, Brown.

Squire, L.F. & Novelline, R.A. (1988). *Fundamentals of radiology* (4th ed.). Cambridge: Harvard University Press.

Theorell, C.J. (1993). Diagnostic imaging (pp. 846–871). In C. Kenner, A. Brueggemeyer, & L.P. Gunderson (eds.), *Comprehensive neonatal nursing: A physiologic perspective*. Philadelphia: W.B. Saunders.

252. Answer: (**B**) Cord care should involve the use of antimicrobial agents such as triple dye or bacitracin.

REFERENCES

Gunderson, L.P. & Gumm, B. (1993). Neonatal acquired immunodeficiency syndrome: Human immunodeficiency virus infection and acquired immunodeficiency syndrome in the infant (pp. 940–967). In C. Kenner, A. Brueggemeyer, & L.P. Gunderson (eds.), *Comprehensive neonatal care: A physiologic perspective*. Philadelphia: W.B. Saunders.

Mendez, H. & Jule, J.E. (1990). Care of the infant born exposed to human immunodeficiency virus. *Obstetrics and Gynecology Clinics of North America,* 17(3), 637–649.

253. Answer: (**A**) Parents of NICU infants played a role in creating the imperative for pain management for infants. They advocated the use of anesthetics during surgery on infants, a practice that was not the standard of care even as late as the middle 1980s.

REFERENCES

Franck, L.S. (1993). Identification, management, and prevention of pain in the neonate (pp. 913–925). In C. Kenner, A. Brueggemeyer, & L.P. Gunderson (eds.), *Comprehensive neonatal nursing: A physiologic perspective*. Philadelphia: W.B. Saunders.

Lawson, J.R. (1988). Pain in the neonate and fetus. *New England Journal of Medicine, 318,* 1398.

Shearer, M.H. (1986). Surgery on the paralyzed, unanesthetized newborn. *Birth, 15,* 36–38.

254. Answer: (**C**) Infants and children should be immunized according to the American Academy of Pediatrics recommendations. The AAP recommends that the diphtheria, tetanus, and pertussis (DTP); inactivated polio (IP); measles, mumps, rubella (MMR); and *Haemophilus influenzae b* (Hib) vaccines be administered to infants and children who are known to be either asymptomatic or symptomatic.

REFERENCES

American Academy of Pediatrics (AAP). (1988). *Report of the Committee on Infectious Disease.* (21st ed., pp. 91–115). Elk Grove, IL: Author.

American Academy of Pediatrics and American College of Obstetricians and Gynecologists. (1988). Guidelines for perinatal care (2nd ed.). Elk Grove, IL: American Academy of Pediatrics.

Gunderson, L.P. & Gumm, B. (1993). Neonatal acquired immunodeficiency syndrome: Human immunodeficiency virus infection and acquired immunodeficiency syndrome in the infant (pp. 940–967). In C. Kenner, A. Brueggemeyer, & L.P. Gunderson (eds.), *Comprehensive neonatal care: A physiologic perspective*. Philadelphia: W.B. Saunders.

Mendez, H. & Jule, J.E. (1990). Care of the infant born exposed to human immunodeficiency virus. *Obstetrics and Gynecology Clinics of North America,* 17(3), 637–649.

255. Answer: (**B**) Mask ventilation is contraindicated when a tracheoesophageal fistula with esophageal atresia is present. Rupture of the esophageal pouch and overdistention of the stomach could occur. As a result, reflux of stomach contents can occur through the fistula into the trachea, causing pneumonia. Proper positioning of the endotracheal tube, if needed, and the use of minimal ventilator pressure will minimize these complications.

REFERENCES

Harjo, J. & Jones, M.A. (1993). The surgical neonate (pp. 903–912). In C. Kenner, A. Brueggemeyer, & L.P. Gunderson (eds.), *Comprehensive neonatal nursing: A physiologic perspective.* Philadelphia: W.B. Saunders.

Kenner, C., Brueggemeyer, A., & Harjo, J. (1988). *Neonatal surgery: A nursing perspective.* Orlando, FL: Grune & Stratton.

256. Answer: (**A**) In the infant, the manifestations of the signs and symptoms of HIV can range from subclinical, mild moderate, and severe. Symptoms usually do not present as a single entity; instead, manifestations of HIV involve multiple organ systems. The multiple organ involvement leads to progressive clinical deterioration and, eventually, immune dysfunction, opportunistic infections, and secondary cancers.

REFERENCES

Gunderson, L.P. & Gumm, B. (1993). Neonatal acquired immunodeficiency syndrome: Human immunodeficiency virus infection and acquired immunodeficiency syndrome in the infant (pp. 940–967). In C. Kenner, A. Brueggemeyer, & L.P. Gunderson (eds.), *Comprehensive neonatal care: A physiologic perspective.* Philadelphia: W.B. Saunders.

Mendez, H. & Jule, J.E. (1990). Care of the infant born exposed to human immunodeficiency virus. *Obstetrics and Gynecology Clinics of North America,* 17(3), 637–649.

257. Answer: (**A**) Pregnant women are more sensitive to inhalation anesthetics because their endorphin level is elevated, therefore they are more susceptible to overdosing. Regional anesthetics also require special attention, because with the increase in femoral venous and intra-abdominal pressure, the epidural veins are enlarged, which decreases the epidural space, thus decreasing the amount of anesthetic needed.

REFERENCES

Bergman, K., Kenner, C., Levine, A.H., & Inturrisi, M. (1993). Fetal therapy (pp. 887–902). In C. Kenner, A. Brueggemeyer, & L.P. Gunderson (eds.), *Comprehensive neonatal nursing: A physiologic perspective.* Philadelphia: W.B. Saunders.

Harrison, M.R., Golbus, M.S., & Filly, R.A. (1989). *The unborn patient: Prenatal diagnosis and treatment.* Orlando, FL: Grune & Stratton.

258. Answer: (**A**) Respiratory infections such as *Pneumocystis carinii* are the most common type of infection contracted by the HIV-infected infant.

REFERENCES

Gunderson, L.P. & Gumm, B. (1993). Neonatal acquired immunodeficiency syndrome: Human immunodeficiency virus infection and acquired immunodeficiency syndrome in the infant (pp. 940–967). In C. Kenner, A. Brueggemeyer, & L.P. Gunderson (eds.), *Comprehensive neonatal care: A physiologic perspective.* Philadelphia: W.B. Saunders.

Mendez, H. & Jule, J.E. (1990). Care of the infant born exposed to human immunodeficiency virus. *Obstetrics and Gynecology Clinics of North America,* 17(3), 637–649.

Harrison, C.J. (1990). Pediatric AIDS: Pediatric Grand Rounds, March 8, 1990. Cincinnati, Children's Hospital Medical Center.

Hart, C., Schoechetman, G., & Spira, T. (1988). Direct detection of HIV RNA expression in seropositive subjects. *Lancet, 2,* 596–599.

259. Answer: (**C**) Electroencephalogram examination records the electrical activity of the brain. Numerous electrodes are placed at precise locations on the infant's head to record electrical impulses from various parts of the brain. This procedure can be important in diagnosing lesions or tumors, identifying nonfunctional areas of the brain, or pinpointing the focus of seizure activity.

REFERENCES

Gomella, T.L., Cunningham, M.D., & Eyal, F.G. (1992). *Neonatology: Management, procedures, oncall problems, diseases, drugs.* Norwalk, CT: Appleton & Lange.

Harjo, J. & Jones, M.A. (1993). Diagnostic tests and laboratory values (pp. 872–884). In C. Kenner, A. Brueggemeyer, & L.P. Gunderson (eds.), *Comprehensive neonatal nursing: A physiologic perspective.* Philadelphia: W.B. Saunders.

260. Answer: (**C**) The role of myelin as insulation, affecting the speed of impulse conduction and not necessary for nerve function, has been proven. However, it was not until the discovery that as many as 80 percent of the

fibers that transmit pain information in the adult remain unmyelinated.

REFERENCES

Franck, L.S. (1993). Identification, management, and prevention of pain in the neonate (pp. 913–925). In C. Kenner, A. Brueggemeyer, & L.P. Gunderson (eds.), *Comprehensive neonatal nursing: A physiologic perspective*. Philadelphia: W.B. Saunders.

Price, D.D. & Dubner, R. (1977). Neurons that subserve the sensory-discriminative aspects of pain. *Pain, 3,* 307–338.

Schulte, F.C. (1975). Neurophysiological aspects of brain development. *Mead-Johnson Symposia on Perinatal Development, 6,* 34–47.

261. Answer: (**B**) The use of expert systems present some concerns for the nursing profession. Several authors caution that nurses must not see the computer as having reasoning skills superior to their own. As dependence on computer systems grows, there is a tendency for users to be unaware of the criteria or logic of the program's algorithms (decision pathways). Nurses must understand clearly that expert systems can supplement but never replace their own knowledge and expertise.

Reference information, communication of policies and changes in procedures as well as other routine communication are facilitated by use of computer. NICU nurse managers are often frustrated by the difficulty in communicating with a large and increasingly part-time nursing staff. Use of computer applications (i.e., electronic mail, on-line reference information, remote access from home, etc.) can improve communication and ensure all staff receive information and have the opportunity to participate in unit planning and decision making. Nurses participating in QI monitoring must ensure that the data represent important aspects of patient care outcome and are meaningful to the practice of nursing.

REFERENCES

Andreoli, K. & Musser, L.A. (1985). Computers in nursing care: The state of the art. *Nursing Outlook, 33,* 16–21.

Franck, L.S. (1993). Use of computers in neonatal nursing (pp. 1034–1045). In C. Kenner, A. Brueggemeyer, & L.P. Gunderson (eds.), *Comprehensive neonatal care: A physiologic perspective*. Philadelphia: W.B. Saunders.

Greer, J. & Hexum, J. (1987). Dimensions of computerized quality assurance systems. *Journal of Nursing Quality Assurance, 1*(4), 9–14.

Joint Commission on Accreditation of Hospitals. (1990). *Accreditation manual for hospitals*. Oakbrook Terrace, IL; JCAHO.

Sinclair, V.G. (1988). High technology in critical care: Implications for nursing's role and practice. *Focus on Critical Care, 15*(4), 36–41.

Tamarisk, N.K. (1982). The computer as a clinical tool. *Nursing Management, 13*(8), 46–49.

262. Answer: (**A**) Pharmacologic intervention is indicated if there has been (1) weight loss from gastrointestinal symptoms and/or hyperactivity associated with withdrawal; (2) inability of the infant to rest; (3) fever unrelated to infection; or (4) seizures. Paregoric is the drug of choice as it improves the sucking ability and is correlated with a weight gain. Paregoric is an opiate and provides direct relief by its cross-dependence with heroin. It also exerts a direct effect on the gastrointestinal system to reduce diarrhea. Another drug that may help is Valium. However, Valium depresses sucking, heart rate, and respirations and is contraindicated with an infant who is jaundiced. Late onset seizures after Valium's discontinuance have been reported. Phenobarbital also can be used to ease irritability. However, it has little effect on relieving the vomiting and diarrhea and may depress sucking and cause the infant to be sedated. Care should be taken to maintain universal isolation precautions as there is an increased incidence of hepatitis and HIV among the women and their infants.

REFERENCES

Chasnoff, I. (1988). Newborn infants with drug withdrawal symptoms. *Pediatrics in Review, 9*(9), 273–277.

Flandermeyer, A.A. (1993). The drug-exposed neonate (pp. 997–1033). In C. Kenner, A. Brueggemeyer, & L.P. Gunderson (eds.), *Comprehensive neonatal care: A physiologic perspective*. Philadelphia: W.B. Saunders.

Schneider, J. & Chasnoff, I. (1987) Cocaine abuse during pregnancy: Its effects on infant motor development-A clinical perspective. *Topics in Acute Care, Trauma, & Rehabilitation, 2*(1), 59–69.

263. Answer: (**A**) Closed procedures (percutaneous, catheter placements) carry fewer risks to the mother but may be less beneficial to the fetus. The risks to the mother undergoing a closed proce-

dure include minor discomfort (procedure is done under local and intravenous sedation with a narcotic or benzodiazepine); preterm labor (mild to moderate, usually amenable to bed rest or oral tocolytic agents, or both); premature rupture of membranes (infrequent); and chorioamnionitis (infrequent but would require premature delivery). The risks to the fetus include injury to a fetal part (done under ultrasonographic guidance) and lack of successful placement owing to fetal position or dislodging of catheter from the fetal bladder by fetal movement during or after the procedure. Open procedures (hysterotomy) carry greater risks to the mother and the fetus yet if successful result in amelioration of the in utero condition. Maternal risks include those of general anesthesia and cesarean section. In addition, there is the risk of premature rupture of membranes, chorioamnionitis, and preterm labor.

REFERENCES

Bergman, K., Kenner, C., Levine, A.H., & Inturrisi, M. (1993). Fetal therapy (pp. 887–902). In C. Kenner, A. Brueggemeyer, & L.P. Gunderson (eds.), *Comprehensive neonatal nursing: A physiologic perspective.* Philadelphia: W.B. Saunders.

Harrison, M.R., Golbus, M.S., & Filly, R.A. (1989). *The unborn patient: Prenatal diagnosis and treatment.* Orlando, FL: Grune & Stratton.

264. Answer: (**A**) Potential for the technology to redesign nursing workflow and restructure nursing priorities is great. Early studies of computerized nursing documentation systems are promising. The ultimate advancement is for computers to possess artificial intelligence (the ability to learn) to actually make decisions. The other advance is to have computer technology at the "point of care," the bedside.

REFERENCES

Duncan, R.G. & Pomerance, J.J. (1982). Computer assistance in delivery of patient care in a neonatal intensive care unit (pp. 337–351). In T.R. Harris & J.P. Bahr (eds.), *The uses of computers in perinatal medicine.* New York: Praeger.

Franck, L.S. (1993). Use of computers in neonatal nursing (pp. 1034–1045). In C. Kenner, A. Brueggemeyer, & L.P. Gunderson (eds.), *Comprehensive neonatal care: A physiologic perspective.* Philadelphia: W.B. Saunders.

Harper, R.G., Carrera, E., Weiss, S., & Luongo, M. (1985). A complete computerized program for nutritional management in the neonatal intensive care nursery. *Journal of Perinatology, 2*(2), 161–162.

Prophet, C.M. (1989). Patient care planning: An interdisciplinary approach (pp. 827–833). In L. Kingsland (ed.), *Proceedings, Thirteenth annual symposium on computer applications in medical care.* Washington, DC: IEEE Computer Society Press.

Simpson, R.L. (1991). The joint commission did what you wouldn't. *Nursing Management, 22*(10), 26–27.

Thomas, L.W. (1987). Computerized order calculation and label generation for neonatal parenteral nutrient solutions. *Journal of Medical Systems, 12*(2), 115–120.

265. Answer: (**C**) Third-spacing of fluids, or capillary leak syndrome, is a result of the trauma to the GI system in which the capillary membrane permeability is changed. The body's compensatory response to this trauma is a movement of fluid across this "leaky" membrane. Fluid moves out of the vascular compartment and into the tissues. The infant becomes swollen with generalized ascites.

REFERENCES

Harjo, J. & Jones, M.A. (1993). The surgical neonate (pp. 903–912). In C. Kenner, A. Brueggemeyer, & L.P. Gunderson (eds.), *Comprehensive neonatal nursing: A physiologic perspective.* Philadelphia: W.B. Saunders.

Kenner, C., Brueggemeyer, A., & Harjo, J. (1988). *Neonatal surgery: A nursing perspective.* Orlando, FL: Grune & Stratton.

266. Answer: (**B**) Dysmorphic characteristics of FAS include a series of facial anomalies, abnormal palmar creases, and congenital heart disease. Facial anomalies include microcephaly, short palpebral fissures, flat midface, indistinct philtrum, thin upper lip, epicanthal folds, low nasal bridge, minor ear anomalies, short nose, and micrognathia (Streissguth, Clarren, & Jones, 1985). A quantifiable result of FAS is cognitive impairment. Cognitive impairment can be categorized as (1) minimally brain damaged, (2) mildly to moderately retarded, and (3) severely to profoundly retarded.

REFERENCES

Flandermeyer, A.A. (1993). The drug-exposed neonate (pp. 997–1033). In C. Kenner, A. Brueggemeyer, & L.P. Gunderson (eds.), *Comprehensive neonatal care: A physiologic perspective.* Philadelphia: W.B. Saunders.

Harwood, H. & Napolitano, D. (1985). Economic implications of the fetal alcohol syndrome. *Alcohol Health and Research World,* Fall, 38–43.

Streissguth, A., Clarren, S., & Jones, K. (1985). A natural history of the fetal alcohol syndrome: A 10-year follow-up of 11 patients. *Alcohol Health and Research World,* Fall, 13–19.

267. Answer: (**A, B, & C**) Fear of addiction and disproportionate concern for side effects have resulted in severe underutilization of narcotic analgesics for acute postoperative pain. Assessment criteria must be standardized and tested for reliability and validity in various subpopulations of neonates.

REFERENCES

Franck, L.S. (1993). Identification, management, and prevention of pain in the neonate (pp. 913–925). In C. Kenner, A. Brueggemeyer, & L.P. Gunderson (eds.), *Comprehensive neonatal nursing: A physiologic perspective.* Philadelphia: W.B. Saunders.

Schechter, N.L. (1989). The undertreatment of pain in children: An overview. *Pediatric Clinics of North America, 36*(4), 781–794.

268. Answer: (**B**) Glucose metabolism may be altered as a response to surgery. Dextrostix should be monitored every one to two hours after surgery.

REFERENCES

Harjo, J. & Jones, M.A. (1993). The surgical neonate (pp. 903–912). In C. Kenner, A. Brueggemeyer, & L.P. Gunderson (eds.), *Comprehensive neonatal nursing: A physiologic perspective.* Philadelphia: W.B. Saunders.

Kenner, C., Harjo, J., & Brueggemeyer, A. (1988). *Neonatal surgery: A nursing perspective.* Orlando: Grune & Stratton.

269. Answer: (**A**) Environmental stimuli are problems for the VLBW. Strategies to developmentally support these infants include reduce light (cover all bedsides, tablebeds, cribs, etc., with dark cloths or covers), reduce noise (implement quiet hour and post signs at bedside to remind staff; pad trash cans, doors, drawers; pad loudspeakers at bedside).

REFERENCES

Blackburn, S.T. & VandenBerg, K.A. (1993). Assessment and management of neonatal neurobehavioral development (pp. 1094–1133). In C. Kenner, A. Brueggemeyer, & L.P. Gunderson (eds.), *Comprehensive neonatal care: A physiologic perspective.* Philadelphia: W.B. Saunders.

VandenBerg, K.A. (1990). Behaviorally supportive care for the extremely premature infant. In L.P. Gunderson & C. Kenner (eds.), *Care of the 24–25 gestational age infant (small baby protocol).* Petaluma, CA: Neonatal Network.

270. Answer: (**C**) Many complications after liver transplantation are heralded by an increase in hepatocellular enzymes, often associated with malaise, fever, leukocytosis, and jaundice. This clinical picture defines hepatic allograft dysfunction but does not separate allograft rejection from other allograft complications such as primary nonfunction, bile duct abnormalities, hepatic artery thrombosis, or allograft infection.

REFERENCES

A-Kader, H.H., Ryckman, F.C., & Balistreri, W.F. (1991). Liver transplantation in the pediatric population: Indications and monitoring. *Clinical Transplant, 5,* 161.

Ryckman, F.C. & Pedersen, S.H. (1993). Hepatic and renal transplantation in infants and children (pp. 968–980). In C. Kenner, A. Brueggemeyer, & L.P. Gunderson (eds.), *Comprehensive neonatal care: A physiologic perspective.* Philadelphia: W.B. Saunders.

Ryckman, F.C., Schroeder, T.J., Pedersen, S.H., Fisher, R.A., Farrell, M.K., Heubi, J.E., Ziegler, M.M., & Balistreri, W.F. (1991). The use of monoclonal immunosuppressive therapy in pediatric renal and liver transplantation. *Clinical Transplantation, 5,* 189.

Starzl, T.E. & Demetris, A.J. (1990). Liver transplantation. A 31-year perspective. Part III. In S.A. Wells, Jr. (ed.), *Current problems in surgery.* Chicago: Year Book Medical Publishers.

Todo, S., Fung, J.J., Starzl, T.E., Tzakis, A., Demetris, A.J., Kormos, R. Jain, A., Alessiani, M., Takaya, S., & Shapiro, R. (1990). Liver kidney, and thoracic organ transplantation under FK 506. *Annals of Surgery, 212,* 295–307.

271. Answer: (**B**) The term neonatal abstinence syndrome was coined due to the consistent pattern of symptoms. The triad of findings among heroin-exposed infants are SGA, CNS, and GI symptoms. CNS symptomatology is the first to appear and includes such behaviors as hyperactivity, irritability, tremors, high-pitched cry, hypertonicity, and convulsions.

REFERENCES

Boobis, S. & Sullivan, F. (1986). Effects of life-style on reproduction (pp. 373–425). In S. Fabro & A. Sciall (eds.), *Drug and chemical action in pregnancy: Pharmacologic and toxicologic principles.* New York: Marcel Dekker.

Flandermeyer, A.A. (1993). The drug-exposed neonate (pp. 997–1033). In C. Kenner, A. Brueggemeyer, & L.P. Gunderson (eds.), *Comprehensive neonatal care: A physiologic perspective.* Philadelphia: W.B. Saunders.

Glass, L. & Evans, H. (1977). Physiological effects of intrauterine exposure to narcotics (pp. 108–115). In J.L. Rementeria (ed.), *Drug abuse in pregnancy and neonatal effects.* St. Louis: C.V. Mosby.

Glass, L., Rajegowda, B., & Evans, H. (1971). Absence of respiratory distress syndrome in the premature infants of heroin-addicted mothers. *Lancet, 2,* 685.
Naeye, R., Blanc, W., LeBlanc, W., & Khatamee, M. (1973). Fetal complications of maternal heroin addiction: Abnormal growth, infections, and episodes of stress. *Journal of Pediatrics, 83*(96), 1055–1061.
Phillips, K. (1986). Neonatal drug addicts. *Nursing Times,* March, 19, 36–38.
Reddy, A., Harper, R., & Stern, G. (1971). Observations on heroin and methadone withdrawal in the newborn. *Pediatrics, 48*(3), 353–358.
Zelson, C., Rubio, E., & Wasserman, E. (1971). Neonatal narcotic addiction: 10 year observation. *Pediatrics, 48*(2), 178–189.

272. Answer: (**B**) The process of neuronal competition for synaptic connections (particularly during the third trimester) results in a large amount of cell death and remodeling of the neuronal structure.

REFERENCES

Franck, L.S. (1993). Identification, management, and prevention of pain in the neonate (pp. 913–925). In C. Kenner, A. Brueggemeyer, & L.P. Gunderson (eds.), *Comprehensive neonatal nursing: A physiologic perspective.* Philadelphia: W.B. Saunders.
Volpe, J.J. (1987). Neuronal proliferation, migration, organization and myelination. *Neurology of the newborn* (2nd ed.). Philadelphia: W.B. Saunders.

273. Answer: (**B**) After a period of use of specialized formula for low birth weight infants, reports began to surface about the formation of lactobezoars in these infants. The lactobezoar formed in the gastrointestinal tract of premature infants and created large, hard curds that in serious cases had to be surgically removed. When formula companies changed to whey-predominant premature formula, this problem was essentially eliminated (Tsang & Nichols, 1988). This bezoar formation was a direct result of intolerance to the formula ingredients by some premature infants.

REFERENCES

Bassen, J.I. (1986). From problem reporting to technological solutions. *Medical Instrumentation, 20,* 17–26.
Golonka, L. (1986). Trends in health care and use of technology by nurses. *Medical Instrumentation, 20,* 8–10.
Jelliffe, E.F.P. (1977). Infant feeding practices: Associated iatrogenic and commerciogenic diseases. *Pediatric Clinics of North America, 24,* 49–61.
Lefrak-Okikawa, L. (1993). Iatrogenic complications of the neonatal intensive care unit (pp. 981–996). In C. Kenner, A. Brueggemeyer, & L.P. Gunderson (eds.), *Comprehensive neonatal care: A physiologic perspective.* Philadelphia: W.B. Saunders.

274. Answer: (**A**) Assessment of splenic sequestration of blood components can be recognized by leukopenia, thrombocytopenia, or anemia. Most will resolve with transplantation and portal hypertension reversal. When severe leukopenia (white blood cell count <3000) or thrombocytopenia (platelet count <50,000) occurs, splenectomy may be necessary at the time of transplantation. This is very rarely, if ever, necessary in infants and small children owing to the increased risks of sepsis and the likelihood of resolution after transplantation. Dietary salt restriction, caloric support, and occasional albumin supplementation in association with diuretics are used to control ascites.

REFERENCES

A-Kader, H.H., Ryckman, F.C., & Balistreri, W.F. (1991). Liver transplantation in the pediatric population: Indications and monitoring. *Clinical Transplant, 5,* 161.
Kalayoglu, M., Stratta, R.J., Sollinger, H.W., Hoffmann, R.M., D'Alessandro, A.M., Pirsch, J.D. & Belzer, F.O. (1989). Liver transplantation in infants and children. *Journal of Pediatric Surgery, 24,* 70–76.
Ryckman, F.C. & Pedersen, S.H. (1993). Hepatic and renal transplantation in infants and children (pp. 968–980). In C. Kenner, A. Brueggemeyer, & L.P. Gunderson (eds.), *Comprehensive neonatal care: A physiologic perspective.* Philadelphia: W.B. Saunders.

275. Answer: (**B**) Positioning of the sick or immature infant includes consideration of the effects of gravity along with neuromuscular characteristics such as variable weak muscle tone and decreased flexion in the limbs, trunk, and pelvis. These infants are at risk for positioning disorders such as widely abducted hips (frog-leg position), retracted and abducted shoulders, ankle and foot eversion, increased neck extension with a right-sided head preference, and increased trunk extension with arching of the neck and back. These positioning disorders affect later development because of their impact on the ability of the child to bear weight, bring the shoulders forward and hands to midline, and rotate the head. Therefore, in addition to improved physiologic status, developmental goals of positioning

include enhancement of flexion in the limbs and trunk, extensor balance, and facilitation of midline skills.

REFERENCES

Blackburn, S.T. & VandenBerg, K.A. (1993). Assessment and management of neonatal neurobehavioral development (pp. 1094–1133). In C. Kenner, A. Brueggemeyer, & L.P. Gunderson (eds.), *Comprehensive neonatal care: A physiologic perspective.* Philadelphia: W.B. Saunders.

Updike, C., Schmidt, R.E., Macke, C., Cahoon, J., & Miller, M. (1986). Positional support for premature infants. *American Journal of Occupational Therapy, 40,* 712–715.

276. Answer: (**A**) During pregnancy, maternal heroin ingestion creates a passive fetal addiction. When the mother's heroin supply is erratic or if she tries to "kick the habit," the fetus mirrors its mother's withdrawal response. Withdrawal symptoms of an adult consist of irritability, anxiety, tremulousness, and abdominal cramping. The fetus, too, becomes agitated, which expends energy and increases oxygen demands. However, during this time of enhanced metabolic needs, there is an actual reduction in uteroplacental exchange secondary to uterine cramping. This results in fetal hypoxia, which in turn induces deep breathing movements and fetal straining. During straining, meconium can be passed and subsequently aspirated. This has been deduced from an increased incidence of aspiration pneumonia and meconium aspiration.

REFERENCES

Connaughton, J., Finnegan, L., Schut, J., & Emich, J. (1975). Current concepts in the management of the pregnant opiate addict. *Addictive Diseases: An International Journal, 2*(1), 21–35.

Flandermeyer, A.A. (1993). The drug-exposed neonate (pp. 997–1033). In C. Kenner, A. Brueggemeyer, & L.P. Gunderson (eds.), *Comprehensive neonatal care: A physiologic perspective.* Philadelphia: W.B. Saunders.

Ostrea, E. & Chavez, C. (1979). Perinatal problems (excluding neonatal withdrawal) in maternal drug addiction: A study of 830 cases. *Journal of Pediatrics, 94*(2), 292–295.

277. Answer: (**B**) A systematic review of unusual incidents can determine what led to a particular complication. Another way to assist in the reduction of human error is to inform the staff about mistakes that have been made by others. To accomplish this, managers and QA/QI committee members must share information about errors.

REFERENCES

Bassen, J.I. (1986). From problem reporting to technological solutions. *Medical Instrumentation, 20,* 17–26.

Golonka, L. (1986). Trends in health care and use of technology by nurses. *Medical Instrumentation, 20,* 8–10.

Lefrak-Okikawa, L. (1993). Iatrogenic complications of the neonatal intensive care unit (pp. 981–996). In C. Kenner, A. Brueggemeyer, & L.P. Gunderson (eds.), *Comprehensive neonatal care: A physiologic perspective.* Philadelphia: W.B. Saunders.

Raju, T.N., Thornton, J.P., Kecskes, S., Perry, M., & Geldman, S. (1989). Medication errors in neonatal and paediatric intensive-care units. *Lancet, 2,* 374–376.

278. Answer: (**A**) Potential complications of cocaine specific to pregnancy are spontaneous abortion, increased rate of placental abruption associated with stillbirths, and elevated incidence of prematurity. Cocaine has been implicated as inducing placental vasoconstriction associated with an abrupt hypertensive episode, precipitating placental separation from the uterine lining. Once this occurs, there is a significant incidence of associated fetal death, thus contributing to the reported number of stillbirths.

REFERENCES

Acker, D., Sachs, B., Tracey, K., & Wise, W. (1983). Abruptio placentae associated with cocaine use. *American Journal of Obstetrics & Gynecology, 146*(2), 220–221.

Chasnoff, I., Burns, W., Schnoll, S., & Burns, K. (1985). Cocaine use in pregnancy. *New England Journal of Medicine, 313*(11), 660–669.

Chasnoff, I., Burns, K., & Burns, W. (1987). Cocaine use in pregnancy: Perinatal morbidity and mortality. *Neurotoxicology and Teratology, 9*(4), 291–293.

Flandermeyer, A.A. (1993). The drug-exposed neonate (pp. 997–1033). In C. Kenner, A. Brueggemeyer, & L.P. Gunderson (eds.), *Comprehensive neonatal care: A physiologic perspective.* Philadelphia: W.B. Saunders.

MacGregor, S., Keith, L., Chasnoff, I., Rosner, M., Chisum, G., Shaw, P., & Minogue, J. (1987). Cocaine use during pregnancy: Adverse perinatal outcome. *American Journal of Obstetrics and Gynecology, 157*(3), 686–690.

Oro, A. & Dixon, S. (1987). Perinatal cocaine and methamphetamine exposure: Maternal and neonatal correlates. *Journal of Pediatrics, 11*(4), 571–578.

Townsend, R., Laing, F., & Jeffrey, Jr., B. (1988). Placental abruption associated with cocaine abuse. *AJR, 150*(6), 1339–1340.

279. Answer: (**A**) Boarder babies present different challenges for nurses. They do not usually require intensive medical

care, and the focus shifts to normalizing their environment and fostering growth and development. Some problems boarder babies encounter in the hospital are nosocomial infections with resistant organisms, fresh air deprivation, inappropriate developmental stimulation, and inappropriate housing (environmental light, sounds, and smells).

REFERENCES

Boarder Babies: Winning the Battle. (1991, January-February). *Discharge Planning Update,* p. 15.

Gunderson, L.P. & Gumm, B. (1993). Neonatal acquired immunodeficiency syndrome: Human immunodeficiency virus infection and acquired immunodeficiency syndrome in the infant (pp. 940–967). In C. Kenner, A. Brueggemeyer, & L.P. Gunderson (eds.), *Comprehensive neonatal care: A physiologic perspective.* Philadelphia: W.B. Saunders.

Mendez, H. & Jule, J.E. (1990). Care of the infant born exposed to human immunodeficiency virus. *Obstetrics and Gynecology Clinics of North America,* 17(3), 637–649.

280. Answer: (**B**) It has been well documented by many studies, that maternal smoking is responsible for causing infants to weigh less than infants born to nonsmoking mothers. With this reduced birth weight found among infants of comparable gestation, an underlying mechanism other than prematurity was felt to be responsible. Smoking also places the woman at risk for prematurity and pregnancy related complications (e.g., placental previa and abruptio) versus direct fetal complications such as birth anomalies.

REFERENCES

Buchan, P. (1983). Cigarette smoking in pregnancy and fetal hyperviscosity. *British Medical Journal, 286,* 1315.

Curet, L., Rao, A., Zachman, R., Morrison, J., Burkett, G., Poole, K., & the Collaborative Group on Antenatal Steroid Therapy (1983). *American Journal of Obstetrics and Gynaecology, 95*(2), 195–196.

Crosby, W., Metcoff, J., Costiloe, J., Mameesh, M., Sandstead, H., Jacob, R., McClain, P., Jacobson, G., Reid, W., & Burns, G. (1977). Fetal malnutrition: An appraisal of correlated factors. *American Journal of Obstetrics and Gynecology, 140*(4), 446–450.

Flandermeyer, A.A. (1993). The drug-exposed neonate (pp. 997–1033). In C. Kenner, A. Brueggemeyer, & L.P. Gunderson (eds.), *Comprehensive neonatal care: A physiologic perspective.* Philadelphia: W.B. Saunders.

Guyton, A. (1981). *Textbook of medical physiology* (6th ed.). Philadelphia: W.B. Saunders.

Longo, L. (1976). Carbon monoxide: Effects on oxygenation of the fetus in utero. *Science, 194,* 523–525.

Meyer, M., Jonas, B., & Tonascia, J. (1976). Perinatal events associated with maternal smoking during pregnancy. *American Journal of Epidemiology, 103*(5), 464–476.

U.S. Department of Health and Human Services (1980). *The health consequences of smoking for women.* Washington DC: Public Health Service, Office on Smoking and Health.

281. Answer: (**C**) Indications for transplantation in children include (1) progressive end-stage liver disease, (2) stable liver disease with a known lethality, (3) fatal hepatic-based metabolic disease, (4) metabolic disease correctable by liver cell replacement, and (5) social invalidism (A-Kader, Ryckman, & Balistreri, 1991).

REFERENCES

A-Kader, H.H., Ryckman, F.C., & Balistreri, W.F. (1991). Liver transplantation in the pediatric population: Indications and monitoring. *Clinical Transplant, 5,* 161.

Ryckman, F.C. & Pedersen, S.H. (1993). Hepatic and renal transplantation in infants and children (pp. 968–980). In C. Kenner, A. Brueggemeyer, & L.P. Gunderson (eds.), *Comprehensive neonatal care: A physiologic perspective.* Philadelphia: W.B. Saunders.

282. Answer: (**C**) The infant cues include state and behavioral capabilities, responses to stimuli, and signs of stress, overstimulation, and stability. Caregiving based on infant cues involves attention to messages from the infant that may indicate timing for interventions, such as when to provide care or opportunities for sensory input and interaction.

REFERENCES

Als, H. (1982). Toward a synactive theory of development: Promise for the assessment and support of infant individuality. *Infant Mental Health Journal, 3,* 229–243.

Als, H., Lester, B.M., Tronick, E.Z., & Brazelton, T.B. (1982). Assessment of preterm infant behavior (APIB). In H.E. Fitzgerald & M. Yogman (eds.), *Theory and research in behavioral pediatrics.* New York: Plenum Press.

Blackburn, S.T. & VandenBerg, K.A. (1993). Assessment and management of neonatal neurobehavioral development (pp. 1094–1133). In C. Kenner, A. Brueggemeyer, & L.P. Gunderson (eds.), *Comprehensive neonatal care: A physiologic perspective.* Philadelphia: W.B. Saunders.

283. Answer: (**A**) Three factors are repeatedly cited as increasing the likelihood of user acceptance: (1) involvement of uses in system development and implementation; (2) immediate, tangible

benefit; and (3) ease of system use (not requiring extensive training).

Computers are also not infallible, and the failure rate (down time) can be high, especially during implementation of new applications. While computers may save time, most hospital computer applications have not been demonstrated to save paper.

Finally, experience has shown that two key elements determine the successful implementation of computerized patient management systems. The first is that the project has the full support of administration, and second, that the system facilitates patient care in obvious and tangible ways.

REFERENCES

Ball, M.J. & Hannah, K.J. (1988). What is informatics and what does it mean for nursing? (pp. 260–266). In M.J. Ball, K.J. Hannah, U. Gerdin-Jelger, & H. Peterson (eds.), *Nursing informatics: Where care and technology meet.* New York: Springer-Verlag.

Franck, L.S. (1993). Use of computers in neonatal nursing (pp. 1034–1045). In C. Kenner, A. Brueggemeyer, & L.P. Gunderson (eds.), *Comprehensive neonatal care: A physiologic perspective.* Philadelphia: W.B. Saunders.

Sivak, E.D., Gochberg, J.S., & Frank, D.M. (1989). Lessons to be learned from the continuing epic of computerizing the intensive care unit (pp. 827–833). In L. Kingsland (ed.), *Proceedings, Thirteenth annual symposium on computer applications in medical care.* Washington, DC: IEEE Computer Society Press.

284. Answer: (**B**) First, preterm infants as a group are found to be less neurologically mature than full-term infants. This lack of maturity produces infants who are less regulatory (organized) and more unpredictable in their behavior, making it harder to understand and predict how they will behave. This lack of neurologic maturity is directly related to how premature they are—the younger the preterm infant gestationally, the less mature and the more disorganized the infant. Second, preterm infants as a group exhibit a lower level of behavioral social responsiveness, are less persistent and adaptable, and tend to respond in more negative ways than full-term infants.

REFERENCES

Anders, T.F. & Keener, F. (1985). Developmental course of night-time sleep-wake patterns in full-term and premature infants during the first year of life. *Sleep, 8,* 173–192.

Barnard, K.E. (1980). Sleep organization and motor development in prematures. In E.J. Sell (ed.), *Follow-up of high risk newborn: A practical approach.* Springfield, IL: Charles C Thomas.

Barnard, K.E. & Bee, H.L. (1981). *Premature infant refocus project.* School of Nursing and the Child Development and Mental Retardation Center, University of Washington, Seattle, WA.

Bennett, F.C. (1984). Neurodevelopmental outcome of low birth weight infants. In V.C. Kelby (ed.), *Practice of pediatrics.* (Vol 2). New York: Harper & Row.

Johnson-Crowley, N. (1993). Systematic assessment and home follow-up: A basis for monitoring the neonate's integration into the family unit (pp. 1055–1076). In C. Kenner, A. Brueggemeyer, & L.P. Gunderson (eds.), *Comprehensive neonatal care: A physiologic perspective.* Philadelphia: W.B. Saunders.

Tekolste, K.A. & Bennett, F.C. (1987). State of the art, the high risk infant: Transitions in health, development, and family during the first years of life. *Journal of Perinatology, VII*(4), 368–377.

Telzrow, R.W., Kang, R., Mitchell, S.K., Ashworth, C.D., & Barnard, K.E. (1982). An assessment of the behavior of the premature infant of 40 weeks conceptual age. In L.P. Lipsitt & T.M. Field (eds.), *Perinatal risk and newborn behavior.* Norwood, NJ: Ablex.

285. Answer: (**C**) Preterm infants, sensitive to stimuli and limited in energy reserves, respond to their parents' attempt to interact by turning away, dropping off to sleep, or crying inconsolably. Parents see this behavior as negative and difficult to cope with and understand. If we think of parent–infant interaction as a sort of "dance" in which each participant (here, parent and infant) must give clear and readable cues that can be read by the partner, be motorically and neurologically alert to respond quickly and positively to the partner's cues, and retain enough energy to keep the dance going in a smooth and rhythmical way, we can see why interacting (dancing) with a preterm infant may not be the positive experience most parents expect it to be.

REFERENCES

Barnard, K.E. (1987). *Nursing child assessment learner manual.* Seattle, WA: NCAST Publications.

Johnson-Crowley, N. (1993). Systematic assessment and home follow-up: A basis for monitoring the neonate's integration into the family unit (pp. 1055–1076). In C. Kenner, A. Brueggemeyer, & L.P. Gunderson (eds.), *Comprehensive neonatal care: A physiologic perspective.* Philadelphia: W.B. Saunders.

286. Answer: (**B**) The assessment of the family's commitment to home care is perhaps the most critical factor determining the success or failure of home health care. After extensive discharge

teaching, skills development, and repetitive occasions of caregiving, the family must want the child at home and under their care. They must be willing to devote the time and energy required to meet the physical and emotional needs of the child.

REFERENCES

Ballard, R.A. (1988). *Pediatric care of the ICN graduate.* Philadelphia: W.B. Saunders.

Hall, L.H. (1993). Home care (pp. 1148–1158). In C. Kenner, A. Brueggemeyer, & L.P. Gunderson (eds.), *Comprehensive neonatal care: A physiologic perspective.* Philadelphia: W.B. Saunders.

Thilo, E.M., Comito, J., & McCulliss, D. (1987). Home oxygen therapy in the newborn. Costs and parental acceptance. *American Journal of Diseases of Children, 14,* 766–768.

Vohr, B., Chen, A., Coll, C., & Oh, W. (1988). Mothers of preterm and full term infants on home apnea monitors. *American Journal of Diseases of Children, 142,* 229–231.

Wasserman, A. (1984). A prospective study—The impact of home monitoring on the family. *Pediatrics, 74,* 323–329.

Young, L., Creighton, D., & Sauve, R.S. (1988). The needs of families of infants discharged home with continuous oxygen therapy. *Journal of Obstetric, Gynecologic, and Neonatal Nursing, 17*(3), 187–193.

287. Answer: (**C**) Important components for any follow-up program include home visiting to monitor and provide support; measures for systematically assessing the infant and family for identification of problem areas, providing intervention, and evaluating outcomes; protocols of care that are structured, flexible, and consistent from visit to visit; parent involvement in all aspects of care, including assessment, intervention, and evaluation; content encompassing important areas for normal growth and development, yet specific to the needs and problems of preterm infants; and research based and supported.

REFERENCES

Johnson-Crowley, N. & Sumner, G.A. (1987a). *Concept manual: Nursing systems toward effective parenting-preterm.* Seattle, WA: NCAST Publications.

Johnson-Crowley, N. & Sumner, G.A. (1987b). *Protocol manual: Nursing systems toward effective parenting-preterm.* Seattle, WA: NCAST Publications.

Johnson-Crowley, N. (1993). Systematic assessment and home follow-up: A basis for monitoring the neonate's integration into the family unit (pp. 1055–1076). In C. Kenner, A. Brueggemeyer, & L.P. Gunderson (eds.), *Comprehensive neonatal care: A physiologic perspective.* Philadelphia: W.B. Saunders.

288. Answer: (**A**) The NIDCAP incorporates several levels of developmental training in assessment techniques and intervention planning for high-risk preterm and full-term infants. Included in this program is an observation tool (level 1 NIDCAP-naturalistic behavioral observation), which is extremely useful for the NICU nurse. This assessment involves an observation of the infant before, during, and after a routine caregiving episode.

REFERENCES

Als, H. (1982). Toward a synactive theory of development: Promise for the assessment and support of infant individuality. *Infant Mental Health Journal, 3,* 229–243.

Als, H., Lester, B.M., Tronick, E.Z., & Brazelton, T.B. (1982). Assessment of preterm infant behavior (APIB). In H.E. Fitzgerald & M. Yogman (eds.), *Theory and research in behavioral pediatrics.* New York: Plenum Press.

Blackburn, S.T. & VandenBerg, K. A. (1993). Assessment and management of neonatal neurobehavioral development (pp. 1094–1133). In C. Kenner, A. Brueggemeyer, & L.P. Gunderson (eds.), *Comprehensive neonatal care: A physiologic perspective.* Philadelphia: W.B. Saunders.

289. Answer: (**B**) They found the mothers of premature infants expected them to be different from full-term infants and that they actually shaped their maternal responses to their infant based more on their expectations than of actual behavior of the infant. In part, this discrepancy between the actual infant behavior and the expected behavior may come from the lack of experience on the part of the mothers. If one does not know what to expect, then it is difficult to plan or respond in less than an anticipatory or contrived manner.

REFERENCES

Kemp, V.H. & Page, C.K. (1987). Maternal prenatal attachment in normal and high-risk pregnancies. *JOGNN, 16*(3), 179–184.

Kenner, C. & Bagwell, G.A. (1993). Assessment and management of the transition to home (pp. 1134–1147). In C. Kenner, A. Brueggemeyer, & L.P. Gunderson (eds.), *Comprehensive neonatal care: A physiologic perspective.* Philadelphia: W.B. Saunders.

Mehren, E. (1991). *Born too soon: The story of Emily.* New York: Doubleday Book.

Sammons, W.A.H. & Lewis, J.M. (1985). *Premature babies: A different beginning.* St. Louis: C.V. Mosby.

290. Answer: (**A**) While time of NICU discharge, then, is the overriding goal for the health professional and family, the

actual transition to home can bring a time of crisis to the family. The actual assumption of the new parent role can be overwhelming. Some researchers and clinicians view this transition as a crisis rather than a developmental passage to a new functional level.

REFERENCES

Kemp, V.H. & Page, C.K. (1987). Maternal prenatal attachment in normal and high-risk pregnancies. *JOGNN, 16*(3), 179–184.

Kenner, C. & Bagwell, G.A. (1993). Assessment and management of the transition to home (pp. 1134–1147). In C. Kenner, A. Brueggemeyer, & L.P. Gunderson (eds.), *Comprehensive neonatal care: A physiologic perspective.* Philadelphia: W.B. Saunders.

Mehren, E. (1991). *Born too soon: The story of Emily.* New York: Doubleday Book.

Sammons, W.A.H. & Lewis, J.M. (1985). *Premature babies: A different beginning.* St. Louis: C.V. Mosby.

291. Answer: (**C**) The informational needs of parents include how to provide routine newborn care, normal newborn care; how to recognize normal newborn characteristics, both physical and behavioral; how to keep the infant healthy after discharge; their own responsibilities about how to provide care; the equipment used on their infant while in the NICU; and a complete explanation of the medical diagnosis and the expected prognosis.

REFERENCES

Kemp, V.H. & Page, C.K. (1987). Maternal prenatal attachment in normal and high-risk pregnancies. *JOGNN, 16*(3), 179–184.

Kenner, C. & Bagwell, G.A. (1993). Assessment and management of the transition to home (pp. 1134–1147). In C. Kenner, A. Brueggemeyer, & L.P. Gunderson (eds.), *Comprehensive neonatal care: A physiologic perspective.* Philadelphia: W.B. Saunders.

Mehren, E. (1991). *Born too soon: The story of Emily.* New York: Doubleday Book.

Sammons, W.A.H. & Lewis, J.M. (1985). *Premature babies: A different beginning.* St. Louis: C.V. Mosby.

292. Answer: (**C**) Short-term care is considered by many health care providers to be less than six months in duration. In general, long-term care indicates that the duration of the condition and the need for care will exceed six months. Hospice care is a type of caring when cure is no longer a reasonable expectation.

REFERENCES

Ballard, R.A. (1988). *Pediatric care of the ICN graduate.* Philadelphia: W.B. Saunders.

Hall, L.H. (1993). Home care (pp. 1148–1158). In C. Kenner, A. Brueggemeyer, & L.P. Gunderson (eds.), *Comprehensive neonatal care: A physiologic perspective.* Philadelphia: W.B. Saunders.

Thilo, E.M., Comito, J., & McCulliss, D. (1987). Home oxygen therapy in the newborn. Costs and parental acceptance. *American Journal of Diseases of Children, 14*, 766–768.

Vohr, B., Chen, A., Coll, C., & Oh, W. (1988). Mothers of preterm and full term infants on home apnea monitors. *American Journal of Diseases of Children, 142*, 229–231.

Wasserman, A. (1984). A prospective study—The impact of home monitoring on the family. *Pediatrics, 74*, 323–329.

Young, L., Creighton, D., & Sauve, R.S. (1988). The needs of families of infants discharged home with continuous oxygen therapy. *Journal of Obstetric, Gynecologic, and Neonatal Nursing, 17*(3), 187–193.

293. Answer: (**C**) Short-term care of an infant at home can include phototherapy for hyperbilirubinemia, administration of supplemental oxygen for respiratory distress, medication administration for various neonatal conditions, and alternative feeding methods such as gavage for nutritional support. Long-term home care addresses situations for children with disease processes such as bronchopulmonary dysplasia, short bowel or gut syndrome, congenital heart disease, physical and cosmetic defects, neurologic and metabolic disorders, and numerous other prolonged pathologic conditions.

REFERENCES

Ballard, R.A. (1988). *Pediatric care of the ICN graduate.* Philadelphia: W.B. Saunders.

Hall, L.H. (1993). Home care (pp. 1148–1158). In C. Kenner, A. Brueggemeyer, & L.P. Gunderson (eds.), *Comprehensive neonatal care: A physiologic perspective.* Philadelphia: W.B. Saunders.

Thilo, E.M., Comito, J., & McCulliss, D. (1987). Home oxygen therapy in the newborn. Costs and parental acceptance. *American Journal of Diseases of Children, 14*, 766–768.

Vohr, B., Chen, A., Coll, C., & Oh, W. (1988). Mothers of preterm and full term infants on home apnea monitors. *American Journal of Diseases of Children, 142*, 229–231.

Wasserman, A. (1984). A prospective study—The impact of home monitoring on the family. *Pedatrics, 74*, 323–329.

Young, L., Creighton, D., & Sauve, R.S. (1988). The needs of families of infants discharged home with continuous oxygen therapy. *Journal of Obstetric, Gynecologic, and Neonatal Nursing, 17*(3), 187–193.

ANNOTATED BIBLIOGRAPHY

Assessment

Daze, A.M. & Scanlon, J.W. (1985). *Neonatal nursing: A practical guide*. Gaithersburg, MD: Aspen.
A book that presents assessment methods, protocols, and strategies for managing the neonate. It is a practical guide that uses neonatal physiology and pathophysiology as a foundation for nursing practice.

O'Doherty, N. (1985). *Atlas of the newborn*. Lancaster, England: MTP Press Limited.
This 412-page text has excellent color plates of a variety of different normal and abnormal findings for the infant. The text is divided into six sections that deal with the normal infant; low birth weight; trauma; infection; congenital abnormality; and skin defects. The textbook is useful for teaching, especially in the area of physical assessment.

Perlman, M. & Kirpalani, H. (1992). *Residents handbook of neonatology*. St. Louis: C.V. Mosby.
As the title implies, this is a quick reference book that easily fits into a lab coat pocket. The authors have condensed neonatally focused material into a 8 × 5, 304-page book that is easy to use. The text is a wonderful reference for the clinical setting. Most of the information is easy to access and use in the day-to-day management of the neonate.

Biophysical Monitoring

Gomella, T.L., Cunningham, M.D., & Eyal, F.G. (1992). *Neonatology: Management, procedures, on-call problems, diseases, drugs*. Norwalk, CT: Appleton & Lange.
Includes many sections on monitoring of specific types of neonates. Quick reference; not a lot of detail.

Cardiac System

Beachy, P. & Deacon, J. (eds.). (1993). *Core curriculum for neonatal intensive care*. Philadelphia: W.B. Saunders.
A good, quick review reference of the major neonatal topics.

Long, W.A. (1990). *Fetal and neonatal cardiology*. Philadelphia: W.B. Saunders.
One of the most comprehensive textbooks dealing with the topic of neonatal cardiology. The text provides the reader with both the physiologic foundations and embryologic reasons for cardiovascular defects. The text uses numerous contributing authors to present this information-filled work. It is recommended for all advanced practitioners and those interested in neonatal cardiovascular problems.

Critical Periods of Development

England, M.A. (1990). *Color atlas of life before birth: Normal fetal development*. Chicago: Year Book.
Easy-to-use text covering the topic of fetal development. The book has numerous, excellent color plates and good black and white pictures illustrating the phases of normal fetal development.

Grahm, J.M. (1988). *Smith's recognizable patterns of human deformation*. Philadelphia: W.B. Saunders.
This 182-page book uses numerous photographs to illustrate the common deformations that may occur from positioning in utero. The text is wonderful for those working with infants and trying to understand what is a variation of normal in the physical assessment simply due to forces applied in utero. The book is a wonderful reference for all students of neonatal physical assessment.

Moore, K.L. (1989). *The developing human* (4th ed.). Philadelphia: W.B. Saunders.
Excellent review of critical periods of development. Contains common medical conditions that result from genetic and environmental influences.

Sadler, T.W. (1985). *Langman's medical embryology* (5th ed.). Baltimore: Williams & Wilkins.
Good review of embryologic development. Emphasis on medical application.

Gastrointestinal/Nutrition

Beachy, P. & Deacon, J. (eds.). (1993). *Core curriculum for neonatal intensive care*. Philadelphia: W.B. Saunders.
A good, quick review reference of the major neonatal topics.

Lebenthal, E. (ed.). (1989). *Textbook of gastroenterology and nutrition in infancy* (2nd ed.). New York: Raven Press.
Reviews physiologic principles of nutrition from a perinatal, neonatal, infant, and child perspective. It covers in detail the most common neonatal/infant nutrition problems. The text presents the medical model of treatment of nutritional deficiencies.

Genetics

Cohen, F.L. (1984). *Clinical genetics in nursing practice*. Philadelphia: J.B. Lippincott.
Good overview of nursing implications of genetic testing and diagnosis. Out of print but still available in health science and nursing libraries.

Connor, J., & Ferguson-Smith, M. (1987). *Essential medical genetics*. Oxford: Blackwell Scientific.
Describes basic genetics and common medical conditions resulting from a genetic defect.

Cummings, M. (1988). *Human heredity: Principles and issues*. New York: West Publishing.
Basic genetic information; easy to understand.

Thompson, S., & Thompson, M. (1986). *Genetics in medicine* (4th ed.). Philadelphia: W.B. Saunders.
Describes basic genetics and common medical conditions resulting from a genetic defect.

Genitourinary

Avery, G.B. (1987). *Neonatology: Pathophysiology and management of the newborn*.
Excellent general neonatology text. It covers diagnosis and treatment from the medical perspective.

Daze, A.M. & Scanlon, J.W. (1985). *Neonatal nursing: A practical guide*. Gaithersburg, MD: Aspen.
A book that presents assessment methods, protocols, and strategies for managing the neonate. It is a prac-

tical guide that uses neonatal physiology and pathophysiology as a foundation for nursing practice.

Home Care/Follow Up

Bernbaum, J.C. & Hoffman-Williamson, M. (1991). *Primary care of the preterm infant*. St. Louis: C.V. Mosby.
Excellent review of discharge planning and primary care follow-up that is needed for the premature infant and family. The book discusses the medical issues of follow-up with special emphasis on neurologic development and concerns. There is a section devoted to parent concerns after discharge.

Ballard, R.A. (1988). *Pediatric care of the ICN graduate*. Philadelphia: W.B. Saunders.
Good text that describes the problems the infant who has been in an intensive care unit will face after discharge. It depicts the management necessary for follow-up.

Wasik, B.H., Bryant, D.M., & Lyons, C.M. (1990). *Home visiting: Procedures for helping families*. Newbury Park, CA: Sage Publications.
Text reviews issues facing home visitors—professionals and paraprofessionals. Interventions for helping stressed families are outlined. Infant health and developmental records are included. Is a good resource of information for follow-up care.

Immunology

Krugman, S., Katz, S.L., Gershon, A.A. & Wilfert, C. (1992). *Infectious diseases of children*. St. Louis: C.V. Mosby.
The ninth edition of this reference has been reorganized and updated. The text now addresses complete coverage of new developments in pediatric infectious diseases and strategies for treating them. From AIDS to sepsis in the newborn, acute respiratory failure to tuberculosis. The text presents a complete spectrum of conditions. It does have content specific to the neonatal group although the age range covered by the text goes through adolescence.

Remington, J.S. & Klein, J.O. (eds.). (1990). *Infectious diseases of the fetus and newborn infant* (3rd ed.). Philadelphia: W.B. Saunders.
Excellent text covering all the commonly known fetal/neonatal infections. The newer, less common "bugs" that cause infections and sepsis are included. Details laboratory tests, clinical considerations, treatments, and long-term outcomes. Special emphasis is placed on a description of the underlying pathology of the infectious process and mode of transmission.

Shulman, S.T., Kim, J. & MacKendrick, W. (1992). *Handbook of pediatric infectious disease and antimicrobial therapy*. St. Louis: C.V. Mosby.
The text is a wonderful reference guide that gives the reader quick access to common and uncommon pediatric infectious diseases, with the appropriate antimicrobial treatment. The text is loaded with essential information, in a user-friendly handbook style organized by disease entity, microorganisms, and symptom complex, then illustrated by the corresponding table for selecting the appropriate antibiotic or anti-infective. The text incorporates diagnostic commentary with the appropriate antibiotic tables. The text has 51 tables in its 450 pages. It also has some of the most up-to-date information on pediatric AIDS.

Sweet, A.Y & Brown, E.G. (1991). *Fetal and neonatal effects of maternal disease*. St. Louis: C.V. Mosby.
This text book is a wonderful reference book for those individuals interested in the impact that the mother may have on the neonate and the neonates outcome after birth. Over 28 contributors have helped to write this work. The table of contents for the 17 chapters is nicely subdivided into headings that make scanning the table for specific topics extremely easy. The material is well organized and comprehensive. Another plus to this work is that excellent bibliographies are after each topic. This makes it easy for the reader to access further information on a given topic.

Neurology

Beachy, P. & Deacon, J. (eds.). (1993). *Core curriculum for neonatal intensive care*. Philadelphia: W.B. Saunders.
A good quick review reference of the major neonatal topics.

Fenichel, G.M. (1990). *Neonatal neurology*. New York: Churchill Livingstone.
The purpose of this book according to the authors is to provide information to the clinician and not to serve as a comprehensive reference book. The authors have achieved their objective. The text is easy to use and divided into logical sections. The information is easy to read and a highlight of things that can be seen in the nursery. It would be highly recommended for the libraries of any nursery.

Nutrition

Hay, W.W. (1991). *Neonatal nutrition and metabolism*. St. Louis: C.V. Mosby.
A wonderful reference of 558 pages from various contributors with expertise in neonatal nutrition. The text is a must for anyone interested in the care and management of the neonate. The chapters are divided into categories such as growth and energy; specific nutrients; nutrient mixtures and methods of feeding; and disorders. The organization of the sections and chapters makes the book easy to use and apply the information contained within the chapters.

Tsang, R.C. & Nichols, B.L. (1988). *Nutrition during infancy*. St. Louis: C.V. Mosby.
The textbook has a wealth of useful information. The organization of the book takes a developmental approach to neonatal nutritional needs. Each area in nutrition receives a separate section. For example, an entire chapter is dedicated to the topic of vitamin A. In the closing portions of the book, all the information is synthesized into approaches for dealing with neonatal nutrition.

Parenting

Hynan, M.T. (1987). *The pain of premature parents: A psychological guide for coping*. Lanham, MD: University Press of America, Inc.
This book discusses the pain of having a premature infant. It details the perspective of the parents after the birth and after the infant's discharge or death. A good review of parenting issues.

Perinatal/Neonatal Care

Avery, G.B. (1987). *Neonatology: Pathophysiology and management of the newborn*. Philadelphia: J.B. Lippincott.
A 1432-page text that covers a wide variety of perinatal and neonatal topics. The comprehensive text is currently under revision with new editions expected in the future. The book always has been considered a gold standard for the resident and practitioner in the

NICU setting. The chapters are easy to read and understand.

Ballard, R.A. (1988). *Pediatric care of the ICN graduate*. Philadelphia: W.B. Saunders.
Good text that describes the problems the infant who has been in an intensive care unit will face after discharge. It depicts the management necessary for follow-up.

Beachy, P. & Deacon, J. (eds.). (1993). *Core curriculum for neonatal intensive care*. Philadelphia: W.B. Saunders.
A good, quick review reference of the major neonatal topics.

Blackburn, S.T. & Loper, D.L. (1992). *Maternal, fetal, and neonatal physiology: A clinical perspective*. Philadelphia: W.B. Saunders.
Good overview of maternal and neonatal physiology. Covers the topics in a system-by-system review.

Creasy, R. & Resnick, M. (1989). *Maternal-fetal medicine: Principles and practice*. Philadelphia: W.B. Saunders.
A good review of perinatal physiology. It is from the medical model.

Fanaroff, A.A. & Martin, R.J. (1992). *Neonatal-perinatal medicine* (5th ed.). St. Louis: C.V. Mosby.
The revised, fifth edition is a gold standard for neonatal care. Over 100 contributors detail the broad spectrum of clinical problems found in neonatal-perinatal medicine. The comprehensive reference provides exhaustive coverage of disorders and diseases that affect the infant in utero and during the early weeks of life. New sections of genetics and molecular biology, antenatal diagnosis, epidemiology, pain management, and fetal diagnosis and management are incorporated into the latest edition.

Gilbert, E. & Harmon, J. (1993). *High risk pregnancy and delivery* (2nd ed.). St. Louis: C.V. Mosby.
A good review book of common high risk perinatal conditions. Includes nursing management of the clients.

Goetzman, B.W. & Wennberg, R.P. (1991). *Neonatal intensive care handbook (2nd ed.)*. St. Louis: C.V. Mosby.
As the publishers describe this book, it is a practical and portable reference manual. The text is easy to use and provides quick references for the management of the infant. The text includes information on neonatal AIDS, ECMO, metabolic acidosis, drug addiction/withdrawal, emergency drugs, and heart disease to name a few sections. It would be excellent for a quick reference for students, practitioners, and physicians.

Gunderson, L.P. & Kenner, C.A. (1990). *Care of the 24–25 week gestational age infant (small baby protocol)*. Petaluma, CA: Neonatal Network.
The monograph was designed to provide the neonatal nurse and practitioner with practical information about the care of the extremely premature infant. This is the first work that pulls together a variety of topics, both physiological and behavioral, into one quick and easy-to-use text.

Herbst, A.L., Mishell, D.R., Stenchever, M.A. & Droegemuller, W. (1992). *Comprehensive gynecology*. St. Louis: C.V. Mosby.
Considered the "bible" of gynecology, the new second edition remains the single best reference to the broad spectrum of gynecologic issues. The text is extremely comprehensive and is supported by over 850 illustrations and extensive references.

Kenner, C.A. (1992). *Neonatal care*. Springhouse, PA: Springhouse Publishing.
A quick reference book that covers the entire range of neonatal care. The text is easy to use and incorporates principles of family dynamics. The text is a good reference for individuals just learning about the provision of care for the neonate.

Klaus, M.Y & Fanaroff, A.A. (1990). *Care of the high-risk neonate*. Philadelphia: W.B. Saunders.
This book has long been a standard book for practitioners and residents. The material is easy and simple to understand. It is excellent for a reference text and overview in the clinical setting. The reader is directed to other texts for a more in-depth understanding. However, in the 454 pages the authors have filled their work with the facts and figures necessary to survive on a day-to-day basis in the nursery.

Krones, S.B. & Y. Bada-Elizey, H.S. (1993). *Neonatal decision making*. St. Louis: C.V. Mosby.
The text is designed to help individuals select the best therapeutic direction for the management of the neonate. The book is divided into eight sections that cover the fetus, labor and delivery, heat and water balance, physical signs, infections, organ system disorders, and more. The text is 304 pages in length and includes 120 algorithms.

Mattson, S. & Smith, J.E. (1993). *Core curriculum for maternal-newborn nursing*. Philadelphia: W.B. Saunders.
Quick reference for maternal–newborn care. There is not a lot of details but will provide readers with a good list of topics and brief review of each.

Merenstein, G.B. & Gardner, S.L. (1993). *Handbook of neonatal intensive care* (2nd ed.). St. Louis: C.V. Mosby.
Comprehensive text that incorporates both a medical and nursing perspective into the provision of care to the neonate. The latest approaches and techniques have been incorporated into this edition. It is a must for those in the neonatal field. It is also appropriate for the novice-to-intermediate practitioner.

Nelson, N.M. (ed.). (1990). *Current therapy in neonatal-perinatal medicine-2*. Philadelphia: B.C. Decker.
Emphasis on perinatal conditions such as diabetes that affect neonatal outcomes. Highlights antenatal testing and screening. Reviews of pertinent perinatal history that impact neonatal health. Includes sections on DRGs, computers in neonatal medicine, immunizations, use of nurse clinicians, and transport. Neonatal conditions are discussed in less detail than a neonatal text but give appropriate information to assess and management of care.

Polin, R.A. & Fox, W.W. (1992). *Fetal and neonatal physiology*. Philadelphia: W.B. Saunders.
Details fetal and neonatal physiology. It describes all of the most common neonatal problems and their medical management. Especially well-done descriptions of the physiologic principles underlying the pathology of fetal/neonatal problems.

Pharmacology

Pawlak, R.P. & Herfert, L.A.T. (1990). *Drug administration in the NICU: A handbook for nurses* (revised, 2nd edition). Petaluma, CA: Neonatal Network.
A comprehensive quick reference spiral-bound text dealing with pharmacology. The text is easy to use and practical for the clinical setting.

Neonatal Pharmacology Quarterly. Petaluma, CA: NICU, Ink.

A new journal that reviews pharmacology principles and applications with the neonatal population. This is a multidisciplinary journal.

Yeh, T.F. (1991). *Neonatal therapeutics*. St. Louis: C.V. Mosby.
The book is an easy to read and understand presentation dealing with neonatal pharmacology. Numerous contributors have come together to help write this book. The text is organized around topics versus specific classifications of drugs. This organizational presentation makes it easy to use and understand and to apply the principles to the clinical setting.

Young, R.E. & Mangum, O.B. (1990). *Neofax*. Columbus, OH: Ross Labs.
A quick reference text covering drugs that are routinely used in the NICU. The text is easy to use and a required reference for any nursery across the country.

Pulmonary

Aloan, C.A. (1987). *Respiratory care of the newborn: a clinical manual*. Philadelphia: J.B. Lippincott.
As the title reflects, this book is designed to be used by the clinician interested in physiologic alterations of the pulmonary system. The book is divided into easy-to-read chapters that cover topics from gestational maturation to the dynamics of ventilator management. This book does not go into detail on the topics. It would be an excellent resource for an individual just beginning a career in the realm of neonatal management and care.

Blackburn, S. R. & Loper, D.L. (1992). *Maternal, fetal and neonatal physiology: A clinical perspective*. Philadelphia: W.B. Saunders.
This is one of the best texts to be published. It covers the spectrum of mother and infant physiology, pathophysiology and approaches to management. The text is a must for any individual involved in maternal infant care. The chapters are easy to read and understand. The authors have included wonderful bibliographies at the end of each chapter that provide the reader with additional information on each topic.

Carlo, W.A. & Chatburn, R.L. (1988). *Neonatal respiratory care*. Chicago: Year Book.
A text that explains some basic principles underlying respiratory management. The text covers topics of ventilation principles, physiology of air exchange, and respiratory assist devices.

Goldsmith, J.P. & Karotkin, E.H. (1988). *Assisted ventilation of the neonate*. Philadelphia: W.B. Saunders.
A comprehensive text dealing with neonatal management of ventilation. The book has numerous contributors that help make this a gold standard in ventilation techniques. The text progresses from basic principles of management, physiological principles, to the latest in management from both a nursing and medical perspective. It is highly recommended for the libraries of all nurseries.

Nugent, J. (ed.). (1991). *Acute respiratory care of the neonate*. Petaluma, CA: NICU, Ink.
This text covers the newer therapies in respiratory management and the standard modes of treatment. It outlines the nursing responsibilities of the ECMO infant and the one undergoing high-frequency ventilation. Also, it is a study guide with questions that serve as good practice for test taking.

Polin, R.A. & Burg, F.D. (1983). *Workbook in practical neonatology*. Philadelphia: W.B. Saunders.
Practical approach for caring for the high-risk newborn infant. Uses physiology and clinical examples for patient management. The text is no longer in print, however, it is still available in many libraries.

The Journal of Perinatal & Neonatal Nursing, Aspen Publishers.
Journal dealing with a wide variety of neonatal and perinatal topics. Good reference for cutting-edge advances in nursing care.

Sibling Adaptation

Feetham, S.L., Meister, S.B., Bell, J.M., & Gilliss, C. (eds.) (1993). *The nursing of families*. Newbury Park, CA: Sage Publications.
Good reference for family theory/research/education/practice issues. Text is research based and reports findings to support theoretical perspectives and issues on families.

Lansky, V. (1990). *Welcoming your second baby*. Deephaven, MN: Book Peddlers.
Good book for parents welcoming a new baby; assists nurse to view new arrival from family perspective.

Surgical Neonate

Kenner, C., Harjo, J., & Brueggemeyer, A. (eds.) (1988). *Neonatal surgery: A nursing perspective*. Orlando, FL: Grune & Stratton.
A quick reference book covering the common surgical anomalies found in the NICU. It outlines the embryology, pathophysiology, transport considerations, pre- and postoperative care and long-term consequences.

Filston, H.C. & Izant, R.J. (1985). *The surgical neonate: Evaluation and care*. Norwalk, Connecticut: Appleton-Century-Crofts.
This reliable source provides concise information on the rudiments of surgical care for the newborn. Written specifically for the pediatric and general surgeon house officer rotating through the pediatric surgical service, the new edition has been completely revised. Serving as a hands-on reference, information on how to care for an infant with a surgical illness, how to recognize the major congenital anomalies and how to manage each surgical entity can be located and learned quickly. More detailed than handbooks of pediatric surgery, yet efficiently organized to provide the reader with a ready and readable companion during rotations through pediatric services and NICU settings.

Transition to Home

Ballard, R.A. (1988). *Pediatric care of the ICN graduate*. Philadelphia: W.B. Saunders.
Good text that describes the problems the infant who has been in an intensive care unit will face after discharge. It depicts the management necessary for follow-up.

Bernbaum, J. & Hoffman-Williamson, M. (1991). *Primary care of the preterm infant*. St. Louis: C.V. Mosby.
The text is organized in four sections that offer a practical team approach to the special considerations of effective preterm infant care. Part 1 starts with post-ICU treatment and gives the reader practical approaches to planning a smooth transition from the hospital to home. Parts 2 and 3 cover everything from immunizations to neuromuscular assessments. Part 4 addresses the realities of long-term care for the developmentally disabled child. The book is 240 pages with 82 illustrations.

Coen, R.W. & Koffler, H. (1987). *Primary care of the newborn*. Boston: Little, Brown.
This is one of the first books to deal with the management of the infant from a primary care perspective. It

is filled with excellent information from the initial history, physical examination to the problems that may be routine and not so routine. It provides a wonderful balance to the numerous texts on the market that are focused on the critically ill neonate. It is a must read for an practitioner program.

Sammons, W.A.H. & Lewis, J.M. (1985). *Premature babies: A different beginning*. St. Louis: C.V. Mosby.
Although an older book in the age of neonatal practice, this book is packed with information about the infant, the environment, and the family. It is a wonderful introduction for the novice NICU individual. The information, though not highly referenced, is practical and important. The high technology and skills required for caring for the neonate are important, yet only a part of the equation of comprehensive neonatal care. This book picks up where most others leave off. It is an excellent text. Although the material is more than five years old, most of the principles and approaches in the book have not changed drastically.

Seidel, H.M., Rosenstein, B.J. & Pathak, A. (1992). *Primary care of the newborn*. St. Louis: C.V. Mosby.
A pocket style reference book. The quick reference text is focused on the treatment and management of the full-term newborn. The text is 425 pages and follows the sequence of full-term newborn from prenatal visits and examinations to delivery and/or discharge. High-risk care of the infant is briefly addressed. The book is packed with helpful charts, tables, graphs of normal values, color photographs of skin conditions, and appendices covering everything from pharmacology to newborn nursery policy statements.

Children's Hospital of
Michigan's NICU